Autoimmune Diseases: Autoimmune Hepatitis PBC and PSC

Editor

DAVID BERNSTEIN

CLINICS IN LIVER DISEASE

www.liver.theclinics.com

Consulting Editor
NORMAN GITLIN

February 2024 • Volume 28 • Number 1

ELSEVIER

1600 John F. Kennedy Boulevard • Suite 1800 • Philadelphia, Pennsylvania, 19103-2899

http://www.theclinics.com

CLINICS IN LIVER DISEASE Volume 28, Number 1
February 2024 ISSN 1089-3261, ISBN-13: 978-0-443-12145-6

Editor: Kerry Holland
Developmental Editor: Akshay Samson

Clinics in Liver Disease (ISSN 1089-3261) is published quarterly by Elsevier Inc., 360 Park Avenue South, New York, NY 10010-1710. Months of issue are February, May, August, and November. Business and Editorial Offices: 1600 John F. Kennedy Blvd., Ste. 1800, Philadelphia, PA 19103-2899. Customer Service Office: 3251 Riverport Lane, Maryland Heights, MO 63043. Periodicals postage paid at New York, NY and additional mailing offices. Subscription prices are $339.00 per year (U.S. individuals), $100.00 per year (U.S. student/resident), $447.00 per year (international individuals), $200.00 per year (international student/resident), $405.00 per year (Canadian individuals), $100.00 per year (Canadian student/resident). For institutional access pricing please contact Customer Service via the contact information below. Foreign air speed delivery is included in all *Clinics* subscription prices. All prices are subject to change without notice. **POSTMASTER:** Send address changes to *Clinics in Liver Disease*, Elsevier Health Sciences Division, Subscription Customer Service, 3251 Riverport Lane, Maryland Heights, MO 63043. **Customer Service: Telephone: 1-800-654-2452 (U.S. and Canada); 314-447-8871 (outside U.S. and Canada). Fax: 314-447-8029. E-mail: journalscustomerservice-usa@ elsevier.com (for print support); journalsonlinesupport-usa@elsevier.com (for online support).**

Reprints. For copies of 100 or more of articles in this publication, please contact the Commercial Reprints Department, Elsevier Inc., 360 Park Avenue South, New York, NY 10010-1710. Tel.: 212-633-3874; Fax: 212-633-3820; E-mail: reprints@elsevier.com.

Clinics in Liver Disease is covered in *MEDLINE/PubMed (Index Medicus)*, Science Citation Index Expanded, Journal Citation Reports/Science Edition, and Current Contents/Clinical Medicine.

Contributors

CONSULTING EDITOR

NORMAN GITLIN, MD, FRCP (London), FRCPE (EDINBURGH), FAASLD, FACP, FACG
Head of Hepatology, Southern California Liver Centers, San Clemente, California, USA

EDITOR

DAVID BERNSTEIN, MD, MACG, FAASLD, AGAF, FACP
Professor of Medicine, NYU Grossman School of Medicine, Director, GI and Liver Ambulatory Network-Long Island, NYU Langone Health, New York, New York, USA

AUTHORS

KAMAL AMER, MD
Rutgers New Jersey Medical School, Newark, New Jersey, USA

MEHAK BASSI, MD
Division of Gastroenterology and Hepatology, Saint Peter's University Hospital, New Brunswick, New Jersey, USA

AMARPREET BHALLA, MD
Albert Einstein College of Medicine, Department of Pathology, Montefiore Medical Center, Bronx, New York, USA

CHRISTOPHER L. BOWLUS, MD
Lena Valente Professor and Chief, Division of Gastroenterology and Hepatology, University of California, Davis School of Medicine, Sacramento, California, USA

ERICA CHUNG, MD
Division of Gastroenterology, Montefiore Medical Center, Bronx, New York, USA

DOUGLAS T. DIETERICH, MD
Professor of Medicine, Division of Liver Diseases, Institute for Liver Medicine, and Director, Continuing Medical Education, Department of Medicine, Icahn School of Medicine at Mount Sinai, New York, New York, USA

MUHAMMAD SALMAN FAISAL, MD
Department of Gastroenterology and Hepatology, Henry Ford Health, Detroit, Michigan, USA

STEVEN L. FLAMM, MD
Professor of Medicine, Rush University Medical School, Chicago, Illinois, USA

BEN FLIKSHTEYN, MD
Fellow, Rutgers New Jersey Medical School, Newark, New Jersey, USA

BRETT E. FORTUNE, MD, MSc
Division of Hepatology, Montefiore Medical Center, Albert Einstein College of Medicine, Bronx, New York, USA

MERRILL ERIC GERSHWIN, MD
Chief, Division of Rheumatology, Department of Medicine, Allergy and Clinical Immunology, University of California, Davis, Davis, California, USA

APARNA GOEL, MD
Division of Gastroenterology and Hepatology, Stanford University, Palo Alto, California, USA

HUMBERTO C. GONZALEZ, MD
Department of Gastroenterology and Hepatology, Henry Ford Health, Wayne State University School of Medicine, Detroit, Michigan, USA

STUART C. GORDON, MD
Department of Gastroenterology and Hepatology, Henry Ford Health, Wayne State University School of Medicine, Detroit, Michigan, USA

JACQUELINE B. HENSON, MD
Fellow, Division of Gastroenterology, Department of Medicine, Duke University School of Medicine, Durham, North Carolina, USA

GIDEON M. HIRSCHFIELD, MB BChir, PhD, FRCP
Professor of Medicine, Staff Hepatologist, Division of Gastroenterology and Hepatology, Toronto Centre for Liver Disease, University of Toronto, Toronto, Ontario, Canada

BRIAN H. HORWICH, MD, MS
Division of Gastroenterology, Icahn School of Medicine at Mount Sinai, New York, New York, USA

INBAL HOURI, MD
Division of Gastroenterology and Hepatology, Toronto Centre for Liver Disease, University of Toronto, Toronto, Ontario, Canada

BINDU KAUL, MD
Albert Einstein College of Medicine, Department of Radiology, Montefiore Medical Center, Bronx, New York, USA

SANYA KAYANI, MD
Avera McKennan Hospital and University Health Center, Sioux Falls, South Dakota, USA

LINDSAY Y. KING, MD, MPH
Assistant Professor of Medicine, Division of Gastroenterology, Department of Medicine, Duke University School of Medicine, Durham, North Carolina, USA

KRIS V. KOWDLEY, MD, FACG, FAASLD, AGAF
Director, Liver Institute Northwest, Seattle, Washington; Professor of Medicine, Elson Floyd College of Medicine, Spokane, Washington, USA

PAUL KWO, MD
Professor of Medicine, Division of Gastroenterology and Hepatology, Stanford University, Palo Alto, California, USA

MARLYN J. MAYO, MD
Professor of Internal Medicine, Division of Digestive and Liver Diseases, The University of Texas Southwestern Medical Center, Dallas, Texas, USA

YASAMEEN MUZAHIM, MD
Division of Gastroenterology and Hepatology, Rutgers New Jersey Medical School, Newark, New Jersey, USA

HENDRICK PAGAN-TORRES, MD
Fellow of Transplant Hepatology, Division of Digestive and Liver Diseases, The University of Texas Southwestern Medical Center, Dallas, Texas, USA

NIKOLAOS PYRSOPOULOS, MD, PhD, MBA
Professor of Medicine, Division of Gastroenterology and Hepatology, Rutgers New Jersey Medical School, Newark, New Jersey, USA

TANG RUQI, PhD
Division of Gastroenterology and Hepatology, Key Laboratory of Gastroenterology and Hepatology, Ministry of Health, NHC Key Laboratory of Digestive Diseases, State Key Laboratory for Oncogenes and Related Genes, Renji Hospital, School of Medicine, Shanghai Jiao Tong University, Shanghai Institute of Digestive Disease, Shanghai, China

MARK W. RUSSO, MD, MPH
Clinical Professor of Medicine, Medical Director, Liver Transplantation, Atrium Health Wake Forest, Wake Forest School of Medicine-Charlotte Campus, Charlotte, North Carolina, USA

DANIEL SACA, MD
Gastroenterology and Hepatology Division, Rush University Medical School, Chicago, Illinois, USA

SHIVANI K. SHAH, MD
Fellow, Division of Gastroenterology and Hepatology, University of California, Davis School of Medicine, Sacramento, California, USA

MITCHELL L. SHIFFMAN, MD, MACG, AASLDF
Director, Liver Institute of Virginia, Bon Secours Liver Institute of Richmond, Bon Secours Liver Institute of Hampton Roads, Bon Secours Mercy Health System, Richmond, Virginia, USA; Director, Liver Institute of Virginia, Bon Secours Mercy Health, Newport News, Virginia, USA

AALAM SOHAL, MD
Hepatology Fellow, Liver Institute Northwest, Seattle, Washington, USA

ZAID TAFESH, MD, MSc
Assistant Professor, Department of Medicine, Rutgers New Jersey Medical School, Newark, New Jersey, USA

CLARA Y. TOW, MD
Associate Professor, Department of Medicine, Division of Hepatology, Montefiore Medical Center, Albert Einstein College of Medicine, Bronx, New York, USA

ALI WAKIL, MD
Assistant Professor of Medicine, Division of Gastroenterology and Hepatology, Rutgers New Jersey Medical School, Newark, New Jersey, USA

WILLIAM H. WHELESS, MD
Transplant Hepatology Fellow, Division of Hepatology, Atrium Health Wake Forest, Charlotte, North Carolina, USA

MA XIONG, MD, PhD
Division of Gastroenterology and Hepatology, Key Laboratory of Gastroenterology and Hepatology, Ministry of Health, NHC Key Laboratory of Digestive Diseases, State Key Laboratory for Oncogenes and Related Genes, Shanghai Institute of Digestive Disease, Institute of Aging and Tissue Regeneration, Renji Hospital, School of Medicine, Shanghai Jiao Tong University, Shanghai, China

ZHOU YUMING, MD
Division of Gastroenterology and Hepatology, Key Laboratory of Gastroenterology and Hepatology, Ministry of Health, NHC Key Laboratory of Digestive Diseases, State Key Laboratory for Oncogenes and Related Genes, Renji Hospital, School of Medicine, Shanghai Jiao Tong University, Shanghai Institute of Digestive Disease, Shanghai, China

MARIANA ZAPATA, MD
Fellow of Transplant Hepatology, Division of Digestive and Liver Diseases, The University of Texas Southwestern Medical Center, Dallas, Texas, USA

Contents

Autoimmune hepatitis (AIH) is a chronic immunologic disorder in which the immune system targets the liver. The disease has a genetic basis and this accounts for the epidemiologic variation observed in serologic testing and clinical presentation across different populations. The incidence of AIH increases with age into the 70s and seems to be increasing in prevalence. Most patients test positive for antinuclear antibody, ASMA, or anti-LKM but about 20% of patients do not have these serologic markers. At clinical presentation, patients may be asymptomatic, symptomatic, have acute liver failure, or decompensated cirrhosis.

Genome-wide association analyses suggest that HLA genes including HLA-DRB*0301, HLA-DRB*0401, and HLA-B*3501 as well as non-HLA genes including CD28/CTLA4/ICOS and SYNPR increased AIH susceptibility. The destruction of hepatocytes is the result of the imbalance between proinflammatory cells and immunosuppressive cells, especially the imbalance between Tregs and Th17 cells. The microbiome in patients with AIH is decreased in diversity with a specific decline in Bifidobacterium and enrichment in Veillonella and Faecalibacterium. Recent evidence has demonstrated the pathogenic role of E. gallinarum and L.reuteri in inducing autoimmunity in the liver.

Autoimmune hepatitis (AIH) presents a diagnostic challenge because it is relatively rare and heterogenous in presentation. This article presents the currently adopted approach to AIH diagnosis and explores the challenges with accurately identifying this disease entity. AIH offers no pathognomonic findings, instead relies on clinical presentation, serology, and histology to make the diagnosis. Diagnostic scoring systems support clinical judgment and serve as valuable tools in diagnosis and research. Histological analysis remains the cornerstone of diagnosis and to this day biopsy is essential to make the diagnosis.

rates. Despite the association between PBC and hyperlipidemia, treatment is indicated under specific circumstances with statins and fibrates being safe options. Osteoporosis, which is frequently seen, is usually managed based on data from postmenopausal women. Sicca syndrome is treated similarly to its standalone condition with the use of hydroxypropyl methyl-cellulose eye drops and anticholinergic drugs.

leading to biliary strictures, cholangitis, and cirrhosis. Early in presentation, patients may have normal liver tests, though over time develop a cholestatic pattern of liver injury. Diagnosis is made radiographically with magnetic resonance or endoscopic cholangiography. While several autoantibodies are associated with PSC, none have proven to have adequate diagnostic utility. Liver biopsy is rarely recommended unless to evaluate for small-duct PSC or overlap syndrome. Elastography, in various forms, is an effective, non-invasive modality to evaluate liver fibrosis in PSC.

Primary sclerosing cholangitis is a progressive cholestatic liver disease that causes stricturing of the intra and extrahepatic bile ducts that can lead to cirrhosis and end stage liver disease. Effective medical therapy has been elusive, but a course of ursodeoxycholic acid may be prescribed at doses of 17-23 mg/kg/day for up to a year to determine if a reduction in serum alkaline phosphatase is observed. A number of drugs are under investigation, including FXR agonists with choleretic and antimicrobial properties. Liver transplantation for PSC has one of the highest survival rates, but recurrent PSC is seen in up to 25% of recipients.

Cholangiocarcinoma (CCA) is a deadly complication observed in the setting of primary sclerosing cholangitis (PSC). When symptoms develop and CCA is diagnosed, it is usually at an advanced stage. Median survival is less than 12 months. Early identification of CCA leads to improved outcomes. Although diagnostic tests have excellent specificity, they are plagued by low sensitivity. No surveillance strategies have been widely agreed upon, but most societies recommend measurement of serum carbohydrate antigen 19-9 and MRCP every 6 to 12 months in patients with PSC. Advances in understanding of the genetic factors that lead to CCA are awaited.

Autoimmune liver diseases have unique post-transplant considerations. These recipients are at increased risk of rejection, and recurrent disease may also develop, which can progress to graft loss and increase mortality. Monitoring for and managing these complications is therefore important, though data on associated risk factors and immunosuppression strategies has in most cases been mixed. There are also other disease-specific complications that require management and may impact these decisions, including inflammatory bowel disease in PSC. Further work to better understand the optimal management strategies for these patients post-transplant is needed.

CLINICS IN LIVER DISEASE

SERIES OF RELATED INTEREST

Gastroenterology Clinics of North America
https://www.gastro.theclinics.com

THE CLINICS ARE AVAILABLE ONLINE!
Access your subscription at:
www.theclinics.com

Preface

Autoimmune Hepatitis Including Primary Biliary Cholangitis and Primary Sclerosing Cholangitis

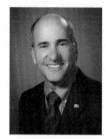

David Bernstein, MD, MACG, FAASLD, AGAF, FACP
Editor

Autoimmune hepatitis, Primary Biliary Cholangitis (PBC), and Primary Sclerosing Cholangitis (PSC) are all chronic, progressive, noncurable conditions affecting the liver, whose pathogenesis remains incompletely understood and whose diagnosis is often delayed or missed in our patient population.

Autoimmune hepatitis, the most common of the three conditions, has been recognized for over 50 years, and when recognized, can be successfully treated. This condition may present as acute hepatitis or as chronic liver disease. As many as half of newly diagnosed patients will have significant fibrosis on initial presentation. Failure to recognize autoimmune hepatitis can delay the administration of potentially life-saving medications and place the patient at risk of more rapidly developing cirrhosis and its complications. Autoimmune hepatitis should be considered in all patients with acute or chronic hepatitis, regardless of age, gender, or ethnic background.

PBC is an autoimmune disorder that leads to the destruction of the small bile ducts within the liver that can progress to the development of significant fibrosis, cirrhosis, and its complications and ultimately, require a liver transplantation. While PBC is not curable, current treatments, including ursodeoxycholic acid and obeticholic acid, are effective in decreasing the abnormal alkaline phosphatase seen in PBC in approximately 80% of patients. Research is continuing to develop better therapies for this condition. Despite better therapies, symptoms and signs of PBC, such as pruritus and fatigue, continue to be challenging to manage. While several new strategies are being developed, continued research is needed so that we can better serve our patients.

PSC is a chronic cholestatic condition characterized by inflammation and fibrosis of the bile ducts that can lead to cirrhosis and its complications as well as predispose

Clin Liver Dis 28 (2024) xiii–xiv
https://doi.org/10.1016/j.cld.2023.07.012
1089-3261/24/© 2023 Published by Elsevier Inc.

liver.theclinics.com

patients to the development of malignancies, such as cholangiocarcinoma, gallbladder cancer, hepatocellular carcinoma, and colon cancer. PSC has a strong association with inflammatory bowel disease (IBD), and patients with IBD should be evaluated for PSC. There are currently no approved medical therapies for PSC, and treatment is driven by symptom management as well as endoscopic intervention. Liver transplantation remains the ultimate treatment for PSC, so there is considerable unmet need to develop medical treatments for this condition.

I hope that you will enjoy this issue, and I believe that it contains pearls to help recognize and manage these patients. Each contributor to this issue has had a career interest in autoimmune liver disease, PBC, or PSC. Each article conveys not only the authors' expertise but also their enthusiasm and determination to extend their knowledge of these conditions to others. I truly hope that you, the readers, will find this issue comprehensive, state-of-the-art, clinically relevant, and most importantly, useful.

David Bernstein, MD, MACG, FAASLD, AGAF, FACP
Professor of Medicine
Division of Gastroenterology
NYU-Grossman School of Medicine
East 38th Street, 23rd Floor
New York, NY 10016, USA

E-mail address:
david.bernstein@nyulangone.org

Autoimmune Hepatitis
Epidemiology, Subtypes, and Presentation

Mitchell L. Shiffman, MD, MACG, AASLDF[a,b,*]

KEYWORDS

- Autoimmune hepatitis • Autoimmune diseases • Epidemiology • Subtypes
- Clinical presentation

KEY POINTS

- Autoimmune hepatitis is an autoimmune disease that targets the liver and is associated with specific genetic markers affecting the immune response.
- The incidence of autoimmune hepatitis increases with age into the 70s. The prevalence of the disease seems to be increasing over time.
- About 20% to 50% of patients with autoimmune hepatitis have coexistent extrahepatic immune disease.
- Autoimmune hepatitis is divided into 2 subtypes based on serologic markers. Subtype 1 is associated with ANA and ASMA. Subtype 2 is associated with anti-LKM. About 20% of patients have no serologic markers.
- The clinical presentation of autoimmune hepatitis varies considerably and includes patients who are asymptomatic, symptomatic, have acute liver failure, or decompensated cirrhosis.

INTRODUCTION

Autoimmune hepatitis (AIH) is a chronic liver disease in which the host immune response targets the liver. The first cases were reported in the 1950s and described patients who developed jaundice, had high serum levels of gamma globulins, a positive lupus erythematosus preparation and liver histology showing severe inflammation with plasma cells.[1,2] The disorder was originally referred to as "lupoid hepatitis" and thought to be part of the spectrum of systemic lupus erythematosus (SLE). The disease was subsequently recognized to be a distinct independent autoimmune disorder and the name AIH was adopted in the 1960s.[3]

AIH can be seen in children and adults of any age, any gender, and any ethnicity or race throughout the world. Most patients already have, will develop, or have a family

[a] Bon Secours Liver Institute of Richmond, Bon Secours Mercy Health, 5855 Bremo Road, Suite 509, Richmond, VA 23226, USA; [b] Bon Secours Liver Institute of Hampton Roads, Bon Secours Mercy Health, 12720 Mc Manus Boulevard, Suite 313, Newport News, VA, 23602, USA
* Liver Institute of Virginia, Bon Secours Mercy Health, Richmond and Newport News, VA.
E-mail address: Mitchell_shiffman@bshsi.org

Clin Liver Dis 28 (2024) 1–14
https://doi.org/10.1016/j.cld.2023.06.002
1089-3261/24/© 2023 Elsevier Inc. All rights reserved.

history of nonhepatic autoimmune disorders and have serologic markers of autoimmune disease.[4–7] AIH, similar to all immune disorders, requires there to be specific genetic alterations in Human Lymphocyte Antigen (HLA) haplotypes and/or mutations in various non-HLA proteins that modulate the immune response.[8] These genetic modifications increase the susceptibility for the patient to develop various immune diseases including AIH but by itself this genetic foundation does not cause an immune disorder until the immune system is "triggered" and the AIH phenotype is expressed. "Triggers" can be any environmental factor that interacts with the host immune response including chemicals, medications, and proteins produced by bacterial, fungal, and viral organisms.[9,10]

AIH is highly heterogenous and variable degrees of hepatic inflammation leads to variable rates of liver injury and fibrosis progression.[4–6] For example, very severe, aggressive immunologic liver injury may result in massive hepatic necrosis, lobular collapse of the hepatic architecture, acute liver failure (ALF), and death without emergent liver transplantation (LT). Alternatively, immune targeting of the liver and hepatic inflammation may be so mild that liver repair is able to keep up with liver injury and fibrosis progression simply does not occur. The severity of the immune response can be modulated by, and in many cases completely suppressed by, immune suppression, which is the primary treatment of AIH. Treatment reduces the risk of disease progression in most patients with AIH. End-stage liver disease develops and the need for LT is only required in about 4% to 6% of patients with AIH.[11]

AIH is a relatively uncommon cause of liver disease and accounts for approximately 5% of patients seen at Liver Institute of Virginia and other Liver Centers worldwide.[4–6] The limited number of patients available for investigation, the genetic-environmental interaction required for disease onset and the varied clinical presentation of the disease has resulted in variable often contradictory data regarding the incidence, prevalence, and natural history of AIH. This article will review data regarding the epidemiology, clinical subtypes, and describe the varied clinical presentations of patients with AIH.

EPIDEMIOLOGY

Although AIH occurs in patients throughout the world, in all ages, genders, ethnicity, and races, there does seem to be subtle differences in the incidence, prevalence, and severity of the disease in various population subgroups. The primary epidemiologic features of AIH are summarized in **Box 1**. The initial epidemiologic data describing AIH were collected in the Scandinavian countries of northwestern Europe and date back to the 1970 to 1990s when formal diagnostic criteria for AIH had not yet been developed. At that time, chronic hepatitis C virus (HCV) could not yet be diagnosed, nonalcoholic fatty liver was uncommon and not recognized as a separate clinical entity, and access to health care and early diagnosis were not as readily available

---

Box 1
Epidemiology of autoimmune hepatitis

- The onset of disease seems to increase with age. Patients may present in their 70s
- Women are affected more commonly but men account for 25% of patients
- The prevalence of all immune disorders, including AIH seems to be increasing over time
- Coexistent autoimmune disease or a family history of autoimmune disorders is present in up to 50% of patients

as they are today. The incidence of new cases of AIH was estimated to be 0.83 to 1.9 per 100,000 persons with a prevalence of 16 to 18 per 100,000.[12,13] Similar estimates for incidence and prevalence were observed in the United States of America (USA).[5,7]

More recent studies have evaluated the incidence of AIH in additional European countries, Israel, Japan, and New Zealand.[14–17] The estimated incidence ranged from 0.67 to 2.0 in Europe with lower rates seen in Israel and the United Kingdom. The highest rates of AIH, 2 per 100,000 were reported from New Zealand and the lowest rates, only 0.05 per 100,000 were in Japan. The prevalence of AIH ranges from 4 to 25 per 100,000. The lowest prevalence seems to be in Asian countries and highest rates seem to be in Denmark and New Zealand.[18] The lower incidence of AIH in the more recent studies is almost certainly due to identification and exclusion of HCV. In contrast, the higher prevalence of AIH is likely due to the development of a formal diagnostic scoring system for AIH, which allowed better recognition and reporting of patients.[19,20] The largest study to estimate the incidence and prevalence for AIH was conducted in the USA and recently published.[21] The study included more than 18 million adults with available data during a mean of 6.7 years. The prevalence of AIH was 26.5 per 100,000. The incidence of a new AIH diagnosis was 4.0 per 100,000. Women accounted for 77% of AIH cases and 75% of new diagnoses. Both the incidence and prevalence of AIH were higher in persons identified as Black race, lowest in Asian race, and similar in Caucasians and Hispanics. The geographic distribution of AIH prevalence and incidence was similar across the USA, except for slightly lower rates in the Pacific region. This is probably due to the higher percentage of Asians in this part of the USA and is consistent with the data reported from that part of the world.[6]

Impact of Age

The age at which AIH was first recognized has historically been described as bimodal with peak incidence of disease onset and diagnosis in the late teens—early 20s and in the 40 to 50s.[22] However, in a large recent study in the USA, the incidence of AIH increased from a low of 1.9 cases per 100,000 in persons aged 18 to 29 years to a high of 8.4 per 1000,000 in persons aged 70 to 79 years.[21] This observation is consistent with other more recent studies in several other countries that have also reported that the onset of AIH increases with age with peak incidence in the range of 50s years or older.[15,23] The frequency of a positive antinuclear antibody (ANA) and the onset of many autoimmune disorders including SLE, multiple sclerosis, and type 1 diabetes mellitus are also increasing in incidence with age.[24–26] This trend in autoimmune disorders may explain the apparent shift in the incidence of AIH to an older age group. The reason for this shift is unclear. However, improved longevity of the elderly population and an increase in exposure to environmental antigens that could "trigger" the immune response and lead to the development of AIH is a likely explanation. The responsiveness of the immune system also changes with age. There is reduced expression of major histocompatibility complex proteins, a decline in the production of cytotoxic T cells, and an increase in autoantibody production by B cells.[27–29]

Racial and Ethnic Differences

The largest study to evaluate racial and ethnic differences in AIH at diagnosis was from a single center in California.[30] This included 183 patients of whom 11% were of Hispanic ethnicity and 9% were Asian. Hispanics had the highest rate of biopsy proven cirrhosis at diagnosis, 55% compared with 29% for Caucasians and 30% for Asians. A similar study from a single center in Baltimore evaluated the severity of AIH at diagnosis in 101 patients.[31] In this study, Black patients had a significantly greater fibrosis score compared with Caucasians, 3.6 versus 2.1; were significantly more likely to have cirrhosis, 57% versus 36%; liver failure, 38% versus 9%; and to be referred for LT, 51% versus 23%. A study in Alaskan natives demonstrated that 35% of this population had jaundice at the time of AIH diagnosis but that patients who were identified with asymptomatic AIH were more likely to have moderate-to-severe fibrosis on biopsy than patients with jaundice.[32] It is difficult to know if these data support true racial and ethnic differences in the onset and natural history of AIH or simply reflect disparities in access to health care that are frequently seen in minority and rural populations.

Genetics and triggers for autoimmune hepatitis

Patients with AIH have specific alterations in genes that modulate the immune response. The most commonly recognized and studied are those alleles, which code for the HLA complex. In Europe and North America, approximately 80% to 85% of patients with AIH have DR3 and/or DR4 haplotypes.[33,34] In addition, 38% of patients with AIH had the specific HLA haplotype A1-B8-DR3 compared with only 11% of patients without AIH.[35] Genetic alterations may also influence the severity of AIH and response to treatment. For example, patients with the A1-B8-RD3 haplotype had more severe AIH and were less responsive to immune suppression than patients without this haplotype.[35,36]

In Japan where the prevalence of AIH is lower than seen in North America and Europe, HLA A1-B8-DR3 is rare. In contrast, HLA DR 4, and DRB1 is the most common haplotype associated with AIH in Japan. DR4 is present in 90% of Japanese patients with AIH compared with only 39% of patients without the disorder.[37,38] In Argentina, AIH is also associated with HLA DR4 and DRB1 but also A11.[39,40] HLA DRB1 is also associated with a protracted form of hepatitis A virus and it has been speculated that HAV may a viral "trigger" for the development of AIH in Argentina.[41] If this is true, vaccination of the population against HAV at birth may reduce the risk AIH.

AIH also has associations with non-HLA proteins involved in the immune response. Tumor necrosis factor, T lymphocyte antigen-4, apoptosis antigen-1, the vitamin D receptor, and interleukin-23 are only some of the many immune modulating proteins in which polymorphisms have been observed in patients with AIH.[5] These genetic changes may alter the way in which the immune system responds to "trigger" antigens to initiate AIH disease, affect the inflammatory severity, which leads to fibrosis progression in AIH, and/or response to treatment.

Various environmental toxins can act as "triggers," initiate the immune response and cause AIH disease in genetically susceptible persons. "Triggers" for AIH can be chemical agents, medications, and proteins from infectious agents including fungus, bacterial, and viruses. The 2 most widely used medications that have been implicated in AIH include nitrofurantoin and minocycline, which together account for 90% of reported cases of drug-induced AIH.[42] Several viruses have been implicated as "triggers" for AIH including Cytomegalovirus, Epstein-Barr,[43] hepatitis E virus,[44] and most recently severe acute respiratory syndrome coronavirus 2 (SARS-CoV-2), which stimulates the immune response to causes coronavirus disease 2019 (COVID-19). Many case reports have described persons who developed AIH during or following COVID-19. AIH has also been reported to appear in patients weeks to months following vaccination against SARS-CoV-2.[45] Despite these observations, proving what the specific "triggering" agent is in any given patient is difficult. The process is almost certainly idiosyncratic and dependent on the presence of a specific polymorphism in one of the many immune-mediating proteins that is unique to that patient, allowing the binding of the "trigger" antigen and leading to a cascade of events resulting in the emergence of AIH. Genetic differences in the frequency of immune polymorphisms may be one explanation for the geographic variation in AIH epidemiology.

Coexistent immune disorders

Approximately 20% to 50% of persons with AIH have coexistent nonhepatic autoimmune disorders.[46,47] Extrahepatic autoimmune diseases are more common in women, in patients with a family history of autoimmune disease and in patients with HLA DRB1.[48,49] Autoimmune diseases may develop in persons who already have well-established AIH or the rheumatologic disorder may precede the development of AIH.[50] The 2 most common extrahepatic diseases observed include thyroid disease and rheumatoid arthritis. Either hyperthyroidism or hypothyroidism occurs in approximately 10% to 20% of patients.[51,52] Rheumatoid arthritis has been observed in up to 40% of patients with AIH, particularly in women aged older than 60 years.[53] Celiac disease is more common in patients with AIH than in the general population, 3.5 versus 2.8%. However, identifying coexistent AIH and celiac disease can be challenging because both can cause gastrointestinal symptoms and elevations in liver enzymes. Approximately 10% to 60% of patients with celiac disease have elevated liver enzymes but only 5% to 15% of patients with celiac disease have coexistent AIH. Resolution of liver enzymes to normal with a strict gluten free diet strongly suggests that the patient does not have coexistent AIH.[54] Almost any rheumatologic disorder can be observed in patients with AIH.

Approximately 20% to 60% of patients with a rheumatologic disease will develop an elevation in liver enzymes.[55,56] The most common cause for this is medications used for the treatment of the immune disease.[50,55] Approximately half of the liver enzyme elevations in patients with rheumatologic diseases are due to drug-induced liver injury (DILI). Discontinuing medications that cause DILI should therefore be the first step in the evaluation and management of patients with a rheumatologic disease who develop an elevation in liver enzymes.[55] However, an elevation in liver transaminases in a patient with a rheumatologic disease should also initiate an evaluation for AIH. Identifying AIH in a patient with a coexistent rheumatologic disease can be challenging because overlapping autoantibodies can be observed in both disorders. Many patients with rheumatologic diseases will test positive for ANA, smooth muscle antibody (SMA) and other serologic markers seen in patients with AIH but have persistently normal liver enzymes. These patients are likely to be at genetic risk to develop AIH in the future but do not have AIH now.[50,55]

Patients with a rheumatologic disease can develop chronic elevations in liver transaminases without progressive liver injury. This syndrome has been referred to autoimmune-associated hepatitis. It can be seen in almost any rheumatologic disorder and was first described in patients with SLE.[50,55,56] Approximately 20% to 60% of patients with SLE will develop elevated liver enzymes. The most common cause for this is DILI, which accounts for about 30% of these patients. Although true AIH and SLE can coexist, about 25% of patients with SLE and persistent elevations in liver transaminases have SLE-associated hepatitis. The serologic and histologic features that differentiate SLE-associated hepatitis from AIH are summarized in **Table 1**. Histologically these patients have mild nonspecific portal inflammation, no interface activity, no piecemeal necrosis and no fibrosis. A fibroscan showing normal liver stiffness, which does not increase over time would be equally convincing. Because autoimmune-associated hepatitis does not typically cause progressive liver injury, treatment with additional immune suppression is not usually required.

SUBTYPES OF AUTOIMMUNE HEPATITIS

Two subtypes of AIH have been described: type 1 and type 2.[5,7] The differentiating factor for these subtypes is the pattern of autoantibodies present in the sera of

Table 1 Characteristics of immune-associated hepatitis compared with autoimmune hepatitis		
	Immune-Associated Hepatitis	**Autoimmune Hepatitis**
Immune markers		
Low compliment 3 or 4	Common	Normal
ANA	90%	60% (Type 1)
ASMA	Negative	90% (Type 1)
Anti-LKM	Negative	5%–10% (Type 2)
Anti-ribosomal P	Positive	Negative
Liver histology		
Portal inflammation	Mild	Moderate–severe
Interface hepatitis	None	Common
Piecemeal necrosis	None	Frequent
Lobular inflammation	None–mild	Common
Fibrosis	None–mild	Variable. Usually greater than stage 1

affected individuals (**Table 2**). Classic type 1 AIH is the most common type of AIH found throughout the world and up to 80% of these patients test positive for ANA and 66% for SMA (referred to in some laboratories as antiactin). In contrast, patients with type 2 AIH are positive for antibodies to liver-kidney microsome 1 (anti-LKM1) and negative for ANA and ASMA. Type 2 AIH is rare, accounts for less than 5% of patients with AIH and most of these patients are diagnosed as children. Type 2 AIH is primarily found in specific geographic regions of the world including Canada, England, Southern Europe, New Zealand, and Australia.[5,7,57,58] These populations are historically related keeping with the strong genetic predisposition for AIH. Type 2 AIH is very rare in Japan.[6,59] Although initial studies suggested that patients with type 2 AIH may have a more aggressive course and be less responsive to treatment, more recent data suggested that the clinical course of types 1 and 2 AIH are similar.[58,59] The titer of ANA, ASMA or anti-LKM does not correlate with disease activity or risk of fibrosis progression.[60,61] About 20% of patients with AIH will be negative for ANA, ASMA, and anti-LKM1.[62–65] The clinical presentation and response to treatment of patients with seronegative AIH seems to be similar to the other subtypes.

ANA and ASMA are not unique to AIH and can be found in patients with many other systemic and hepatic immune disorders.[57] Similarly, autoantibodies seen in other liver

Table 2 Autoantibodies seen in patients with autoimmune hepatitis	
Type 1	**Type 2**
Most commonly seen: ANA SMA	Most commonly seen: Anti-liver-kidney-microsome 1 (anti-LKM1)
Less commonly seen: ANCA AMA IGG4 Soluble liver antigen SLA	Less commonly seen: Anti-liver cytosol 1 (anti-LC1) Anti-liver-kidney-microsome 3 (anti-LKM3)

immune diseases including antinuclear cytoplasmic antibody (ANCA), antimitochondrial antibody (AMA), and immune-gamma globulin 4 (IGG4) can also be seen in patients with AIH and this has led to the term "overlap syndrome."[66] Antisoluble liver antigen (anti-SLA) is the most specific single immune marker for type 1 AIH with a positive predictive value of 99% but is only present in 20% to 30% of these patients.[57,67,68] Anti-SLA has been associated with more severe AIH and a higher risk of relapse following withdrawal of immune suppression. Antibodies to liver cytosol are present in about 33% of patients with anti-LKM1 and may represent a more severe form of type 2 AIH in children.[69,70] Anti-LKM3 is present in 17% of patients with type 2 AIH and may be positive in patients negative for anti-LKM1.[71] Anti-LKM1 and anti-LC1 can be found in 5% to 10% of patients with HCV and 13% of patients with hepatitis D virus (HDV) test positive for anti-LKM3.[72,73] These patients likely have specific genetic polymorphisms, which share affinity for proteins from HCV or HDV and type 2 AIH.[74]

CLINICAL PRESENTATION

The clinical presentation of AIH is highly variable, spans the clinical spectrum of disease and includes patients with mild elevations in liver transaminases with or without cirrhosis, moderate-to-severe elevations in liver transaminases with or without jaundice, marked elevations in liver transaminases with jaundice and ALF, and decompensated cirrhosis (**Table 3**). Patients who are suspected to have AIH should be questioned about coexistent autoimmune disorders. Laboratory testing should include serologic markers of autoimmune liver disease, viral hepatitis, and other markers of chronic liver disease, liver chemistries, serum gamma globulins, and a complete blood count. Liver imaging with ultrasound should be performed. If AIH is strongly suspected, the patient should then undergo liver biopsy. The diagnostic criteria for AIH was developed in 1999 and simplified for clinical use in 2008.[19,20] The later includes an assessment for serologic markers of autoimmune disease (ANA, ASMA, anti-LKM in children, and anti-SLA if negative for ANA and ASMA), the level of gamma globulins in serum, liver histology, and excluding viral hepatitis by

Table 3
Clinical presentations in autoimmune hepatitis

Description	Liver Transaminases	Serology	Histology or Elastography
No AIH Genetic susceptibility	Normal	Positive	Normal
Asymptomatic	Mild elevation Typically <150	Positive or negative	Normal—stage 1
Symptomatic	Mild–moderate elevation Typically <250	Positive or negative	Variable Cirrhosis may be present
Severe	Marked elevation Typically >500	Positive or negative	Severe inflammation Marked interface activity, piecemeal necrosis, and lobular inflammation Cirrhosis may be present
ALF	Marked elevation Typically >500	Positive or negative	Sever inflammation Lobular collapse Cirrhosis may be present
Decompensated cirrhosis	Normal–mild elevation	Positive or negative	Cirrhosis

---

Box 2
Diagnostic criteria for autoimmune hepatitis

- Positive ANA, ASMA and/or anti-SLA in adults. Positive Anti-LKM3 and/or anti-LC1 in children.
- Elevation in serum gamma globulins.
- Negative serologic markers or viral polymerase chain reaction (PCR) testing for viral hepatitis.
- A liver biopsy that demonstrates active hepatitis typically with plasma cells that is consistent with an immune etiology. A liver biopsy is essential, unless contraindicated, prior to initiating treatment.

---

serologic testing.[20] Clinical Care Points that are essential for diagnosis of AIH are listed in **Box 2**.

The treatment of AIH is immune suppression. This foundation of treatment is a corticosteroid such as prednsione at doses of 20-60 mg/day. The starting dose of prednsione can be adjusted based upon the level of the serum liver transamaisnes and the severity of the inflammation on liver biopsy. Patients with contraindications to prednisone can be treated with Budesonide at a dose of 9 mg/day, Budesonide appears to be no better at controlling AIH than proper doses of prednsione, but is associated with less weight gain and bone mineral density loss. As liver enzymes come down the dose of prednsione is tapered slowly. Second line treatment for AIH is with an anti-metabolite such as azathioprine typically prescribed at a dose of 1.0-1.5 mg/kg/day or mycophenolate mofetil at a doses of 250-1000 mg twice daily. Like prednisone, the starting dose utilized is typically based upon the severity of the AIH. The second medication can be started simultaneously with prednisone or delayed until the liver enzymes are coming down, or in the normal range but should be started at least 3-6 months prior to to stopping prednsione. The vast majority of patients with AIH respond to immune suppression and can maintain normal liver enzymes and disease suppression for decades without prednisone as long as they remain on maintenance treatment with a second line agent. Patients who cannot tolerate a second line agent are best switched from prednsione to Budesonide. The treatment of AIH is discussed in more detail in a later contribution to this volume of Clinics in Liver Disease.[75,76,77]

Asymptomatic Autoimmune Hepatitis

About 25% to 33% of patients with AIH are asymptomatic when first recognized.[78,79] Most of these patients will have persistently mild elevations in liver transaminases with normal tests of liver function and platelet count. About 10% to 15% of these patients will have fluctuations in liver transaminases to variable degrees, greater than and less than the limits of normal for variable periods, which may last months to years, before the liver transaminases become persistently elevated.[80] Despite this seemingly benign clinical course, liver histology is actually similar in patients with asymptomatic and symptomatic disease.[81] In addition, about 26% to 70% of patients who are asymptomatic at presentation will develop symptoms during the next decade.[79,81] One study has suggested that the 10-year survival of asymptomatic patients is reduced compared with patients with symptoms, 67% versus 98%, and this is primary because asymptomatic patients are less likely to be treated with immune suppression and experience disease progression despite being asymptomatic.[80] It is therefore imperative that all patients with confirmed or suspected AIH be fully evaluated, for disease activity and severity with either liver histology, and/or vibration controlled (Fibroscan) or Ultrasound shear wave elastography. Patients with an increased liver stiffness by elastography should undergo liver biopsy to confirm histologic severity and offered treatment for AIH if liver injury is significant. Patients who are thought to have liver histology that is "too mild" for treatment must be monitored at periodic intervals with biochemical tests of liver inflammation and tests of liver function and liver histology. The latter is best accomplished by annual or semiannual Fibroscan or Ultrasound shear wave elastography. A sustained increase in liver stiffness should prompt the initiation of treatment. A liver biopsy should be performed prior to initiating treatment if not done preiously. However, it is not essential that liver biopsy be repeated if this had been performed previously and the histogy was consistent with AIH.

Symptomatic Autoimmune Hepatitis

Most patients with AIH present clinically because they have symptoms of chronic liver disease with mild-moderate persistent elevations in liver transaminases. The most common symptom is fatigue, which is present in 85% of patients at diagnosis.[82] Laboratory data may demonstrate either normal liver function and platelet count or a decline in hepatic function and platelet count. The later suggests that the patient may have already developed cirrhosis. A liver biopsy to confirm disease severity should be performed in all symptomatic patients. Treatment of AIH should then be initiated.

Severe acute autoimmune hepatitis and acute liver failure

AIH presents as an acute illness with marked elevation in liver transaminases to values of 500 to more than 1000 IU/L and jaundice in about 25% to 75% of patients.[83–85] Diagnostic testing including liver biopsy should be performed in these patients without delay and treatment with high-dose corticosteroids should be promptly initiated. Delays in diagnosis and initiating treatment could result in the patient developing ALF. Patients with severe acute AIH must be monitored closely, even after treatment with immune suppression has been initiated to confirm clinical response and improvement in liver function.

ALF with coagulopathy and hepatic encephalopathy develops in 3% to 6% of patients with severe acute AIH.[85,86] Some patients may be too ill to undergo liver biopsy because of severe coagulopathy. Patients with AIH and ALF should be transferred to an LT center without delay and not be empirically treated with immune suppression because this may increase the risk for infection and delay or prevent the opportunity to receive an LT. Furthermore, it is unlikely that immune suppression would be effective and reverse severe AIH in a patient who has already developed ALF.

Decompensated cirrhosis

Patients with AIH may develop progressive hepatic fibrosis, cirrhosis, and not be clinically recognized until they develop hepatic decompensation with ascites, edema, hepatic encephalopathy, and or variceal hemorrhage.[87] Many of these patients have normal liver transaminases and "burned out" autoimmune disease with none to minimal inflammation on liver biopsy by the time they are diagnosed. Treatment with immune suppression is not indicated because the patient either has no ongoing inflammation and/or is too ill and at increased risk for infection when treated with immune suppression. Such patients should be considered for LT if clinically appropriate.

SUMMARY

The incidence of AIH increases with age and patients may first present in their 70s. The prevalence seems to be increasing over time. The disease is divided into 2 subgroups based on the pattern of serologic markers. Type 1 is associated with ANA and SMA. Type 2 is associated with anti-LKM and most commonly presents in children. Many other autoantibodies may be present as well. Overall, the 2 subtypes seem to have a similar disease severity, natural history, and response to treatment. The clinical spectrum at diagnosis may vary considerably and includes patients who are asymptomatic, symptomatic with or without stable cirrhosis, have severe hepatitis with or without jaundice, ALF, or decompensated cirrhosis. The treatment for AIH is immune suppression, typically prednsione and an anti-metabolite.

DISCLOSURE

The author has not received any commercial, financial support related to the topic of this article.

REFERENCES

1. Zimmerman HJ, Heller P, Hill RP. Extreme hyperglobulinema in subacute hepatic necrosis. N Engl J Med 1951;244:245–9.
2. Cowling DC, Mackay IR, Taft LI. Lupoid hepatitis. Lancet 1956;271(6957):1323–6.
3. Mackay IR, Weiden S, Hasker J. Autoimmune hepatitis. Ann N Y Acad Sci 1965; 124:767–80.
4. European Association for the Study of the Liver. EASL clinical practice guidelines: autoimmune hepatitis. Hepatology 2015;63:971–1004.
5. Mack CL, Adams D, Assis DN, et al. Diagnosis and management of autoimmune hepatitis in adults and children: 2019 practice guidance and guidelines from the American Association for the Study of Liver Diseases. Hepatology 2020;72: 671–722.
6. Ohira H, Takahashi A, Zeniya M, et al. Clinical practice guidelines for autoimmune hepatitis. Hepatol Res 2022;52:571–85.
7. Boberg KM. Prevalence and epidemiology of autoimmune hepatitis. Clin Liver Dis 2002;6:635–47.
8. Price P, Witt C, Allcock R, et al. The genetic basis for the association of the 8.1 ancestral haplotype (A1, B8, DR3) with multiple immunopathological diseases. Immunol Rev 1999;167:257–74.
9. Christen U, Hintermann E. Pathogen infection as a possible cause for autoimmune hepatitis. Int Rev Immunol 2014;33:296–313.
10. Floreani A, Leung PS, Gershwin ME. Environmental basis of autoimmunity. Clin Rev Allergy Immunol 2016;50:287–300.
11. Manns MP, Czaja AJ, Gorham JD, et al. Diagnosis and management of autoimmune hepatitis. Hepatology 2010;51:2193–223.
12. Boberg KM, Aadland E, Jahnsen J, et al. Incidence and prevalence of primary biliary cirrhosis, primary sclerosing cholangitis, and autoimmune hepatitis in a Norwegian population. Scand J Gastroenterol 1998;33:99–9103.
13. Werner M, Prytz H, Ohlsson B, et al. Epidemiology and the initial presentation of autoimmune hepatitis in Sweden: a nationwide study. Scand J Gastroenterol 2008;43:1232–40.
14. Feld JJ, Heathcote EJ. Epidemiology of autoimmune liver disease. J Gastroenterol Hepatol 2003;18:1118–28.
15. Ngu JH, Bechly K, Chapman BA, et al. Population-based epidemiology study of autoimmune hepatitis: a disease of older women? J Gastroenterol Hepatol 2010; 25:1681–6.

16. Delgado J-S, Vodonos A, Malnick S, et al. Autoimmune hepatitis in southern Israel: a 15-year multicenter study. J Dig Dis 2013;14:611–8.
17. van Gerven NMF, Verwer BJ, Witte BI, et al. Epidemiology and clinical characteristics of autoimmune hepatitis in The Netherlands. Scand J Gastroenterol 2014; 49:1245–54.
18. Czaja AJ. Global disparities and their implications in the occurrence and outcome of autoimmune hepatitis. Dig Dis Sci 2017;62:227–2292.
19. Alvarez F, Berg PA, Bianchi FB, et al. International autoimmune hepatitis group report: review of criteria for diagnosis of autoimmune hepatitis. J Hepatol 1999; 31:929–38.
20. Hennes EM, Zeniya M, Czaja AJ, et al. Simplified criteria for the diagnosis of autoimmune hepatitis. Hepatology 2008;48:169–76.
21. Bittterman T, Lewis JD, Levy C, et al. Sociodemographic and geographic differences in the US epidemiology of autoimmune hepatitis with and without cirrhosis. Hepatology 2023;77:367–78.
22. McFarlane IG. The relationship between autoimmune markers and different clinical syndromes in autoimmune hepatitis. Gut 1998;42:599–602.
23. Gronbaek L, Vilstrup H, Jepsen P. Autoimmune hepatitis in Denmark: incidence, prevalence, prognosis, and causes of death. A nationwide registry-based cohort study. J Hepatol 2014;60:612–7.
24. Lerner A, Matthias T. The world incidence and prevalence of autoimmune diseases is increasing. Int J Celiac Dis 2015;3. 151–5.5.
25. Fatoye F, Gebrye T, Svenson LW. Real-world incidence and prevalence of systemic lupus erythematosus in Alberta, Canada. Rheumatol Int 2018;38:1721–6.
26. Dinse GE, Parks CG, Weinberg CR, et al. Increasing prevalence of antinuclear antibodies in the United States. Arthritis Rheum 2022;74:2032–41.
27. Schwab R, Russo C, Weksler ME. Altered major histocompatibility complex-restricted antigen recognition by T cells from elderly humans. Eur J Immunol 1992;22:2989–93.
28. De Paoli P, Battistin S, Santini GF. Age-related changes in human lymphocyte subsets: progressive reduction of the CD4 CD45R (suppressor inducer) population. Clin Immunol Immunopathol 1988;48:290–6.
29. Rowley MJ, Buchanan H, Mackay IR. Reciprocal change with age in antibody to extrinsic and intrinsic antigens. Lancet 1968;2:24–6.
30. Wong RJ, Gish R, Frederick T, et al. The impact of race/ethnicity on the clinical epidemiology of autoimmune hepatitis. J Clin Gastroenterol 2012;46:155–61.
31. Verma S, Torbenson M, Thuluvath PJ. The impact of ethnicity on the natural history of autoimmune hepatitis. Hepatology 2007;46:1828–35.
32. Hurlburt KJ, McMahon BJ, Deubner H, et al. Prevalence of autoimmune liver disease in Alaska Natives. Am J Gastroenterol 2002;97:2402–7.
33. Czaja AJ, Donaldson PT. Genetic susceptibilities for immune expression and liver cell injury in autoimmune hepatitis. Immunol Rev 2000;174:250–9.
34. Czaja AJ, Strettell MDJ, Thomson LJ, et al. Associations between alleles of the major histocompatibility complex and type 1 autoimmune hepatitis. Hepatology 1997;25:317–23.
35. Donaldson PT, Doherty DG, Hayllar KM, et al. Susceptibility to autoimmune chronic active hepatitis: human leukocyte antigen DR4 and A1–B8-DR3 are independent risk factors. Hepatology 1991;13:701–6.
36. Strettell MDJ, Donaldson PT, Thomson LJ, et al. Allelic basis for HLA-encoded susceptibility to type 1 autoimmune hepatitis. Gastroenterology 1997;112:2028–35.

37. Seki T, Kiyosawa K, Inoko H, et al. Association of autoimmune hepatitis with HLA-Bw54 and DR4 in Japanese patients. Hepatology 1990;12:1300–4.

38. Seki T, Ota M, Furuta S, et al. HLA class II molecules and autoimmune hepatitis susceptibility in Japanese patients. Gastroenterology 1992;103:1041–7.

39. Marcos Y, Fainboim HA, Capucchio M, et al. Two-locus involvement in the association of human leukocyte antigen with the extrahepatic manifestations of autoimmune chronic active hepatitis. Hepatology 1994;19:1371–4.

40. Pando M, Larriba J, Fernandez GC, et al. Pediatric and adult forms of type 1 autoimmune hepatitis in Argentina: evidence for differential genetic predisposition. Hepatology 1999;30:1374–80.

41. Fainboim L, Velasco VCC, Marcos CY, et al. Protracted, but not acute, hepatitis Avirus infection is strongly associated with HLA-DRB1*1301, a marker for pediatric autoimmune hepatitis. Hepatology 2001;33:1512–7.

42. Björnsson E, Talwalkar J, Treeprasertsuk S, et al. Drug induced autoimmune hepatitis: clinical characteristics and prognosis. Hepatology 2010;51:2040–8.

43. Vento S, Guella L, Mirandola F, et al. Epstein-Barr virus as a trigger for autoimmune hepatitis in susceptible individuals. Lancet 1995;346:608–9.

44. Pischke S, Gisa A, Suneetha PV, et al. Increased HEV seroprevalence in patients with autoimmune hepatitis. PLoS One 2014;9:e85330.

45. Sgamato C, Rocco A, Compare D, et al. Autoimmune liver diseases and SARS-CoV-2. World J Gastroenterol 2023;29:1838–51.

46. Muratori P, Fabbri A, Lalanne C, et al. Autoimmune liver disease and concomitant extrahepatic autoimmune disease. Eur J Gastroenterol Hepatol 2015;27:1175–9.

47. Bittencourt PL, Farias AQ, Porta G, et al. Frequency of concurrent autoimmune disorders in patients with autoimmune hepatitis: effect of age, gender, and genetic background. J Clin Gastroenterol 2008;42:300–5.

48. Czaja AJ, Carpenter HA, Santrach PJ, et al. Significance of HLA DR4 in type 1 autoimmune hepatitis. Gastroenterology 1993;105:1502–7.

49. Fogel R, Comerford M, Chilukuri P, et al. Extrahepatic autoimmune diseases are prevalent in autoimmune hepatitis patients and their first-degree relatives: survey study. Interact J Med Res 2018;7:e18.

50. Gebreselassie A, Aduli F, Howell CD. Rheumatologic diseases and the liver. Clin Liver Dis 2019;23:247–61.

51. Teufel A, Weinmann A, Kahaly GJ, et al. Concurrent autoimmune diseases in patients with autoimmune hepatitis. J Clin Gastroenterol 2010;44:208–13.

52. Wong GW, Yeong T, Lawrence D, et al. Concurrent extrahepatic autoimmunity in autoimmune hepatitis: implications for diagnosis, clinical course and long-term outcomes. Liver Int 2017;37:449–57.

53. Czaja AJ, Carpenter HA. Distinctive clinical phenotype and treatment outcome of type 1 autoimmune hepatitis in the elderly. Hepatology 2006;43:532–8.

54. Rubio-Taia A, Murray JA. The liver and celiac disease. Clin Liver Dis 2019;23:167–76.

55. Selmi C, Generali E, Gershwin ME. Rheumatic manifestations in autoimmune liver disease. Rheum Dis Clin North Am 2018;44:65–87.

56. Takahashi A, Abe K, Saito R, et al. Liver dysfunction in patients with systemic lupus erythematosus. Intern Med 2013;52:1461–5.

57. Terziroli Beretta-Piccoli B, Mieli-Vergani G, Vergani D. Autoimmune hepatitis: serum autoantibodies in clinical practice. Clin Rev Allergy Immunol 2022;63:124–37.

58. Homberg JC, Abuaf N, Bernard O, et al. Chronic active hepatitis associated with antiliver/kidney microsome antibody type 1: a second type of "autoimmune" hepatitis. Hepatology 1987;7:1333–9.
59. Gregorio GV, Portmann B, Reid F, et al. Autoimmune hepatitis in childhood: a 20-year experience. Hepatology 1997;25:541–7.
60. Czaja AJ. Behavior and significance of autoantibodies in type 1 autoimmune hepatitis. J Hepatol 1999;30:394–401.
61. Gregorio GV, McFarlane B, Bracken P, et al. Organ and non-organ specific auto-antibody titres and IgG levels as markers of disease activity: a longitudinal study in childhood autoimmune liver disease. Autoimmunity 2002;35:515–9.
62. Czaja AJ, Hay JE, Rakela J. Clinical features and prognostic indications of severe corticosteroid treated cryptogenic chronic active hepatitis. Mayo Clin Proc 1990; 65:23–30.
63. Johnson PJ, McFarlane IG, McFarlane BM, et al. Auto-immune features in patients with idiopathic chronic active hepatitis who are seronegative for conventional autoantibodies. J Gastroenterol Hepatol 1990;5:244–51.
64. Kaymakoglu S, Cakaloglu Y, Demir K, et al. Is severe cryptogenic chronic hepatitis similar to autoimmune hepatitis? J Hepatol 1998;28:78–83.
65. Mehendiratta V, Mitroo P, Bombonati A, et al. Serologic markers do not predict histologic severity or response to treatment in patients with autoimmune hepatitis. Clin Gastroenterol Hepatol 2009;7:98–103.
66. Kerkar N, Chan A. Autoimmune hepatitis, sclerosing cholangitis, and autoimmune sclerosing cholangitis overlap syndrome. Clin Liver Dis 2018;22:689–702.
67. Kanzler S, Weidemann C, Gerken G, et al. Clinical significance of autoantibodies to soluble liver antigen in autoimmune hepatitis. J Hepatol 1999;31:635–40.
68. Efe C, Ozaslan E, Wahlin S, et al. Antibodies to soluble liver antigen in patients with various liver diseases: a multicentre study. Liver Int 2013;33:190–6.
69. Martini E, Abuaf N, Cavalli F, et al. Antibody to liver cytosol (anti-LC1) in patients with autoimmune chronic active hepatitis type 2. Hepatology 1988;8:1662–6.
70. Abuaf N, Johanet C, Chretien P, et al. Characterization of the liver cytosol antigen type 1 reacting with autoantibodies in chronic active hepatitis. Hepatology 1992; 16:892–8.
71. Fabien N, Desbos A, Bienvenu J, et al. Autoantibodies directed against the UDP-glucuronosyltransferases in human autoimmune hepatitis. Autoimmun Rev 2004; 3:1–9.
72. Miyakawa H, Kako M, Nagai K, et al. HCV-RNA in type 2 autoimmune hepatitis. Am J Gastroenterol 1991;86:1688–9.
73. Crivelli O, Lavarini C, Chiaberge E, et al. Microsomal autoantibodies in chronic infection with the HBsAg associated delta (delta) agent. Clin Exp Immunol 1983;54:232–8.
74. Cassani F, Cataleta M, Valentini P, et al. Serum autoantibodies in chronic hepatitis C: c-comparison with autoimmune hepatitis and impact on the disease profile. Hepatology 1997;26:561–6.
75. Kelly C, Zen Y, Heneghan MA. Post-Transplant Immunosuppression in Autoimmune Liver Disease. J Clin Exp Hepatol 2023;13(2):350–9.
76. Manns MP, Woynarowski M, Kreisel W, et al. Budesonide induces remission more effectively than prednisone in a controlled trial of patients with autoimmune hepatitis. Gastroenterology 2010;139:1198–206.
77. Peiseler M, Liebscher T, Sebode M, et al. Efficacy and Limitations of Budesonide as a Second-Line Treatment for Patients With Autoimmune Hepatitis. Clin Gastroenterol Hepatol 2018;16:260–7.

78. Czaja AJ. Diagnosis and management of autoimmune hepatitis: current status and future directions. Gut Liv 2016;10:177–203.

79. Feld JJ, Dinh H, Arenovich T, et al. Autoimmune hepatitis: effect of symptoms and cirrhosis on natural history and outcome. Hepatology 2005;42:53–62.

80. Czaja AJ. Features and consequences of untreated type 1 autoimmune hepatitis. Liver Int 2009;29:816–23.

81. Kogan J, Safadi R, Ashur Y, et al. Prognosis of symptomatic versus asymptomatic autoimmune hepatitis: a study of 68 patients. J Clin Gastroenterol 2002;35:75–81.

82. Czaja AJ. Natural history, clinical features, and treatment of autoimmune hepatitis. Semin Liver Dis 1984;4:1–12.

83. Nikias GA, Batts KP, Czaja AJ. The nature and prognostic implications of autoimmune hepatitis with an acute presentation. J Hepatol 1994;21:866–71.

84. Ferrari R, Pappas G, Agostinelli D, et al. Type 1 autoimmune hepatitis: patterns of clinical presentation and differential diagnosis of the "acute" type. QJM 2004;97: 407–12.

85. Czaja AJ. Acute and acute severe (fulminant) autoimmune hepatitis. Dig Dis Sci 2013;58:897–914.

86. Stravitz RT, Lefkowitch JH, Fontana RJ, et al. Autoimmune acute liver failure: proposed clinical and histological criteria. Hepatology 2011;53:517–26.

87. Wang Z, Sheng L, Yang Y, et al. The management of autoimmune hepatitis patients with decompensated cirrhosis: real-world experience and a comprehensive review. Clin Rev Allergy Immunol 2017;52:424–35.

Autoimmune Hepatitis
Pathophysiology

Zhou Yuming, MD[a], Tang Ruqi, PhD[a], Merrill Eric Gershwin, MD[b],*,
Ma Xiong, MD, PhD[a,c],*

KEYWORDS

- Autoimmune hepatitis • Autoantibodies • T cells • Molecular mimicry
- Immune regulation • Microbiome • Autoimmunity

KEY POINTS

- Genome-wide association analyses suggest that HLA genes including *HLA-DRB*0301*, *HLA-DRB*0401*, and *HLA-B*3501* as well as non-HLA genes including *CD28/CTLA4/ICOS* and *SYNPR* increased AIH susceptibility.
- The destruction of hepatocytes is the result of the imbalance between proinflammatory cells and immunosuppressive cells, especially the imbalance between Tregs and Th17 cells.
- The microbiome in patients with AIH is decreased in diversity with a specific decline in *Bifidobacterium* and enrichment in *Veillonella* and *Faecalibacterium*. Recent evidence has demonstrated the pathogenic role of *E. gallinarum* and *L.reuteri* in inducing autoimmunity in the liver.

INTRODUCTION

Autoimmune hepatitis (AIH) is a chronic inflammatory disease of the liver, characterized by elevated transaminase, high circulating immunoglobin G levels, presence of autoantibodies, and characteristic histological features including interface hepatitis.[1] AIH is classified on the bases of the serum autoantibody profile into AIH-1 and AIH-2. Anti-nuclear antibodies (ANA) and anti-smooth muscle antibodies (SMA) have been identified as markers of AIH-1, whereas anti-liver microsomal type 1 antibodies (anti-LKM1), and anti-liver cytosol type 1 antibodies (anti-LC1) have been recognized

[a] Division of Gastroenterology and Hepatology, Key Laboratory of Gastroenterology and Hepatology, Ministry of Health, NHC Key Laboratory of Digestive Diseases, State Key Laboratory for Oncogenes and Related Genes, Renji Hospital, School of Medicine, Shanghai Jiao Tong University, Shanghai Institute of Digestive Disease, 145 Middle Shandong Road, Shanghai, China; [b] Division of Rheumatology, Department of Medicine, Allergy and Clinical Immunology, University of California at Davis, 451 Health Sciences Drive, Suite 6510, Davis, CA 95616, USA; [c] Institute of Aging & Tissue Regeneration, Renji Hospital, School of Medicine, Shanghai Jiao Tong University, Shanghai, China
* Corresponding authors.
E-mail addresses: megershwin@ucdavis.edu (M.E.G.); maxiongmd@hotmail.com (M.X.)

Clin Liver Dis 28 (2024) 15–35
https://doi.org/10.1016/j.cld.2023.06.003
1089-3261/24/© 2023 Elsevier Inc. All rights reserved.

liver.theclinics.com

as markers of AIH-2.[2] Some individuals only have abnormalities of liver biochemistry in the absence of obvious clinical symptoms, while others manifest with acute liver failure with severe jaundice, fatigue, coagulation dysfunction, and so forth.[1]

The etiology and pathophysiology of AIH are still unclear. The distinguishing histological characteristic of AIH is interface hepatitis with lymphocyte infiltrations. Positive serum autoantibodies and hypergammaglobulinemia in patients with AIH also suggest that a dysregulated immune system is the critical pathobiological change of AIH. Results from twin studies and familial studies on AIH indicated the involvement of genetics in the pathogenesis of AIH.[3,4] Evidence of higher susceptibility to extrahepatic autoimmune diseases in patients with AIH also suggests the importance of genetic changes in the onset of AIH.[5] Environmental factors such as viral infections, drug exposures, microbiome alteration may trigger immune-mediated attacks toward the hepatocytes. Therefore, the initiation of AIH is thought to result from certain environmental triggers-induced immune-mediated attacks against self-antigens in individuals with specific genetic backgrounds. Herein we review the current knowledge on the pathophysiology of AIH and introduce animal models that can enhance our comprehension of AIH pathophysiology (**Fig. 1**).

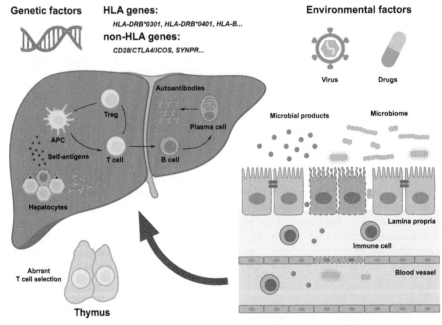

Fig. 1. Pathophysiology of AIH. The initiation of AIH is the result of environmental and genetic factors. HLA genes such as *HLA-DRB*0301*, *HLA-DRB*0401*, and *HLA-B* as well as non-HLA genes such as *CD28/CTLA4/ICOS*, and *SYNPR* increased AIH susceptibility. Environmental factors including viral infections, drug exposures, and microbiome alteration may trigger AIH development. The dysregulated immune system is central to AIH pathophysiology. T cells are selected in the thymus. Failure of positive selection results in the generation of autoreactive T cells which disrupt the immunotolerance towards self-antigens. Interactions between APCs, Tregs, T cells, B cells, plasma cells and other immunocytes are altered in AIH, leading to damage to hepatocytes and autoantibody production. Microbiomes are also involved in the process. The loss of the intestinal barrier, such as tight junctions, leads to bacterial translocation and microbial products entering the blood, followed by immune cell activation and migration, and ultimately disruption of liver homeostasis.

AUTOANTIBODIES
Anti-nuclear Antibodies

ANA are classical antibodies of AIH-1 and are listed in both simplified and comprehensive diagnostic criteria for AIH.[6,7] The positivity of ANA alone exists in 15% of patients with AIH-1.[8] As non-organ-specific autoantibodies, ANA can also be seen in a number of liver pathologies, including primary biliary cholangitis (PBC), viral hepatitis, Wilson disease, and so forth. Indirect immunofluorescence assay on the murine liver, kidney, stomach, and human larynx epithelioma cancer cell line is the most common method to detect ANA.[9] The targets of ANA in AIH-1 include chromatin, ribonucleoproteins, and ribonucleoprotein complexes.[2] However, the liver-specific nuclear targets of ANA in AIH are still unclear.

Smooth Muscle Antibodies

SMA binds to both microfilaments and intermediate filaments such as actin, vimentin and desmin. Actin can be classified into F-actin and G-actin based on its conformations. SMA that targets F-actin is a more specific type of autoantibody in AIH-1. Similar to ANA, SMA is the diagnostic autoantibody for AIH-1. The positivity of SMA alone exists in 35% of patients with AIH. Positivity of ANA and SMA together are present in 60% of patients with AIH-1.[8] Similar to ANA, the presence of SMA also occurs in other liver diseases.

Anti-soluble Liver Antigen

Soluble liver antigen (SLA) exists in the supernatant of liver homogenates. Although SLA is non-organ specific, it is high in the liver and kidney.[10] Liver-pancreas antigen (LP) is detected high in the liver and pancreas.[11] Antibodies to SLA and LP are proven to be identical and positive in patients with AIH.[12] Anti-SLA has the highest specificity for AIH diagnosis and is correlated to the disease severity.[12]

Anti-liver Microsomal Type 1 Antibodies

Anti-LKM1 are specific markers for AIH-2 when hepatitis C virus (HCV) infection is excluded. Anti-LKM1 is present in 5-10% of patients with HCV. The target of anti-LKM1 is CYP2D6. The immunodominant epitope in CYP2D6 is the peptide ranging from amino acids 254-257, which is recognized by most anti-LKM1 positive sera from patients with AIH-2.[13] A CYP2D6 epitope map is well-summarized in a review by U. Chridten and E. Hintermann.[14]

Anti-liver Cytosol Type 1 Antibodies

Anti-LC1 are another type of diagnostic autoantibodies for AIH-2, and sometimes are the only positive autoantibodies present in patients with AIH-2.[15] Anti-LC1 target formiminotransferase cyclodeaminase (FTCD), which is high in the liver. Moreover, anti-LC1 are correlated with disease activity and severity.

Epitope spreading

Epitope spreading, also known as epitope diversification, refers to the immune response towards additional epitopes after the initial epitope triggered immune system activation. Under physiological conditions, epitope spreading allows the identification of more targets on foreign pathogens. In the context of autoimmune diseases, epitope spreading amplifies the immune responses toward self-antigens.[16] The role of epitope spreading has been demonstrated in AIH-2. CYP2D6 mice showed obvious epitope spreading to other regions. In patients with AIH-2, intra-molecular epitope spreading is observed in some patients to a lesser extent. Of note, the initial immunodominant epitope remained to be the strongest epitope throughout the time.[17]

HISTOLOGY OF AUTOIMMUNE HEPATITIS

The key histological features of AIH include interface hepatitis, emperipolesis, and hepatocellular rosettes.[6] The defining histological characteristic of AIH is interface hepatitis, which is the inflammatory infiltration in the interface characterized by plasma cells and lymphocytes along with hepatocyte necrosis.[18] The presence of plasma cells in the infiltrate favors the diagnosis, however, the absence of plasma cells does not rule out the possibility of AIH.[18] The term "hepatocellular rosette" refers to the glandular arrangement of regenerated hepatocytes. Emperipolesis describes the presence of lymphocytes inside the hepatocyte, primarily CD8$^+$ T cells.[19] In contrast to previous understandings, a recent study showed that hepatocellular rosette and emperipolesis are not disease-specific since these features showed no difference in frequencies between HCV and AIH biopsies with matched inflammatory grade.[20] Acute onset AIH has obvious centrilobular necrosis apart from the histological features mentioned above, which makes it hard to distinguish acute onset AIH and drug-induced liver injury.[21] A recent consensus from the International AIH Pathology Group combined both acute and chronic histological features and established new diagnostic criteria for AIH with a dominant pattern of portal hepatitis or lobular hepatitis.[22]

Infiltrated lymphocytes are predominantly CD4$^+$ T cells. The ratio of CD4$^+$/CD8$^+$ T cells in AIH was significantly higher than that in hepatitis B and PBC.[23] Apart from the altered percentages, lymphocytes are distributed differently. CD4$^+$ T cells were distributed in the portal tracts, whereas CD8$^+$ T cells were found in the periportal area.[24] Conversely, in acute onset AIH, CD8$^+$ T cells predominated among other lymphocytes in the interface hepatitis and centrilobular necrosis.[21]

GENETIC FACTORS OF AUTOIMMUNE HEPATITIS

The main genetic regions linked to an elevated risk of AIH are the human leukocyte antigen (HLA) genes. The primary susceptibility genotype in the European populations was HLA-DRB*0301 while the secondary susceptibility genotype was HLA-DRB*0401 according to a genome-wide association analysis by de Boer and colleagues.[25] Furthermore, a genome-wide meta-analysis revealed that HLA-B*3501 was strongly associated with AIH in Chinese populations.[26] Results from studies on single genetic variants of HLA vary across different populations and ethnic groups. HLA-DRB1*1301, HLA-DRB1*0405, HLA-DRB1*13, and HLA-DRB1*03 were associated with AIH-1.[27,28] The detailed associations between AIH and HLA allele or halophyte are summarized elsewhere.[29,30]

In addition to conferring disease susceptibility, HLA gene variations are also associated with disease course and severity. Patients with homozygous HLA-DRB1*03, HLA-DRB1*13, or HLA-DRB1*07 were likely to be suboptimal responders to treatment and develop end-stage liver disease.[31] HLA-DRB1*03 and HLA-DRB1*13 were related to cirrhosis.[31,32] HLA-DRB1*0301 and HLA-DRB1*1301 were correlated with poor treatment response rates.[27,33]

Non-HLA genes were also identified as susceptibility genes of AIH. A genome-wide association study revealed that cluster of differentiation 28/CTLA4/inducible T cell costimulator (CD28/CTLA4/ICOS), and synaptoporin (SYNPR) were significantly associated with AIH-1 in a Chinese population. CD28, CTLA4, and ICOS are all costimulatory molecules on T cells.[26] SYNPR is a membrane protein of synaptic vesicles, suggesting a link between the immune and nervous systems.[26] In the same study,

STAT1/STAT4,LINC00392, IRF8, and *LILRA4/LILRA5* showed a possible association with AIH. The other genome wide study also identified ser homology 2 adaptor protein 3 and caspase recruitment domain family member 10 as likely risk factors for AIH in European populations. Other non-HLA gene polymorphisms have been found such as polymorphisms in various cytokine-related genes.[34–39] These results demonstrated the connections between genetic variants and the dysregulated immune system in AIH.

In conclusion, the results of genetic studies in different populations are heterogeneous. Moreover, further investigations remain to be done to understand the mechanisms of how polymorphisms in HLA and non-HLA genes break the immune tolerance in liver and affect AIH initiation and progression.

ENVIRONMENTAL FACTORS OF AUTOIMMUNE HEPATITIS

In addition to genetic factors, environmental factors, such as viral infections, drug exposures, and gut microbiota, have been implicated in triggering AIH.

Viral Infections and Molecular Mimicry

Evidence suggests that viral infections are potentially a trigger of autoimmune diseases. Subsequent AIH development after hepatitis A virus infections in genetically susceptible individuals has been reported.[40] The presence of typical AIH autoantibodies in patients infected with hepatic viruses has also observed.[41] The most significant association between hepatic virus and AIH belongs to HCV.

The presence of autoantibodies is a common occurrence in patients with chronic hepatitis C. The key autoantibody in AIH-2 is anti-LKM1, which targets CYP2D6, an enzyme in the liver. Proteins of HCV showed similarities with the CYP2D6 epitope sequence.[42] The pathogenic mechanism underlies is molecular mimicry, which refers to the structural similarity between the pathogen and the host. Due to this resemblance, the immune system is fooled and produces antibodies that target both pathogens and self-antigens.[43]

Drugs

Drug-induced liver injury can present similar manifestations to AIH. Despite the fact that drug-induced AIH is distinct from idiopathic AIH, medications still have the potential to induce AIH. Drugs such as halothane, trichloroethylene, dihydralazine, tienilic acid, interferons, and so forth. were reported to cause AIH or AIH-like liver injury.[44,45] Halothane, an inhalation anesthesia, is metabolized by CYP2E1.[46] It can cause hepatitis with necrosis and positive serum autoantibodies.[47,48] The target of these autoantibodies seems to be the neoantigen formed during the trifluoroacetylation of the proteins in the liver.[45] Interferons are used as treatments for hepatitis B virus and HCV. It also boosts immune responses and may cause presentations that are similar to acute hepatitis.

Microbiome

A growing body of evidence points to the microbiome's involvement in immune-mediated diseases.[49] Alterations of the microbiome in patients with AIH and experimental autoimmune hepatitis (EAH) models have been demonstrated.

The alpha diversity of intestinal microbiome in patients with AIH and EAH decreased significantly compared to normal controls.[50–53] The composition changes of AIH microbiome in each study vary (**Table 1**). Thus it is difficult to pinpoint the exact disease-specific microbiome changes. Overall, *Veillonella* and *Faecalibacterium* were enriched in AIH.[50–52,54,55] The specific decline of *Bifidobacterium* was reported in several studies.[52,56,57] The lack of *Bifidobacterium* is also related to failure to achieve remission.[52] A recent study demonstrated the protective functions of *Bifidobacterium animalis* ssp. lactis 420 (B420) in EAH models. B420 strengthened the intestinal barrier and suppressed RIP3 signaling, which is activated by dysbiosis, resulting in the suppression of hepatic macrophages and alleviated liver injury.[58,59]

In AIH, the disrupted bacteria homeostasis in the liver may trigger immune responses. Under normal conditions, *Enterococcus gallinarum* locates in the intestine. The translocation of *E. gallinarum* to the liver has been found in both EAH mice models and patients with AIH, and triggers autoimmunity response.[60] A recent study found that Tet2-deficient mice, which exhibit autoantibody profile and pathological features similar to patients with AIH, showed increased translocated bacteria, especially Lactobacillus reuteri (*L.reuteri*). Indole-3-aldehyde (I3A) produced by *L. reuteri* induces AIH-like liver damage through the upregulation of AhR.[61] This result is contradictory to the previous findings on AhR, which found that AhR activation has immune regulatory effects. To determine the role of different AhR ligands in the pathophysiology of AIH, more research is needed.

Bacterial fermentation products, butyric acids, have anti-inflammatory effects. The ester form of butyric acid, methyl butyrate ameliorates Con-A-induced AIH probably through the inhibition of Th1 cells.[62] The results indicate that microbiome metabolites may also affect AIH.

To sum up, the decreased diversity of microbiome in AIH is observed, together with enriched *Veillonella*, *Faecalibacterium* and decreased *Bifidobacterium*. Recent studies on *E. gallinarum* and *L.reuteri* suggested the pathogenic role of translocated microbiome in AIH.

DYSREGULATED IMMUNE SYSTEM
Regulatory T Cells

Regulatory T cells (Tregs) primarily regulate immune responses and mediate tolerance to self-components (**Fig. 2**).

In general, the frequency of Tregs is decreased in the peripheral blood while increased in the liver of individuals with AIH compared to healthy controls and patients with other chronic liver diseases such as non-alcoholic fatty liver disease.[63–68] However, other evidence suggests that the frequency of Tregs was not different from healthy controls, and the number of intrahepatic Tregs was decreased.[69–71] A significant difference in Treg frequency was observed between patients with AIH in active phase and in remission.[65,69] This indicates that disease activities may account for contradictory results. Also, the inconsistent results may be due to the different markers used to detect Tregs and whether immunosuppressive agents were used in patients with AIH.

It has also been reported that the expansion and immunoregulatory properties of Tregs were impaired in patients with AIH compared to healthy controls.[64,72] The expression of FOXP3 was downregulated in AIH Tregs, resulting in failed suppression of conventional T cells.[70,73] Besides low FOXP3 expression, the poor responsiveness to IL-2 of Tregs lead to decreased IL-10 secretion, which accounts for defected suppressive effects of Tregs.[63] The microenvironment may be accountable for the defected suppressive function of Treg in AIH. The immunosuppressive ability of Tregs was impaired in a proinflammatory microenvironment lacking IL-2. In addition, Tregs were more prone to apoptosis in this microenvironment.[74] Results from a clinical trial showed that low-dose IL-2 activated and expanded Tregs in several autoimmune diseases including AIH.[75] Also, low-dose IL-2 administration restored the equilibrium

Table 1
Studies on microbiome changes in AIH

Country	Groups	Material	Diversity	Enriched Taxa in AIH	Enriched Taxa in Controls	Study
China	AIH(24) vs HC (8)	Stool	NA	None	*Bifidobacterium* and *Lactobacillus*	Lin et al,[56] 2015
Japan	AIH(17) vs HC (15)	Saliva	NS	*Veillonella*	*Streptococcus* and *Fusobacterium*	Abe et al,[54] 2018
China	AIH(91) vs HC(98)	Stool	Decreased	*Veillonella, Klebsiella, Streptococcus,* and *Lactobacillus*	*Clostridiales, RF39, Ruminococcaceae, Rikenellaceae, Oscillospira, Parabacteroides* and *Coprococcus*	Wei et al,[50] 2020
Egypt	AIH(15) vs HC(10)	Stool	Decreased	Phylum level: *Firmicutes, Bacteroides,* and *Proteobacteria;* Genus level: *Faecalibacterium, Blautia, Streptococcus, Haemophilus, Bacteroides,* and *Veillonella*	*Prevotella, Parabacteroides,* and *Dilaster*	Elsherbiny et al,[51] 2020
China	AIH(37) vs HC(78)	Stool	NS	Phylum level: *Verrucomicrobia;* Genus level: 15 genera including *Veillonella, Faecalibacterium, Akkermansia,* and so forth.	Phylum level: *Lentisphaerae* and *Synergistetes;* Genus level: 19 genera including *Pseudobutyrivibrio, Lachnospira, Ruminococcaceae,* and so forth.	Lou et al,[55] 2020
Germany	AIH(72) vs PBC(99) vs UC(81) vs HC(95)	Stool	Decreased (vs HC); NS (vs PBC); increased (vs UC)	*Streptococcus* (vs HC); *Faecalibacterium* (vs PBC)	*Faecalibacterium,* and *Bifidobacterium* (vs HC); *Bifidobacterium* (vs PBC); *Bifidobacterium* (vs UC)	Liwinski et al,[52] 2020

(continued on next page)

Table 1
(continued)

Country	Groups	Material	Diversity	Enriched Taxa in AIH	Enriched Taxa in Controls	Study
NA	HLA-DR3 NOD mice vs wild type NOD mice	Stool	Decreased	Genus level: *Lactobacillus, Lactococcus,* and *Turicibacter*	Phylum level: *Firmicutes*; Genus level: *Allobaculum*	Yuksel et al,[53] 2015
NA	TCE treated MRL+/+ mice vs control mice	Stool	NS	Phylum level: *Verrucomicrobia*; Genus level: *Akkermansia* Species level: *Akkermansia muciniphila*	Phylum level: *Actinobacteria*; Genus level: *Alistipes, Bifidobacterium,* and *Turicibacter*	Wang et al,[57] 2021

Abbreviations: AIH, autoimmune hepatitis; HC, healthy control; NA, not applicable; NS, no significance; PBC, primary biliary cholangitis; UC, ulcerative colitis.

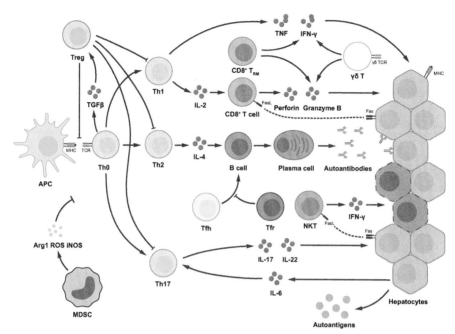

Fig. 2. Dysregulated immune system in AIH. APCs, primarily DCs, uptake autoantigens and present the antigenic peptides to Th0 cells, which subsequently differentiated into Th1, Th1, and Th17 cells. Th1 cells activate CD8$^+$ T cells and secrete TNFα and INF-γ, causing damage to hepatocytes. CD8$^+$ tissue resident memory T cells (T$_{RM}$) and γδ T cells are also involved in liver damage. Th2 cells assist in the activation of B cells, which differentiate into autobody-producing plasma cells. IL-17 and IL-22 secreted by Th17 cells are both proinflammatory in nature. Hepatocytes in AIH produce IL-6, which together with TGF-β promotes the differentiation of Th17 cells. NKT cells affect hepatocytes both in a direct way via FasL and an indirect way via IFN-γ production. Tfh cells promote B cell proliferation and antibody production while Tfr cells played the opposite role. MDSCs inhibit T cells by expression arginase 1, induction of reactive oxygen species (ROS) and inducible nitric oxide synthase (iNOS).

between Tregs and effector T cells in EAH mice.[76] Other studies found that the regulatory effects of Tregs were no different from healthy controls as reflected by the level of IFNγ production, and the proliferative ability of effector T cells.[64,69] However, different Tregs/effector T cell ratios used to assess the function of Tregs in their EAH models may be responsible for conflicting results.[77,78]

The underlying mechanism of Treg dysfunction may relate to CD39 and arylhydrocarbon-receptor (AhR). CD39 is an enzyme that hydrolyzes ATP and produces adenosine, which exhibits immunosuppressive effects.[79] CD39$^+$ Tregs are considered to suppress Th17 cells.[80] A diminution in the frequency of and impeded suppressive ability of CD39$^+$ Tregs was demonstrated in patients with AIH relative to both healthy counterparts and those with other liver diseases.[80] Further study on CD39 revealed the effects of AhR on Tregs. After binding to its ligand, AhR usually binds to AhR nuclear translocator and subsequently upregulates CD39. In AIH, AhR signaling was impaired and caused low levels of CD39 expression in Tregs, thus impairing suppression of effectors T cells.[81,82]

Evidence suggested that the stability of Tregs in AIH is dampened. CD39$^+$ Tregs had increased the production of IL-17 and IFN-γ upon proinflammatory stimulations compared to healthy controls.[80] Therefore, immune dysregulation in AIH may be a result of a switch from Tregs to effector T cells.

The altered frequency, impaired function and signaling as well as impeded stability of Tregs in a proinflammatory microenvironment probably contribute to the pathogenesis of AIH. Therapies based on Tregs may be an effective way to control AIH.

CD4+ T Cells

CD4+ T cells are enriched in the hepatic inflammatory infiltration of patients with AIH.[83–85] A recent study revealed that the AIH patient had an increased number of TNF-producing CD4+ T cells in the liver, and these cells were most likely Th1 cells.[86] Galectin-9 (Gal9) on Tregs binds to T cell immunoglobulin and mucin domain 3 (Tim3) on CD4+ effector T cells and inhibits Th1 immune reaction. Both the numbers of Gal9+ Tregs and Tim3+ CD4+ effectors cells were reduced in AIH, indicating impaired immune regulation.[87]

Among all the helper T cells, the involvement of Th17 cells in the pathophysiology of AIH has been extensively studied. Th17 cells mainly secrete IL-17 and IL-22. Th17-associated cytokines play pathogenic roles in several autoimmune diseases.[88] Both the level of IL-17 and the percentage of Th17 were increased in the serum and liver of patients with AIH compared with healthy controls and patients with chronic viral hepatitis.[89,90] Furthermore, RORγt, the transcriptional factor of Th17 cells, was upregulated in the liver of patients with AIH and EAH models.[65,89]

In juvenile patients with AIH, CD39+ Th17 was lower than in healthy controls, together with impaired production of adenosine.[91] Similar to Tregs, the response of Th17 cells to AhR was impaired in AIH, The disruption of AhR signaling downregulated CD39 and changed the regulatory function of Th17 cells into a pathogenic one.[81]

Hepatocytes are stimulated by IL-17 to produce IL-6.[89] IL-6 together with TGF-β is the key factor of naïve T cells differentiating into Th17 cells. This may form a positive feedback loop to expand Th17 cells. One pathophysiological feature of AIH is hypothesized to be the imbalance between Tregs and Th17 cells. Evidence showed that the number of Th17 cells and Tregs was negatively correlated in patients with AIH.[65] The ratio of FOXP3/RORγt, the transcriptional factors of Tregs and Th17 cells, can be used as a marker to evaluate disease activity.[92]

CD8+ T Cells

CD8+ T cells, also termed killer T cells, attack infected or neoplastic cells by apoptosis. CD8+ T cells are found enriched in the hepatic lobule and are the predominant cells found in emperipolesis in AIH, although the number of infiltrating CD8+ T cells is not as many as CD4+ T cells.[19,93,94]

CD8+ T cell clones from T cells infiltrating AIH livers showed spontaneous cytotoxic activity to autologous B cells.[83] The weapons of CD8+ T cells, granzyme B and perforin both showed higher expressions in the hepatic tissue of patients with AIH.[95] Patients with AIH exhibited a greater proportion of Fas-positive CD8+ T cells in comparison to healthy counterparts.[96,97] In AIH-2, the cytotoxicity of CYP2D6-specific CD8+ T cells was related to disease activity.[98]

Our group found that the number of CD69+CD103+CD8+ tissue resident memory T cells, which secrete granzyme B and IFN-γ, in the AIH liver is higher than in healthy controls and other liver diseases, and it is positively related to ALT and IgG levels.

γδ T Cells

γδ T cell has unconventional γδ T cells receptors (TCRs) rather than the classical αβ TCRs and is negative for both CD4 and CD8. Vδ1 and Vδ2 are the two primary subtypes of γδ T cells. Vδ1 is abundant in the epithelium and has regulatory and effector properties. In contrast, Vδ2 is prevalent in peripheral blood and plays a role in defending against pathogens and neoplastic cells.[70,99]

An elevated number of circulating and hepatic infiltrating γδ T cells was found in both adult and pediatric patients with active AIH.[70,100,101] Additionally, the physiological ratio of Vδ1/Vδ2 was inverted, indicating more INF-γ producing Vδ1[+] cells in γδ T cell population. Granzyme B, an indicator of liver damage, was also upregulated within γδ T cells in AIH. However, other studies demonstrate that increased γδ T level in AIH was indistinguishable from that in viral hepatitis.[102]

Natural Killer T Cells

A subpopulation of T cells known as natural killer T (NKT) cells display both the natural killer cell marker (CD56) and the T cell marker (CD3). Instead of MHC-I or MHC-II molecule, NKT cells identify the glycolipid antigen on the MHC class I-like protein CD1. Based on the α chain of TCR, NKT cells can be divided into invariant NKT (iNKT), also called type 1 NKT and variant NKT, also called type 2 NKT. NKT cells that expressed IL-4 were less frequent in AIH. However, no difference in the frequency of INF-γ expressing NKT cells between patients with AIH and healthy controls was observed.[70] Dividing NKT cells into type 1 and type 2, Sebode and colleagues[103] found that the type 2 NKT cells were more abundant in patients with AIH with a proinflammatory cytokine profile. Increased expression of CD1d on T cells supported the activation and Th1-skewing of type 2 NKT cells in transgenic EAH models. As a result, lymphocyte infiltration and autoantibody production occurred in the models.[104]

B Cells and Plasma Cells

Positive autoantibodies and hypergammaglobulinemia are classical characteristics of AIH. Also, the presence of plasma cells in the inflammatory infiltrates in the liver biopsy supports the diagnosis of AIH.[20] These features indicate of involvement of B cells and plasma cells in AIH pathophysiology.

Depletion of B cells in EAH models resulted in a reduced percentage of experienced CD4[+] and CD8[+] T cells and an elevated proportion of naïve T cells. The proliferation of T cells was also impaired in B cell-depleted mice.[105] However, another study showed contradictory results. EAH mice lacking B cells demonstrated increased CD4[+] T cell proliferation. CD11b was upregulated in B cells and CD11b[+] B cells reduced the inflammatory infiltration and the level of transaminases in the models via downregulating CD4[+] T cells and IFNγ production.[106] The differing B cell populations that were included in the two research might be the cause of the contradictory results. Antigen-presenting B cells are pathological while IL-10-producing B cells are regulatory. Besides, the EAH models used in these studies are different. Validating the roles of various B cell subtypes on AIH needs further studies.

Follicular Helper T and Follicular Regulatory T Cells

Follicular helper T (Tfh) cells provide signals for B cells during antibody production in the germinal center (GC). Follicular regulatory T (Tfr) cells interact with Tfh and B cells in GC and regulate their functions. The number of Tfh cells was reduced while the number of Tfr cells was elevated in the peripheral blood and spleen of patients with AIH and EAH mice.[107–109] In vitro study showed that Tfh cells promoted B cells proliferation and antibody production while Tfr cells played the opposite role.[109] Tfh cells positively correlated with B cells and the level of IgG in patients with AIH.[108,109] This indicates that the imbalance of Tfr/Tfh may participate in the immune dysregulation of AIH. However, another study found the inversed results of the number of Tfh and Tfr in EAH mice livers.[110] More research on Tfh and Tfr cells needs to be undertaken before the association between these cells and AIH development is more clearly understood.

Dendritic Cells

Recent studies have revealed the role of dendritic cells (DCs) in the pathogenesis of AIH. The frequency of circulating mature conventional DCs was elevated in patients with AIH. Excessive maturation of conventional dendritic cells caused by aberrant autophagy regulation contributes to AIH pathogenesis.[111] Moreover, IL-12 production of conventional DCs resulted in the IFN-γ production of NKT cells in Con-A-induced liver injury and depletion of conventional DCs alleviated liver damage.[112] Besides studies on conventional DCs, changes in hepatic DCs have also been investigated. It was suggested that defective Wnt/β-catenin signaling changed the immunotolerant state of hepatic DCs into an immunogenic one.[113]

Myeloid-Derived Suppressor Cells

Myeloid-derived suppressor cells (MDSCs) are a group of heterogenous immature myeloid cells that exhibits immunosuppressive effects. MDSCs inhibit the proliferation and promote the apoptosis of CD4$^+$ and CD8$^+$ T cells in AIH.[114] Non-cirrhotic patients with AIH had higher frequencies of MDSCs compared to controls while cirrhotic AIH did not.[114] The decrease in MDSCs in cirrhotic patients may accelerate liver injury.

ANIMAL MODELS FOR UNDERSTANDING THE PATHOPHYSIOLOGY OF AUTOIMMUNE HEPATITIS

Animal models have been used as effective tools to understand the pathophysiology of human diseases and to evaluate the therapeutic and adverse effects of certain interventions. Although it is hard to develop a model that mimics the exact pathophysiological changes of AIH in humans, various animal models developed still help us discover the underlying mechanisms. Here, we describe several currently utilized animal models.

Liver Antigen-Induced Animal Models

The first EAH model was developed using two fractions of antigens extracted from normal human liver called liver-specific protein 1 and 2 (LP1 and LP2). The injection of LP1 together with LP2 in rabbits resulted in lymphocytes and plasma cell infiltration in the liver, a feature of chronic active hepatitis.[115] Injection of LP2 alone resulted in hepatitis in a small proportion of rabbits with lesser extents compared with LP1. The results indicated the role of LP1, also called liver-specific membrane lipoprotein (LSP), in inducing hepatitis.[116] The injection of liver-specific lipoprotein, which contains LSP, with Klebsiella pneumoniae 03:K1 as adjuvants in SMA mice caused antibody production together with AIH-like pathological features. The transfer of splenocytes from the diseased mice to normal syngeneic mice leads to hepatitis similar to the donor.[117] Another study also developed an EAH model by injecting exogenous antigens. S-100 liver homogenates together with Freund's adjuvant was injected into the peritoneal cavity of male C57BL/6 mice, causing infiltrates around central vein and hepatocyte necrosis.[118] However, the antigens used in these EAH models are a group of heterogeneous proteins, so it is hard to identify the disease-causing antigens. Also, these models only induced acute liver injury rather than chronic hepatitis seen in patients with AIH.

In addition to using exogenous liver homogenates, liver autoantigen exposure is another way to induce models. CYP2D6 and FTCD are the targets of AIH-2-specific autoantibodies anti-LKM1 and anti-LC1, respectively. Models focused on the induction of CYP2D6 and FTCD by adenovirus infections have been developed. CYP2D6 mice exhibit chronic hepatitis with antigen-specific T cell infiltrations. Moreover, hepatic stellate cells are activated, contributing to hepatic fibrosis.[119] These pathological changes are similar to the natural history of AIH. After transient acute hepatitis, FTCD mice showed chronic infiltration and fibrosis driven by CD4$^+$ T cells.[120] In summary, these models mimic the pathophysiology of AIH-2. The development of AIH-1 models is challenging since no disease-specific antigens have been identified.

Spontaneous Autoimmune Hepatitis Developed in Transgenic Animal Models

Transgenic mice are designed to overexpress or be deficient in certain proteins that help us understand the mechanisms and immunopathology of AIH. The first transgenic EAH model is NTxPD-1$^{-/-}$ mice which received both programmed cell death 1 (*PD-1*) gene knockout and thymectomy. PD-1 is a co-inhibitory immunoreceptor that regulates T cell activities and thymectomy results in loss of Tregs. As a result, NTxPD-1$^{-/-}$ mice developed severe hepatitis with CD4$^+$ T cells infiltrating the portal area, CD8$^+$ T cells infiltrating the parenchyma and ANA production. The following transfer studies showed that total transfer of splenocytes induced hepatitis while transfer of CD4$^+$ T cells depleted splenocytes did not, indicating the role of CD4$^+$ T cells in AIH.[121] However, the induced hepatitis in NTxPD-1$^{-/-}$ mice is lethal, shortening their lifespan to less than one month, so it is unlikely to study the chronic course of AIH. Another transgenic model is based on breaking central tolerance in mice. The depletion of *TRAF6* results in the inhibition of medullary thymic epithelial cell development, which is crucial for central tolerance. *Traf6*ΔTEC mice developed inflammatory infiltration with plasma cells in the portal area and interface hepatitis, both are diagnostic histopathological characteristics of AIH. *Traf6*ΔTEC mice also contain positive ANA and anti-SLA in the blood. Further flow cytometry analysis found that CD4$^+$ and CD8$^+$ T cells are increased in the liver resident T cell populations.[122] Both of these transgenic models showed AIH-like autoimmunity that can be used to investigate the pathophysiology of AIH.

A recent study demonstrates that Tet2^{ΔVAV} mice with myelo-expansion have elevated plasma autoantibody and IgG levels and displayed classical AIH histology characteristics including interface hepatitis, lymphocytes and plasma cells infiltration, hepatocellular rosettes and emperipolesis.[61] The I3A producing *L. reuteri* was identified as the trigger of AIH pathology in this transgenic model, linking microbiome to the development of AIH.

Animal Models Induced by Exogenous Compounds

As described in previous sections, exogenous compounds can be the trigger of AIH, such as halothane, trichloroethylene, and interferons. Con A, a kind of plant lectin, is used to induce acute immune-mediated hepatic injury first in 1992 by G. Tiegs.[123] Con A-induced hepatitis is the widely employed animal model for investigations on AIH. Con A binds to the mannose receptor on sinusoidal endothelial cells, breaking down the barrier and further binding to Kupffer cells, which act as APCs to activate T cells. Activated T cells interact with various immune cells and promote proinflammatory cytokine production, resulting in hepatocyte damage.[124] This model is fast and convenient to establish. However, the downside of Con A-induced hepatitis is the short time course of hepatic injuries, making it unsuitable to study the chronic pathophysiological changes of AIH.

SUMMARY

Despite the fact that the pathophysiology of AIH is not clearly understood, studies have revealed the involvement of genetic and environmental factors. HLA genes are the most important genes associated with AIH susceptibility. Environmental factors such as viral infections, drug exposures, and microbiome alteration are likely to trigger AIH. The key to the pathophysiology is the dysregulated immune system. Uncontrolled liver inflammation is a result of increased pathogenic immune cells such as CD4$^+$ and CD8$^+$ T cells as well as impaired immunosuppressive cells such as Tregs. Development of animal models mimicking AIH in humans can help understand the disease pathophysiology and potential therapeutic targets.

CLINICS CARE POINTS

- Autoimmune hepatitis (AIH) is a chronic inflammatory liver disease. The clinical characteristics of AIH include elevated transaminase, high circulating immunoglobin G levels, positive autoantibodies, and key histological features.
- A recent consensus from the International AIH Pathology Group combined both acute and chronic histological features and established new diagnostic criteria for AIH with a dominant pattern of portal hepatitis or lobular hepatitis.
- The pathophysiology of AIH is not clearly understood. Genetic and environmental factors, dysregulated immune system and altered microbiomes may contribute to the development of AIH. Further research into these factors may lead to the development of new therapeutic options.
- Development of animal models mimicking AIH in humans may aid in the understanding of AIH pathophysiology and potential therapeutic targets.

FUNDING

This work was supported by the National Natural Science Foundation of China, China grants (#81830016, 81771732 and 81620108002 to M. Xiong, #81922010, 81873561 and 81570469 to T. Ruqi).

REFERENCES

1. Muratori L, Lohse AW, Lenzi M. Diagnosis and management of autoimmune hepatitis. BMJ 2023;380:e070201.
2. Mieli-Vergani G, Vergani D, Czaja AJ, et al. Autoimmune hepatitis. Nat Rev Dis Primers 2018;4.
3. van Gerven NMF, Verwer BJ, Witte BI, et al. Epidemiology and clinical characteristics of autoimmune hepatitis in The Netherlands. Scand J Gastroenterol 2014;49(10):1245–54.
4. Gronbaek L, Vilstrup H, Pedersen L, et al. Family occurrence of autoimmune hepatitis: a Danish nationwide registry-based cohort study. J Hepatol 2018; 69(4):873–7.

5. Gronbaek L, Vilstrup H, Pedersen L, et al. Extrahepatic autoimmune diseases in patients with autoimmune hepatitis and their relatives: a Danish nationwide cohort study. Liver Int 2019;39(1):205–14.

6. Hennes EM, Zeniya M, Czaja AJ, et al. Simplified criteria for the diagnosis of autoimmune hepatitis. Hepatology 2008;48(1):169–76.

7. Alvarez E, Berg PA, Bianchi FB, et al. International autoimmune hepatitis group report: review of criteria for diagnosis of autoimmune hepatitis. J Hepatol 1999; 31(5):929–38.

8. Bogdanos DP, Invernizzi P, Mackay IR, et al. Autoimmune liver serology: current diagnostic and clinical challenges. World J Gastroenterol 2008;14(21):3374–87.

9. Johanet C, Beleoken E, Ballot E. Autoantibodies in autoimmune hepatitis: anti-nuclear antibodies (ANA). Clin Res Hepatol Gastroenterol 2012;36(4):394–6.

10. Manns M, Gerken G, Kyriatsoulis A, et al. Characterisation of a new subgroup of autoimmune chronic active hepatitis by autoantibodies against a soluble liver antigen. Lancet 1987;1(8528):292–4.

11. Stechemesser E, Klein R, Berg PA. Characterization and clinical relevance of liver-pancreas antibodies in autoimmune hepatitis. Hepatology 1993;18(1):1–9.

12. Wies I, Brunner S, Henninger J, et al. Identification of target antigen for SLA/LP autoantibodies in autoimmune hepatitis. Lancet 2000;355(9214):1510–5.

13. Gueguen M, Boniface O, Bernard O, et al. Identification of the main epitope on human cytochrome P450 IID6 recognized by anti-liver kidney microsome antibody. J Autoimmun 1991;4(4):607–15.

14. Christen U, Hintermann E. Autoantibodies in autoimmune hepatitis: can epitopes Tell Us about the etiology of the Disease? Front Immunol 2018;9:163.

15. Dalekos GN, Gatselis NK. Autoimmune serology testing in clinical practice: an updated roadmap for the diagnosis of autoimmune hepatitis. Eur J Intern Med 2023;108:9–17.

16. Powell AM, Black MM. Epitope spreading: protection from pathogens, but propagation of autoimmunity? Clin Exp Dermatol 2001;26(5):427–33.

17. Hintermann E, Holdener M, Bayer M, et al. Epitope spreading of the anti-CYP2D6 antibody response in patients with autoimmune hepatitis and in the CYP2D6 mouse model. J Autoimmun 2011;37(3):242–53.

18. Tiniakos DG, Brain JG, Bury YA. Role of histopathology in autoimmune hepatitis. Dig Dis 2015;33:53–64.

19. Miao Q, Bian Z, Tang R, et al. Emperipolesis mediated by CD8 T cells is a characteristic histopathologic feature of autoimmune hepatitis. Clin Rev Allergy Immunol 2015;48(2–3):226–35.

20. Gurung A, Assis DN, McCarty TR, et al. Histologic features of autoimmune hepatitis: a critical appraisal. Hum Pathol 2018;82:51–60.

21. Okano N, Yamamoto K, Sakaguchi K, et al. Clinicopathological features of acute-onset autoimmune hepatitis. Hepatol Res 2003;25(3):263–70.

22. Lohse AW, Sebode M, Bhathal PS, et al. Consensus recommendations for histological criteria of autoimmune hepatitis from the international AIH pathology group results of a workshop on AIH histology hosted by the European reference network on hepatological diseases and the European society of pathology. Liver Int 2022;42(5):1058–69.

23. Lohr HF, Schlaak JF, Gerken G, et al. Phenotypical analysis and cytokine release of liver-infiltrating and peripheral blood T lymphocytes from patients with chronic hepatitis of different etiology. Liver 1994;14(3):161–6.

24. De Biasio MB, Periolo N, Avagnina A, et al. Liver infiltrating mononuclear cells in children with type 1 autoimmune hepatitis. J Clin Pathol 2006;59(4):417–23.

25. de Boer YS, van Gerven NMF, Zwiers A, et al. Genome-wide association study identifies variants associated with autoimmune hepatitis type 1. Gastroenterology 2014;147(2):443–52.

26. Li Y, Sun Y, Liu Y, et al. Genome-wide meta-analysis identifies susceptibility loci for autoimmune hepatitis type 1. Hepatology 2022;76(3):564–75.

27. Pando M, Larriba J, Fernandez GC, et al. Pediatric and adult forms of type I autoimmune hepatitis in Argentina: evidence for differential genetic predisposition. Hepatology 1999;30(6):1374–80.

28. Bittencourt PL, Goldberg AC, Cancado ELR, et al. Genetic heterogeneity in susceptibility to autoimmune hepatitis types 1 and 2. Am J Gastroenterol 1999; 94(7):1906–13.

29. Beretta-Piccoli BT, Mieli-Vergani G, Vergani D. HLA gut microbiome and hepatic autoimmunity. Front Immunol 2022;13:980768.

30. Lapierre P, Alvarez F. Type 2 autoimmune hepatitis: genetic susceptibility. *Front Immunol* 2022;13:1025343.

31. Ma Y, Su H, Yuksel M, et al. Human leukocyte antigen profile predicts severity of autoimmune liver disease in children of european ancestry. Hepatology 2021; 74(4):2032–46.

32. Higuchi T, Oka S, Furukawa H, et al. Role of deleterious single nucleotide variants in the coding regions of TNFAIP3 for Japanese autoimmune hepatitis with cirrhosis. *Sci Rep* 2019;9:7925.

33. Czaja AJ, Strettell MDJ, Thomson LJ, et al. Associations between alleles of the major histocompatibility complex and type 1 autoimmune hepatitis. Hepatology 1997;25(2):317–23.

34. Higuchi T, Oka S, Furukawa H, et al. Association of a single nucleotide polymorphism upstream of ICOS with Japanese autoimmune hepatitis type 1. J Hum Genet 2017;62(4):481–4.

35. Migita K, Nakamura M, Abiru S, et al. Association of STAT4 polymorphisms with susceptibility to type-1 autoimmune hepatitis in the Japanese population. PLoS One 2013;8(8):e71382.

36. Yousefi A, Najafi M, Motamed F, et al. Association of interleukin-6 and interleukin-1 family gene polymorphisms in autoimmune hepatitis. Ann Hepatol 2018;17(6):1021–5.

37. Yousefi A, Bidoki AZ, Shafioyoun A, et al. Association of IL-10 and TGF-beta cytokine gene polymorphisms with autoimmune hepatitis. Clin Res Hepatol Gastroenterol 2019;43(1):45–50.

38. Yousefi A, Mahmoudi E, Bidoki AZ, et al. IL4 gene polymorphisms in Iranian patients with autoimmune hepatitis. Expert Rev Gastroenterol Hepatol 2016;10(5): 659–63.

39. Yousefi A, Mahmoudi E, Noveiry BB, et al. Autoimmune hepatitis association with single nucleotide polymorphism of interleukin-2, but not interferon-gamma. Clin Res Hepatol Gastroenterol 2018;42(2):134–8.

40. Vento S, Garofano T, Diperri G, et al. Identification of hepatitis A virus as a trigger for autoimmune chronic hepatitis type 1 in susceptible individuals. Lancet 1991; 337(8751):1183–7.

41. Vergani D, Mieli-Vergani G. Autoimmune manifestations in viral hepatitis. Semin Immunopathol 2013;35(1):73–85.

42. Marceau G, Lapierre P, Beland K, et al. LKM1 autoantibodies in chronic hepatitis C infection: a case of molecular mimicry? Hepatology 2005;42(3):675–82.

43. Christen U, Hintermann E. Pathogens and autoimmune hepatitis. Clin Exp Immunol 2019;195(1):35–51.

44. Webb GJ, Hirschfield GM, Krawitt EL, et al. Cellular and molecular mechanisms of autoimmune hepatitis. Annu Rev Pathol 2018;13:247–92.
45. Sirbe C, Simu G, Szabo I, et al. Pathogenesis of autoimmune hepatitis-cellular and molecular mechanisms. Int J Mol Sci 2021;22(24):13578.
46. Gut J, Christen U, Frey N, et al. Molecular mimicry in halothane hepatitis: biochemical and structural characterization of lipoylated autoantigens. Toxicology 1995;97(1–3):199–224.
47. Neuberger J, Mielivergani G, Tredger JM, et al. Oxidative metabolism of halothane in the production of altered hepatocyte membrane antigens in acute halothane-induced hepatic necrosis. Gut 1981;22(8):669–72.
48. Vergani D, Mielivergani G, Alberti A, et al. Antibodies to the surface of halothane-altered rabbit hepatocytes in patients with severe halothane-associated hepatitis. N Engl J Med 1980;303(2):66–71.
49. Miyauchi E, Shimokawa C, Steimle A, et al. The impact of the gut microbiome on extra-intestinal autoimmune diseases. Nat Rev Immunol 2023;23(1):9–23.
50. Wei Y, Li Y, Yan L, et al. Alterations of gut microbiome in autoimmune hepatitis. Gut 2020;69(3):569–77.
51. Elsherbiny NM, Rammadan M, Hassan EA, et al. Autoimmune hepatitis: shifts in gut microbiota and metabolic pathways among egyptian patients. Microorganisms 2020;8(7).
52. Liwinski T, Casar C, Ruehlemann MC, et al. A disease-specific decline of the relative abundance of Bifidobacterium in patients with autoimmune hepatitis. Aliment Pharmacol Ther 2020;51(12):1417–28.
53. Yuksel M, Wang Y, Tai N, et al. A novel "humanized mouse" model for autoimmune hepatitis and the association of gut microbiota with liver inflammation. Hepatology 2015;62(5):1536–50.
54. Abe K, Takahashi A, Fujita M, et al. Dysbiosis of oral microbiota and its association with salivary immunological biomarkers in autoimmune liver disease. PLoS One 2018;13(7):e0198757.
55. Lou J, Jiang Y, Rao B, et al. Fecal microbiomes distinguish patients with autoimmune hepatitis from healthy individuals. Front Cell Infect Microbiol 2020;10:342.
56. Lin R, Zhou L, Zhang J, et al. Abnormal intestinal permeability and microbiota in patients with autoimmune hepatitis. Int J Clin Exp Path 2015;8(5):5153–60.
57. Wang H, Banerjee N, Liang Y, et al. Gut microbiome-host interactions in driving environmental pollutant trichloroethene-mediated autoimmunity. Toxicol Appl Pharmacol 2021;424:115597.
58. Zhang H, Liu M, Liu X, et al. Bifidobacterium animalisssp. lactis 420 mitigates autoimmune hepatitis through regulating intestinal barrier and liver immune cells. Front Immunol 2020;11:569104.
59. Zhang H, Liu M, Zhong W, et al. Leaky gut driven by dysbiosis augments activation and accumulation of liver macrophages via RIP3 signaling pathway in autoimmune hepatitis. Front Immunol 2021;12:624360.
60. Vieira SM, Hiltensperger M, Kumar V, et al. Translocation of a gut pathobiont drives autoimmunity in mice and humans. Science 2018;359(6380):1156–60.
61. Pandey SP, Bender MJ, McPherson AC, et al. Tet2 deficiency drives liver microbiome dysbiosis triggering Tc1 cell autoimmune hepatitis. Cell Host Microbe 2022;30(7):1003–+.
62. Yang J, Xie W, Yu K, et al. Methyl butyrate attenuates concanavalin A-induced autoimmune hepatitis by inhibiting Th1-cell activation and homing to the liver. Cell Immunol 2022;378:104575.

63. Liberal R, Grant CR, Holder BS, et al. In autoimmune hepatitis type 1 or the auto-immune hepatitis-sclerosing cholangitis variant defective regulatory T-cell responsiveness to IL-2 results in low IL-10 production and impaired suppression. Hepatology 2015;62(3):863–75.

64. Longhi MS, Ma Y, Bogdanos DP, et al. Impairment of CD4+CD25+ regulatory T-cells in autoimmune liver disease. J Hepatol 2004;41(1):31–7.

65. Ma L, Zhang L, Zhuang Y, et al. The imbalance between Foxp3(+)Tregs and Th1/Th17/Th22 cells in patients with newly diagnosed autoimmune hepatitis. J Immunol Res 2018;2018:3753081.

66. Ai G, Yan W, Yu H, et al. Soluble Fgl2 restricts autoimmune hepatitis progression via suppressing Tc17 and conventional CD8+T cell function. J Gene Med 2018; 20(7–8):e3023.

67. Behairy BE, El-Araby HA, Abd El Kader HH, et al. Assessment of intrahepatic regulatory T cells in children with autoimmune hepatitis. Ann Hepatol 2016; 15(5):682–90.

68. Diestelhorst J, Junge N, Schlue J, et al. Pediatric autoimmune hepatitis shows a disproportionate decline of regulatory T cells in the liver and of IL-2 in the blood of patients undergoing therapy. PLoS One 2017;12(7):e0181107.

69. Peiseler M, Sebode M, Franke B, et al. FOXP3+ regulatory T cells in autoimmune hepatitis are fully functional and not reduced in frequency. J Hepatol 2012;57(1): 125–32.

70. Ferri S, Longhi MS, De Molo C, et al. A multifaceted imbalance of T cells with regulatory function characterizes Type 1 autoimmune hepatitis. Hepatology 2010;52(3):999–1007.

71. John K, Hardtke-Wolenski M, Jaeckel E, et al. Increased apoptosis of regulatory T cells in patients with active autoimmune hepatitis. Cell Death Dis 2017;8(12): 3219.

72. Longhi MS, Ma Y, Mitry RR, et al. Effect of CD4+CD25+ regulatory T-cells on CD8 T-cell function in patients with autoimmune hepatitis. J Autoimmun 2005; 25(1):63–71.

73. Longhi MS, Hussain MJ, Mitry RR, et al. Functional study of CD4(+)CD25(+) regulatory T cells in health and autoimmune hepatitis. J Immunol 2006;176(7): 4484–91.

74. Chen Y-Y, Jeffery HC, Hunter S, et al. Human intrahepatic regulatory T Cells are functional, require il-2 from effector cells for survival, and are susceptible to fas ligand-mediated apoptosis. Hepatology 2016;64(1):138–50.

75. Rosenzwajg M, Lorenzon R, Cacoub P, et al. Immunological and clinical effects of low-dose interleukin-2 across 11 autoimmune diseases in a single, open clinical trial. Ann Rheum Dis 2019;78(2):209–17.

76. Buitrago-Molina LE, Pietrek J, Noyan F, et al. Treg-specific IL-2 therapy can reestablish intrahepatic immune regulation in autoimmune hepatitis. J Autoimmun 2021;117:102591.

77. Longhi MS, Ma Y, Mieli-Vergani G, et al. Regulatory T cells in autoimmune hepatitis. J Hepatol 2012;57(4):932–3.

78. Ferri S, Lalanne C, Masi C, et al. Regulatory T cell defects in adult autoimmune hepatitis. J Hepatol 2012;57(5):1154–5.

79. Allard B, Beavis PA, Darcy PK, et al. Immunosuppressive activities of adenosine in cancer. Curr Opin Pharmacol 2016;29:7–16.

80. Grant CR, Liberal R, Holder BS, et al. Dysfunctional CD39(POS) regulatory T cells and aberrant control of T-helper Type 17 Cells in autoimmune hepatitis. Hepatology 2014;59(3):1007–15.

81. Vuerich M, Harshe R, Frank LA, et al. Altered aryl-hydrocarbon-receptor signalling affects regulatory and effector cell immunity in autoimmune hepatitis. J Hepatol 2021;74(1):48–57.

82. Gandhi R, Kumar D, Burns EJ, et al. Activation of the aryl hydrocarbon receptor induces human type 1 regulatory T cell-like and Foxp3(+) regulatory T cells. Nat Immunol 2010;11(9). 846-U103.

83. Lohr H, Manns M, Kyriatsoulis A, et al. Clonal analysis of liver-infiltrating T cells in patients with LKM-1 antibody-positive autoimmune chronic active hepatitis. Clin Exp Immunol. May 1991;84(2):297–302.

84. Wen L, Peakman M, Loboyeo A, et al. T-cell-directed hepatocyte damage in autoimmune chronic active hepatitis. Lancet 1990;336(8730):1527–30.

85. Lohr HF, Schlaak JF, Lohse AW, et al. Autoreactive CD4(+) LKM-specific and anticlonotypic T-cell responses in LKM-1 antibody-positive autoimmune hepatitis. Hepatology 1996;24(6):1416–21.

86. Bovensiepen CS, Schakat M, Sebode M, et al. TNF-producing Th1 cells are selectively expanded in liver infiltrates of patients with autoimmune hepatitis. J Immunol 2019;203(12):3148–56.

87. Liberal R, Grant CR, Holder BS, et al. The impaired immune regulation of autoimmune hepatitis is linked to a defective galectin-9/tim-3 pathway. Hepatology 2012;56(2):677–86.

88. Majumder S, McGeachy MJ. IL-17 in the pathogenesis of disease: good intentions gone awry. Annu Rev Immunol 2021;39:537–56.

89. Zhao L, Tang Y, You Z, et al. Interleukin-17 contributes to the pathogenesis of autoimmune hepatitis through inducing hepatic interleukin-6 expression. PLoS One 2011;6(4):e18909.

90. An J. Expression and Significance of Th17 cells and related factors in patients with autoimmune hepatitis. Comb Chem High Throughput Screen 2019;22(4):232–7.

91. Liberal R, Grant CR, Ma Y, et al. CD39 mediated regulation of Th17-cell effector function is impaired in juvenile autoimmune liver disease. J Autoimmun 2016;72:102–12.

92. Mitra S, Anand S, Das A, et al. A molecular marker of disease activity in autoimmune liver diseases with histopathological correlation; FoXp3/ROR gamma t ratio. Apmis 2015;123(11):935–44.

93. Renand A, Habes S, Mosnier J-F, et al. Immune alterations in patients with type 1 autoimmune hepatitis persist upon standard immunosuppressive treatment. Hepatol Commun 2018;2(8):972–85.

94. Senaldi G, Portmann B, Mowat AP, et al. Immunohistochemical features of the portal tract mononuclear cell infiltrate in chronic aggressive hepatitis. Arch Dis Child 1992;67(12):1447–53.

95. Tordjmann T, Soulie A, Guettier C, et al. Perforin and granzyme B lytic protein expression during chronic viral and autoimmune hepatitis. Liver 1998;18(6):391–7.

96. Zwolak A, Surdacka A, Daniluk J. Bcl-2 and Fas expression in peripheral blood leukocytes of patients with alcoholic and autoimmune liver disorders. Hum Exp Toxicol 2016;35(8):799–807.

97. Ogawa S, Sakaguchi K, Takaki A, et al. Increase in CD95 (Fas/APO-1)-positive CD4(+) and CD8(+) T cells in peripheral blood derived from patients with autoimmune hepatitis or chronic hepatitis C with autoimmune phenomena. J Gastroenterol Hepatol 2000;15(1):69–75.

98. Longhi MS, Hussain MJ, Bogdanos DP, et al. Cytochrome P450IID6-specific CD8 T cell immune responses mirror disease activity in autoimmune hepatitis type 2. Hepatology 2007;46(2):472–84.

99. Rajoriya N, Fergusson JR, Leithead JA, et al. Gamma delta T-lymphocytes in hepatitis C and chronic liver disease. Front Immunol 2014;5:1–9.

100. Martins EBG, Graham AK, Chapman RW, et al. Elevation of gamma delta T lymphocytes in peripheral blood and livers of patients with primary sclerosing cholangitis and other autoimmune liver diseases. Hepatology 1996;23(5):988–93.

101. Wen L, Peakman M, Mielivergani G, et al. Elevation of activated gamma delta T cell receptor bearing T lymphocytes in patients with autoimmune chronic liver disease. Clin Exp Immunol 1992;89(1):78–82.

102. Kasper H-U, Ligum D, Cucus J, et al. Liver distribution of gamma delta-T-cells in patients with chronic hepatitis of different etiology. Apmis 2009;117(11):779–85.

103. Sebode M, Wigger J, Filpe P, et al. Inflammatory phenotype of intrahepatic sulfatide-reactive type II NKT cells in humans with autoimmune hepatitis. *Front Immunol* 2019;10:1065.

104. Weng X, He Y, Visvabharathy L, et al. Crosstalk between type II NKT cells and T cells leads to spontaneous chronic inflammatory liver disease. J Hepatol 2017;67(4):791–800.

105. Beland K, Marceau G, Labardy A, et al. Depletion of B cells induces remission of autoimmune hepatitis in mice through reduced antigen presentation and help to T cells. Hepatology 2015;62(5):1511–23.

106. Liu X, Jiang X, Liu R, et al. B cells expressing CD11b effectively inhibit CD4+T-cell responses and ameliorate experimental autoimmune hepatitis in mice. Hepatology 2015;62(5):1563–75.

107. Ma L, Zhang L, Dai J, et al. Dysregulated TFR and TFH cells correlate with B-cell differentiation and antibody production in autoimmune hepatitis. J Cell Mol Med 2020;24(7):3948–57.

108. Kimura N, Yamagiwa S, Sugano T, et al. Possible involvement of chemokine C-C receptor 7(-)programmed cell death-1(+) follicular helper T-cell subset in the pathogenesis of autoimmune hepatitis. J Gastroenterol Hepatol 2018;33(1): 298–306.

109. Ma L, Qin J, Ji H, et al. Tfh and plasma cells are correlated with hypergammaglobulinaemia in patients with autoimmune hepatitis. Liver Int 2014;34(3): 405–15.

110. Ma L, Zhang L-w, Zhuang Y, et al. Exploration the significance of Tfh and related molecules on C57BL/6 mice model of experimental autoimmune hepatitis. J Microbiol Immunol Infect 2021;54(2):221–7.

111. Fan X, Men R, Huang C, et al. Critical roles of conventional dendritic cells in autoimmune hepatitis via autophagy regulation. *Cell Death Dis* 2020;11(1):23.

112. Wang J, Cao X, Zhao J, et al. Critical roles of conventional dendritic cells in promoting T cell-dependent hepatitis through regulating natural killer T cells. Clin Exp Immunol 2017;188(1):127–37.

113. Tan K, Xie X, Shi W, et al. Deficiency of canonical Wnt/beta-catenin signalling in hepatic dendritic cells triggers autoimmune hepatitis. Liver Int 2020;40(1): 131–40.

114. Li H, Dai F, Peng Q, et al. Myeloid-derived suppressor cells suppress CD4(+) and CD8(+) T cell responses in autoimmune hepatitis. Mol Med Rep 2015; 12(3):3667–73.

115. Meyerzum Kh, Miescher PA, Kossling FK. Experimental chronic active hepatitis in rabbits following immunization with human liver proteins. Clin Exp Immunol 1972;11(1):99–108.
116. McFarlane IG, Wojcicka BM, Zucker GM, et al. Purification and characterization of human liver-specific membrane lipoprotein (LSP). Clin Exp Immunol 1977; 27(3):381–90.
117. Kuriki J, Murakami H, Kakumu S, et al. Experimental autoimmune hepatitis in mice after immunization with syngeneic liver proteins together with the polysaccharide of Klebsiella pneumoniae. Gastroenterology 1983;84(3):596–603.
118. Lohse AW, Manns M, Dienes HP, et al. Experimental autoimmune hepatitis: disease induction, time course and T-cell reactivity. Hepatology 1990;11(1):24–30.
119. Hintermann E, Ehser J, Bayer M, et al. Mechanism of autoimmune hepatic fibrogenesis induced by an adenovirus encoding the human liver autoantigen cytochrome P450 2D6. J Autoimmun 2013;44:49–60.
120. Hardtke-Wolenski M, Fischer K, Noyan F, et al. Genetic predisposition and environmental danger signals initiate chronic autoimmune hepatitis driven by CD4(+) T cells. Hepatology 2013;58(2):718–28.
121. Kido M, Watanabe N, Okazaki T, et al. Fatal autoimmune hepatitis induced by concurrent loss of naturally arising regulatory T cells and PD-1-mediated signaling. Gastroenterology 2008;135(4):1333–43.
122. Bonito AJ, Aloman C, Fiel MI, et al. Medullary thymic epithelial cell depletion leads to autoimmune hepatitis. J Clin Invest 2013;123(8):3510–24.
123. Tiegs G, Hentschel J, Wendel A. A T cell-dependent experimental liver injury in mice inducible by concanavalin A. J Clin Invest 1992;90(1):196–203.
124. Hao J, Sun W, Xu H. Pathogenesis of Concanavalin A induced autoimmune hepatitis in mice. Int Immunopharmacol 2022;102:108411.

Diagnosis of Autoimmune Hepatitis

Ben Flikshteyn, MD*, Kamal Amer, MD, Zaid Tafesh, MD, MSc,
Nikolaos T. Pyrsopoulos, MD, PhD, MBA, AGAF, FRCP

KEYWORDS

- Autoimmune • Hepatitis • Diagnosis • Hepatology • Antibodies

KEY POINTS

- Autoimmune hepatitis (AIH) diagnostic subtypes and scoring systems.
- AIH histological findings.
- AIH-related antibodies.
- AIH and primary biliary cholangitis overlap syndrome.
- AIH and primary sclerosing cholangitis overlap syndrome.

INTRODUCTION

Autoimmune hepatitis (AIH) presents a diagnostic challenge because it is relatively rare and heterogenous in presentation. Furthermore, there is no single pathognomonic finding that can alone be used to make the diagnosis.[1] Instead, AIH is diagnosed because of histological abnormalities, laboratory findings compatible with the diagnosis, and detection of characteristic autoantibodies. Even these criteria are imperfect as 25% to 39% of patients with acute onset AIH have normal immunoglobulin G (IgG) levels[2] and an additional 9% to 17% test negative for circulating autoantibodies.[3] Furthermore, accurate diagnosis requires the exclusion of other disease entities with presentations that may resemble the clinical course and findings seen in AIH, including viral hepatitis, drug-induced liver injury, and metabolic or hereditary liver diseases.[4] AIH can be further divided into subtypes based on the presence or absence of certain autoantibodies. Diagnostic scoring systems support clinical judgment and serve as valuable tools in diagnosis and research. These criteria stratify the likelihood AIH is present and can even help to identify overlap syndromes with primary sclerosing cholangitis (PSC) or primary biliary cirrhosis (PBC). Ultimately, description of histological features and detection of autoantibodies is crucial in diagnosing AIH. The importance of accurate diagnosis of AIH is essential given the risks associated

Rutgers New Jersey School of Medicine, 185 South Orange Avenue, MSB H-538, Newark, NJ 07103, USA
* Corresponding author.
E-mail address: Bf359@njms.rutgers.edu

Clin Liver Dis 28 (2024) 37–50
https://doi.org/10.1016/j.cld.2023.06.004
1089-3261/24/© 2023 Elsevier Inc. All rights reserved.
liver.theclinics.com

with long-term immunosuppression that is often necessary in the management of this condition. This article presents the currently adopted approach to AIH diagnosis and explores the challenges with accurately identifying this disease entity.

DIAGNOSTIC SUBTYPES

AIH can be divided into 2 major subtypes based on the specific autoantibodies that are detected.[5] Type 1 AIH is characterized by the presence of antinuclear antibodies (ANA) and/or smooth muscle antibodies (SMA)/antiactin.[6] Type 1 is the "classic" variety and accounts for 80% of cases and is more commonly seen in adults. Meanwhile, type 2 AIH is characterized by the presence of liver kidney microsome type 1 (anti-LKM1) antibodies, typically without detectable ANA and SMA.[7] This subtype presents at a younger age, mainly affecting children, and portends faster disease progression. Less commonly, patients with type 1 AIH may also present with antibodies against soluble liver antigen (anti-SLA), which is characterized by a more aggressive disease subtype that is resistant to drug withdrawal.[8] An additional subset of cases dubbed seronegative AIH is negative for ANA, SMA, and LKM1. These comprise up to 20% of presentations and can trigger a search for a plethora of other autoantibodies. Generally, the clinical presentation and response to treatment of adults does not vary significantly when stratified by subtype but may be more helpful in children.[9]

DIAGNOSTIC SCORING SYSTEMS

In 1992, a panel of 27 scientists convened a meeting with the goal of creating diagnostic criteria for AIH. This assembly, which would become known as the International Autoimmune Hepatitis Group (IAIHG), put forth a scoring system in 1993.[4] This group reconvened and published the revised AIH criteria in 1999[4] and the simplified AIH criteria in 2008.[10] These scoring systems are designed to be interpreted with data obtained at the time of presentation. There are robust data to support their performance characteristics. Qiu and colleagues[11] tested the simplified criteria in a cohort of Chinese patients and found sensitivity and specificity for probable AIH to be 90% and 95%, respectively. This study also suggested that liver histology was critical to diagnosis, especially when using the simplified criteria. Czaja and colleagues[12] applied both the revised and simplified criteria to a cohort of patients with diverse chronic liver diseases. Compared head-to-head, the revised criteria boast a greater sensitivity (100% vs 95%). Meanwhile, the simplified scoring system is more specific (90% vs 73%) and accurate (92% vs 82%). This study suggested that the revised criteria may fail to identify patients with more mild disease that do not have such marked elevations in IgG, antibody titers, or certain histological features. The simplified criteria perform best in the more classic presentation of AIH, whereas the revised criteria are useful for patients with fewer or more atypical features.[12] Thus, the scoring systems are not interchangeable and should be tailored to the specific clinical scenario. For example, the simplified criteria can be helpful to exclude the diagnosis of AIH in those with concurrent liver diseases with autoimmune features. Meanwhile, the strength of the revised criteria is to identify AIH in patients who may lack expected features (hypergammaglobulinemia and presence of autoantibodies) or those with unexpected manifestations (antimitochondrial antibodies [AMA], features of cholestatic disease, or atypical histology).

The criteria are pictured below (**Tables 1** and **2**).[13]

- Both scoring systems have limitations including[4] the lack of prospective studies for validation

Table 1	
Revised autoimmune hepatitis criteria	
Clinical Feature	**Score**
Female gender	+2
ALP:AST ratio	
<1.5	+2
1.5–3.0	0
>3.0	−2
Serum globulin or IgG above normal	
>2.0	+3
1.5–2.0	+2
1.0–1.5	+1
<1.0	0
ANA, SMA, LKM1	
>1:80	+3
1:80	+2
1:40	+1
<1:40	0
Illicit drug use history	
Positive	−4
Negative	+1
Average alcohol intake per day	
<25 g/d	+2
>60 g/d	−2
Histologic findings	
Interface hepatitis	+3
Lymphoplasmacytic infiltrate	+1
Rosette formation	+1
None of the above	−5
Biliary changes	−3
Other changes	+2
Other autoimmune disease	+2
AMA positivity	−4
Hepatitis viral markers	
Positive	−3
Negative	+3
Aggregate score without treatment	
Definite AIH	≥15
Probable AIH	≥6

- Compromised diagnostic accuracy in the setting of concurrent disease states such as PSC, PBC, and non-alcoholic fatty liver disease/non-alcoholic steatohepatitis (NAFLD/NASH)[14]
- Failure to include other serological markers such as anti-SLA
- Reliance on the detection of autoantibodies by immunofluorescence rather than enzyme-linked immunoassay

Table 2	
Simplified autoimmune hepatitis criteria	
Clinical Feature	**Score**
ANA or SMA	
≥ 1:40	+1
≥ 1:80 or	+2
LKM ≥1:40 or	+2
SLA positive	+2
Serum IgG	
>upper limit of normal	+1
>1.1 × upper limit of normal	+2
Histologic findings	
Compatible with AIH	+1
Typical of AIH	+2
Hepatitis viral markers	
Negative	+2
Aggregate score without treatment	
Definite AIH	≥7
Probable AIH	≥6

- Most suited for defining cohorts of patients with AIH for clinical studies

Diagnostic scoring systems for AIH are useful tools that should be used to support clinical diagnosis in challenging cases or justify the need for more invasive testing such as liver biopsy. They can also be used to define cohorts for clinical studies. However, they are not a surrogate for clinical judgment. The consensus remains that liver biopsy is the gold standard for diagnosis of AIH and preferably should not be omitted in the workup.[15] Other scoring systems, such as the Paris criteria, have a role in overlap syndromes as discussed later in this article.

AUTOIMMUNE HEPATITIS AUTOANTIBODIES

Autoantibodies are detected by immunofluorescence (IF) run on a multiorgan substrate panel that should include kidney, liver, and stomach. This permits the detection of ANA, SMA, anti-LKM1, AMA, and antibodies to liver cytosol type 1 (anti-LC1). Once past this screening stage, further testing is carried out on HEp2 cells to determine the pattern of staining, although the clinical utility of this is unclear. Unlike the aforementioned autoantibodies, anti-SLA/LP require enzyme-linked immunosorbent assay (ELISA) or dot-blot for detection.[16]

Detection of circulating autoantibodies plays a crucial role in the diagnosis of AIH. In fact, they can be detected in up to 95% of cases when tested according to the guidelines set forth by the IAIHG.[17] These autoantibodies also assist to stratify AIH by subtypes, which may have implications for clinical course and treatment. Autoantibodies of interest range from those commonly encountered in the initial diagnostic workup of AIH to those more rarely detected but may predict a different disease course.[18]

ANA, SMA, and anti-LKM1 make up the conventional autoantibodies.[19] Czaja and colleagues evaluated a group of 265 adults meeting codified criteria for AIH. In this mostly North American population, ANA was positive in 80%, SMA was positive in 63%, and anti-LKM1 was positive in 3% of patients meeting criteria for AIH.[20] This same study found that concurrent positivity for ANA and SMA had superior performance characteristics in sensitivity, specificity, accuracy, and both positive and negative predictive values as compared with either antibody alone.

Anti-LKM1 antibodies are directed against cytochrome CYP450 enzymes, CYP2D6 and CYP2C9 in particular.[21] These autoantibodies should be sought in initial workup for pediatric populations but reserved for adults with negative serology for ANA and SMA. It has an exceedingly low sensitivity of 1% in North American adults and is most frequently identified in isolation of ANA and SMA. This justifies the rationale for omitting testing for anti-LKM1 in initial serology in adults. In the pediatric population, however, 12% to 38% of children with AIH test positive for anti-LKM1.[22] Along with anti-LC1, anti-LKM1, and less frequently anti-LKM3 are associated with AIH type 2. A series of 38 patients with AIH type 2 revealed prevalence of 66% and 53% for anti-LKM1 and anti-LC1, respectively.[23] Unfortunately, neither is specific to AIH and has been reported in a small proportion of patients with chronic HCV.[24] Anti-LC1 positivity in isolation does suggest a diagnosis of AIH type 2. The presence of anti-LC1 can actually be masked by concurrent anti-LKM1 positivity as the latter stains throughout the cytoplasm on IF. The molecular target of anti-LC1 has been identified as formino-transferase cyclodeaminase, which should catalyze development of assays to enhance detection.[25]

Anti-SLA/LP is the only AIH-specific autoantibody and as such has high diagnostic value.[26] It is the sole antibody detected in as many as 14% to 20% of patients with AIH.[27] Historically, it has been associated with the third subtype of AIH[28] but is positive in 7% to 22% of patients with AIH type 1.[29] The studies that described AIH type 3 as anti-SLA/LP positivity in isolation of conventional antibodies used older IAIHG recommendations with higher titer cutoffs for ANA and SMA. In fact, it can be positive in patients with AIH type 1, AIH type 2, and even AIH-PSC.[30] The antigen target for anti-SLA and anti-LP alike is synthase (S), which converts O-phosphoseryl-tRNA (Sep) to selenocysteinyl-tRNA (Sec), granting the name SepSecS.[31] This knowledge powered the development of reliable assays in the form of ELISA and dot-blot.[8] Anti-SLA/AP may be associated with the presence of anti-Ro52 antibodies but can found in isolation as well, as previously suggested. Its presence may stratify patients by severity of disease and response to therapy, including a higher risk of relapse after cessation of corticosteroids[32] but this remains a controversial association at this time.[8]

Notably, the absence of antibodies does not preclude a diagnosis of AIH. In a study of 53 patients with AIH, determined by histologic and clinical criteria, 9 patients (17%) were found to be negative for all tested antibodies.[33] Further antibody testing can be undertaken and is most useful in patients who have tested negative on the above assays. Antineutrophil-cytoplasmic antibodies are directed against cytoplasmic components of neutrophils and arranged in either a perinuclear (p-ANCA) or cytoplasmic (c-ANCA) pattern.[34] C-ANCA and p-ANCA react mainly with proteinase 3 and myeloperoxidase, respectively.[35] Interestingly, many patients with AIH type 1 (50%–96%) and exceedingly few with AIH type 2 are seropositive for p-ANCA.[36] P-ANCA in AIH can differ from classic p-ANCA by reacting with nuclear membrane components (perinuclear antineutrophil antibodies, p-ANNA).[37] This "atypical" variant of p-ANCA is also seen in PSC and IBD and may act as an additional indicator of AIH in the absence of other autoantibodies.[38]

If all other antibodies are negative but clinical suspicion remains, autoantibodies against F-actin, gp210, and sp100 can be sought and may support the diagnosis of AIH. F-actin specifically is one of the several potential target antigens of AIH-associated SMA.[39] It is positive in 86% to 100% of patients with ANA and SMA.[40] AMA against the E2 subunit of the pyruvate dehydrogenase complexes are the hallmark of primary biliary cholangitis (PBC), and are present in 90% to 95% of PBC-afflicted individuals.[41] This antibody is atypical in AIH and therefore its presence should trigger suspicion for a concurrent disorder including AIH-PBC overlap syndrome.

In summary, autoantibodies play a critical role in the diagnosis and classification of AIH. There is evidence to suggest that the detection of certain antibodies has prognostic value. Ultimately, the absence of autoantibodies does not exclude AIH. Evolving laboratory techniques and standardization of methodology promise to enhance the diagnostic utility of serologic testing in the diagnosis of AIH.

HISTOLOGICAL FINDINGS

Histological findings are a cardinal aspect in the diagnosis of AIH. In fact, the diagnosis almost universally requires a liver biopsy, which also helps to rule out alternate or concurrent liver disease and to grade the severity of inflammation and fibrosis, if present. However, despite the importance of histology in the diagnosis of AIH, it should be noted that there is no pathognomonic finding for AIH. Instead, there is a characteristic set of findings that help support the diagnosis. To achieve a score of 2 points for histology by the simplified diagnostic criteria, 3 histologic features must be present. These features include the presence of interface hepatitis, emperipolesis, and rosette formation.[42] The latter 2 features are characteristic but not specific. These and other supportive findings are described in detail below.

INTERFACE HEPATITIS

The histological hallmark of AIH is interface hepatitis, which is present in 98% of cases, and it is typically a more prominent feature of AIH as compared with other causes of hepatitis.[43] It refers to the extension of portal inflammation beyond the limiting plate and into the adjacent lobule. There is progressive loss of hepatocytes at the portal–lobular interface.[44] When severe, it is associated with ductular reaction, which is a regenerative phenomenon representing proliferation and differentiation of hepatic stem cells.

Interface hepatitis is accompanied by plasma cell infiltration in 66% of cases.[45] Infiltrates rich in plasma cells are found along portal tracts and lobules. These infiltrates may contain other inflammatory cells, such as eosinophils and neutrophils.[46] Plasma cells are typical of AIH but may be rare or absent in up to one-third of cases. The detection of plasma cells in clusters, defined as a collection of more than 5 plasma cells, is a sensitive diagnostic finding.[47] Immunohistochemical staining for multiple myeloma-1 or CD38 may enhance the detection of plasma cell number and distribution.[48]

Interface hepatitis is accompanied by lobular hepatitis in 47% of cases.[45] It is characterized by the infiltration of inflammatory cells into the hepatic lobules, which can lead to destruction of hepatocytes.[28] The extent of lobular inflammation is also graded based on its severity. Lobular changes may include necrosis with the presence of apoptotic bodies. Confluent necrosis may be seen in perivenular areas and is typically associated with periportal inflammation as well. In the absence of portal tract inflammation, this pattern of necrosis is thought to imply acute disease onset, before the development of portal involvement, and if extensive, can portend to a worse prognosis.[49]

EMPERIPOLESIS

Emperipolesis refers to the presence of one cell (a lymphocyte or plasma cell) within the cytoplasm of another cell (a hepatocyte) without evidence of destruction (which differentiates it from phagocytosis) and may be present in 65% to 78% of patients with AIH.[42] Along with interface hepatitis and rosette formation, this is 1 of the 3 criteria needed to qualify for typical histology according to the simplified diagnostic scoring system. Unfortunately, emperipolesis is difficult to evaluate for in routine practice, as electron microscopy outperforms light microscopy in the identification of this histologic finding.[44]

ROSETTE FORMATION

Rosettes are hepatocytes arranged around a central lumen representing a regenerative response to necro-inflammatory damage. This feature is thought to be due to the binding of anti-SMA to hepatocytes.[33] Along with emperipolesis, this feature is thought to be more predictive of AIH than even plasma cell infiltration and interface hepatitis. De Boer and colleagues[50] systematically compared biopsies between 63 patients with AIH and 62 patients with viral hepatitis. The authors found that plasma cell infiltration and interface hepatitis were indeed more common in AIH but that this was true even more so for rosette formation and emperipolesis.

FEATURES OF AUTOIMMUNE ACUTE LIVER FAILURE

When AIH presents with acute liver failure (ALF), it is especially important to make an accurate diagnosis as autoimmune acute liver failure (AI-ALF) is potentially reversible and prompt recognition may improve survival or obviate liver transplantation. In AI-ALF, there are 4 additional histological findings, which predominate in the centrilobular zone.[51] Central perivenulitis is seen in 65%, plasma cell-enriched inflammatory infiltrate in 63%, massive hepatic necrosis in 42%, and lymphoid follicles in 32%. Sixty-six percent of patients with ALF will have 2 (21%), 3 (26%), or all 4 (19%) of these findings. Central perivenulitis and plasma cell infiltration have been shown to suggest a more chronic course.[51]

GRADING AND STAGING FIBROSIS

When AIH presents chronically, fibrosis can be seen on liver biopsy. There are no specific fibrosis scoring systems validated in the setting of AIH. As such, fibrosis is graded as per standard scoring systems, such as the Ishak, Scheur, or METAVIR scoring systems, at the discretion of the pathologist.[52] Timely recognition of AIH presents an opportunity for medical intervention that may effectively alter disease progression because fibrosis has been shown to be reversible with medical therapy.[53] Borssen and colleagues reviewed 258 liver biopsies from 101 patients examined by a single pathologist. About 94.9% of patients responded to medical therapy and 63 patients (62.4%) demonstrated a reduction in fibrosis stage from the first to last biopsy. Twenty-one patients had cirrhosis (Ishak stage 6) on the first biopsy while only 5 had cirrhosis at the time of the final liver biopsy.

EXCLUSION OF ATYPICAL FINDINGS

Some degree of bile duct injury is present in up to 83% of AIH biopsies, even in the absence of an overlap syndrome. In AIH, the bile ducts are not the target of autoimmune inflammation and the inflammatory changes noted on biopsy likely represent collateral damage secondary to generalized inflammation. Thus, bile duct injury is considered an atypical feature of AIH and can suggest comorbid biliary disease.[44] Unfortunately, the exact degree of bile duct damage deemed more than expected in AIH is not established. Prominent ductopenia, a histological description for destruction of bile ducts, is not a feature of AIH and should trigger a search for PBC.

Accumulation of copper-associated protein and/or cytokeratin 7 (CK7)-positive periportal hepatocytes are other atypical histological findings. They are typical of chronic cholestasis and should prompt consideration of an alternate diagnosis or overlap condition. However, when cirrhosis or advanced fibrosis is present, there is accumulation of copper-associated protein and CK7 independent of cause, so these findings lose diagnostic value in this setting.[42] Balitzer and colleagues[42] tested the clinical utility of including these histologic features and proposed new parameters to add to the 2008 simplified scoring system proposed by the IAIHG. The proposed changes led to a probable/definite diagnosis of AIH in 17% of cases that were classified as non-AIH by the simplified scoring system. This implies augmented sensitivity but these results still need to be validated in prospective studies.

SUMMARY OF HISTOLOGICAL FINDINGS

In summary, the histological features seen in AIH on liver biopsy include interface hepatitis, emperipolesis, rosette formation, plasma cell-rich infiltrates, lobular inflammation, and fibrosis. These features are important and necessary for the diagnosis of AIH and can also provide information regarding disease severity and prognosis. Other findings, such as characteristic centrilobular features or evidence of fibrosis can assist in distinguishing presentations such as ALF or chronic AIH with cirrhosis, respectively. Importantly, hepatic fibrosis in the setting of AIH can regress histologically with medical treatment. The presence of atypical features challenges clinicians to broaden the differential diagnosis and consider alternate, concomitant, or overlap disease. Going forward, a deeper understanding of histology in AIH may help to enhance the diagnostic utility of available scoring systems.

DIAGNOSIS OF OVERLAP SYNDROMES

Features of AIH such as elevated serum IgG, presence of autoantibodies, and even histologically evident interface hepatitis occur in other liver disorders as well including viral hepatitis, PBC, PSC, Wilson disease, and alcohol-associated liver disease. At least occasionally, the presence of overlapping features is due to the presence of a concurrent disorder.[54] The frequency of overlap with PBC and PSC is estimated at 7% to 13% and 6% to 11%, respectively.[55] Presentations of overlap syndromes are homogeneous, creating a diagnostic challenge. Some patients with AIH develop biochemical, serological, or histological findings of PBC or PSC. Conversely, some patients with PBC or PSC can develop features of AIH. It is of tantamount importance to make these diagnoses early and accurately to improve both treatment and prognosis.[56]

AUTOIMMUNE HEPATITIS–PRIMARY BILIARY CIRRHOSIS OVERLAP SYNDROME

AIH-PBC overlap is the most commonly described overlap syndrome but no formal definition exists and the diagnostic criteria for this syndrome are not standardized. As many as 30% to 40% of patients with typical PBC histology have circulating ANA and/or SMA as well as interface hepatitis on biopsy.[4] Identifying overlap syndromes is important because patients with AIH-PBC have been shown to benefit from dual therapy with ursodeoxycholic acid (UDCA) and immunosuppression.[57] Conventional scoring systems have poor performance in the setting of overlap syndromes. Instead, patients with AIH-PBC overlap syndrome can be identified via the "Paris criteria." In this system, 2 of the following 3 criteria must be met in addition to diagnostic criteria for AIH:[58]

- Alkaline phosphatase (ALP) 2× or greater upper limit of normal or GGT 5× or greater upper limit of normal
- Presence of AMA
- Florid bile duct lesions on histological examination

A retrospective single-center study by Chaz comparing the Paris criteria to traditional scoring systems found enhanced sensitivity (92%) and specificity (97%).[59] However, the IAIHG has cautioned that it is difficult to interpret these reported test characteristics.[60] One concern is that the Paris criteria may not capture certain patients with less-pronounced cholestatic features on laboratory studies. Additionally, 8% to 12% of patients with AIH may have circulating antibodies to pyruvate dehydrogenase-E2 (AMA) in the absence of bile duct injury or loss on biopsy.[29] Conversely, some patients with features of AIH-PBC may test negative for AMA. This clinical scenario is thought to be an overlap syndrome of AIH and autoimmune cholangiopathy (AIC). AIC-AIH may respond to combination therapy with UDCA and steroids.[61]

AUTOIMMUNE HEPATITIS–PRIMARY SCLEROSING CHOLANGITIS OVERLAP SYNDROME

An AIH-PSC overlap syndrome, also called autoimmune sclerosing cholangitis, has been described.[62] The diagnosis of this syndrome should be considered in all AIH patients with chronic ulcerative colitis, unexplained cholestatic laboratory findings, or nonresponse to glucocorticoid therapy.[63] Chronic ulcerative colitis is present in up to 16% of patients with AIH. Furthermore, 42% of patients with concurrent ulcerative colitis and AIH have cholangiographic changes consistent with PSC.[64] Despite these described relationships, diagnostic criteria are even less well defined than in AIH-PBC variants. Serology for pANCA is an additional diagnostic test, which may have some utility in this setting. It is present in as many as 70% of patients with PSC, and it is more commonly detected in patients with AIH-PSC than AIH alone.[65] However, it is neither sensitive nor specific. Instead, diagnosis of overlap syndromes is based on the following:

- The presence of typical features of AIH
- Absence of AMA
- Evidence of large-duct PSC by endoscopy or magnetic resonance cholangiopancreatography (MRCP)
- Evidence of small duct PSC with "onion skinning" periductal fibrosis on histology

The revised scoring system by the IAIHG has been evaluated for use in AIH-PSC overlap syndrome and demonstrated increased precision as compared with the original.[66] Kaya and colleagues applied the system to 211 patients with cholangiographically proven PSC and found increased precision in detecting overlap syndromes. Accurate diagnosis is important in this setting because those with overlap syndrome have been shown to carry a better prognosis than classic patients with PSC and treatments differ as well.[67]

SUMMARY

AIH is a perplexing entity to diagnose due to its relative rarity and heterogenous presentation. It can present at varying ages, with varying chronicity, and is even divided into 2 major subtypes. AIH offers no pathognomonic findings, instead relying on clinical presentation, serology, and histology to make the diagnosis. The scoring systems described above are designed as tools to aid in diagnosis as well as to define research cohorts. However, they are not a substitute for clinical judgment. Specifically, in less typical scenarios including concomitant liver disease or the presence of an overlap syndrome, these criteria fail to demonstrate the same diagnostic utility. Detection of autoantibodies is an alternate tool to aid in diagnosis. Typical autoantibodies such as ANA, SMA, and anti-LKM1 have proven utility in diagnosis and even prognosis. Several others provide additional information when typical autoantibodies are absent. A plethora of other markers may rise to clinical importance as standardization of and technologies behind assays improve. Histological analysis remains the cornerstone of diagnosis and to this day biopsy is essential to make the diagnosis. The 3 hallmark features of AIH on biopsy are interface hepatitis, emperipolesis, and rosette formation, which are reflected on diagnostic scoring systems accordingly. Other supportive findings may also have prognostic implications. Overlap syndromes pose additional diagnostic uncertainty because traditional scoring systems demonstrate poor performance characteristics. Recognition is important because clinical courses and response to treatment may vary.

CLINICS CARE POINTS

- AIH is a perplexing entity to diagnose due to its relative rarity and heterogenous presentation. It can present at varying ages, with varying chronicity, and is even divided into 2 major subtypes.
- The 3 hallmark features of AIH on biopsy are interface hepatitis, emperipolesis, and rosette formation, which are reflected on diagnostic scoring systems accordingly.
- Overlap syndromes pose additional diagnostic uncertainty because traditional scoring systems demonstrate poor performance characteristics.

REFERENCES

1. European Association for the Study of the Liver. EASL clinical practice guidelines: autoimmune hepatitis. J Hepatol 2015;63(4):971–1004 [Erratum in: J Hepatol. 2015 Dec;63(6):1543-4. PMID: 26341719].
2. Yasui S, Fujiwara K, Yonemitsu Y, et al. Clinicopathological features of severe and fulminant forms of autoimmune hepatitis. J Gastroenterol 2011;46(3):378–90.
3. Fujiwara K, Fukuda Y, Yokosuka O. Precise histological evaluation of liver biopsy specimen is indispensable for diagnosis and treatment of acute-onset autoimmune hepatitis. J Gastroenterol 2008;43(12):951–8.
4. Alvarez F, Berg PA, Bianchi FB, et al. International Autoimmune Hepatitis Group Report: review of criteria for diagnosis of autoimmune hepatitis. J Hepatol 1999;31(5):929–38.
5. Mieli-Vergani G, Vergani D, Czaja A, et al. Autoimmune hepatitis. Nat Rev Dis Prim 2018;4:18017.
6. Obermayer-Straub P, Strassburg CP, Manns MP. Autoimmune hepatitis. J Hepatol 2000;32(1 Suppl):181–97.
7. Czaja AJ, Manns MP. The validity and importance of subtypes in autoimmune hepatitis: a point of view. Am J Gastroenterol 1995;90(8):1206–11. PMID: 7639216.

8. Baeres M, Harkel J, Czaja AJ, et al. Establishment of standardised SLA/LP immunoassays: specificity for autoimmune hepatitis, worldwide occurrence, and clinical characteristics. Gut 2002;51:259–64.

9. Muratori P, Lalanne C, Fabbri A, et al. Type 1 and type 2 autoimmune hepatitis in adults share the same clinical phenotype. Aliment Pharmacol Ther 2015;41(12): 1281–7. Epub 2015 Apr 19. PMID: 25898847.

10. Ducazu O, Degroote H, Geerts A, et al. Diagnostic and prognostic scoring systems for autoimmune hepatitis: a review. Acta Gastroenterol Belg 2021;84(3): 487–95.

11. Qiu D, Wang Q, Wang H, et al. Validation of the simplified criteria for diagnosis of autoimmune hepatitis in Chinese patients. J Hepatol 2011 Feb;54(2):340–7. Epub 2010 Sep 15. PMID: 21056494.

12. Czaja AJ. Performance parameters of the diagnostic scoring systems for autoimmune hepatitis. Hepatology 2008;48(5):1540–8.

13. Hennes EM, Zeniya M, Czaja AJ, et al. Simplified criteria for the diagnosis of autoimmune hepatitis. Hepatology 2008;48:169–76.

14. Yatsuji S, Hashimoto E, Kaneda H, et al. Diagnosing autoimmune hepatitis in nonalcoholic fatty liver disease: is the International Autoimmune Hepatitis Group scoring system useful? J Gastroenterol 2005;40(12):1130–8.

15. Lohse AW, Sebode M, Bhathal PS, et al. Consensus recommendations for histological criteria of autoimmune hepatitis from the international AIH pathology group. Liver Int 2022. https://doi.org/10.1111/liv.15217.

16. Czaja AJ, Homburger HA. Autoantibodies in liver disease. Gastroenterology 2001;120(1):239–49.

17. Terziroli Beretta-Piccoli B, Mieli-Vergani G, Vergani D. Autoimmune hepatitis: serum autoantibodies in clinical practice. Clin Rev Allergy Immunol 2022;63(2): 124–37.

18. Manns MP, Czaja AJ, Gorham JD, et al. American association for the study of liver diseases. Diagnosis and management of autoimmune hepatitis. Hepatology 2010;51(6):2193–213.

19. Czaja AJ. Diagnosis and management of autoimmune hepatitis: current status and future directions. Gut Liver 2016;10(2):177–203.

20. Czaja AJ. Performance parameters of the conventional serological markers for autoimmune hepatitis. Dig Dis Sci 2011;56(2):545–54.

21. Czaja AJ. Autoimmune hepatitis. In: Feldman M, Friedman LS, Brandt LJ, editors. Sleisenger and fordtran's gastrointestinal and liver disease. 11th ed. Philadelphia, PA: Elsevier; 2021. chap 88.

22. Gregorio GV, Portmann B, Reid F, et al. Autoimmune hepatitis in childhood: a 20-year experience. Hepatology 1997;25(3):541–7.

23. Muratori P, Granito A, Quarneti C, et al. Autoimmune hepatitis in Italy: the Bologna experience. J Hepatol 2009;50(6):1210–8.

24. Cassani F, Cataleta M, Valentini P, et al. Serum autoantibodies in chronic hepatitis C: comparison with autoimmune hepatitis and impact on the disease profile. Hepatology 1997;26(3):561–6.

25. Lapierre P, Hajoui O, Homberg JC, et al. Formiminotransferase cyclodeaminase is an organ-specific autoantigen recognized by sera of patients with autoimmune hepatitis. Gastroenterology 1999;116(3):643–9.

26. Vergani D, Alvarez F, Bianchi FB, et al. International autoimmune hepatitis group. Liver autoimmune serology: a consensus statement from the committee for autoimmune serology of the international autoimmune hepatitis group. J Hepatol 2004;41(4):677–83. PMID: 15464251.

27. Ballot E, Homberg JC, Johanet C. Antibodies to soluble liver antigen: an additional marker in type 1 auto-immune hepatitis. J Hepatol 2000;33(2):208–15.
28. Liberal R, Longhi MS, Mieli-Vergani G, et al. Diagnostic criteria of autoimmune hepatitis. Autoimmun Rev 2014;13(4–5):435–40.
29. Czaja AJ, Carpenter HA, Manns MP. Antibodies to soluble liver antigen, P450IID6, and mitochondrial complexes in chronic hepatitis. Gastroenterology 1993;105(5):1522–8.
30. Ma Y, Okamoto M, Thomas MG, et al. Antibodies to conformational epitopes of soluble liver antigen define a severe form of autoimmune liver disease. Hepatology 2002;35(3):658–64.
31. Wies I, Brunner S, Henninger J, et al. Identification of target antigen for SLA/LP autoantibodies in autoimmune hepatitis. Lancet 2000;355(9214):1510–5.
32. Czaja AJ, Shums Z, Norman GL. Nonstandard antibodies as prognostic markers in autoimmune hepatitis. Autoimmunity 2004;37(3):195–201.
33. Muratori P, Granito A, Pappas G, et al. Uncertainties in the diagnosis of autoimmune hepatitis. Expert Rev Clin Immunol 2018;14(8):677–86.
34. Falk RJ, Jennette JC. Anti-neutrophil cytoplasmic autoantibodies with specificity for myeloperoxidase in patients with systemic vasculitis and idiopathic necrotizing and crescentic glomerulonephritis. N Engl J Med 1988;318(25):1651–7.
35. Targan SR, Landers C, Vidrich A, et al. High-titer antineut/rophil cytoplasmic antibodies in type-1 autoimmune hepatitis. Gastroenterology 1995;108(4):1159–66.
36. Mulder AH, Horst G, Haagsma EB, et al. Prevalence and characterization of neutrophil cytoplasmic antibodies in autoimmune liver diseases. Hepatology 1993;17(3):411–7. PMID: 8444414.
37. Terjung B, Spengler U, Sauerbruch T, et al. "Atypical p-ANCA" in IBD and hepatobiliary disorders react with a 50-kilodalton nuclear envelope protein of neutrophils and myeloid cell lines. Gastroenterology 2000;119(2):310–22.
38. Terjung B, Worman HJ, Herzog V, et al. Differentiation of antineutrophil nuclear antibodies in inflammatory bowel and autoimmune liver diseases from antineutrophil cytoplasmic antibodies (p-ANCA) using immunofluorescence microscopy. Clin Exp Immunol 2001;126(1):37–46.
39. Frenzel C, Herkel J, Lüth S, et al. Evaluation of F-actin ELISA for the diagnosis of autoimmune hepatitis. Am J Gastroenterol 2006;101(12):2731–6.
40. Chretien-Leprince P, Ballot E, Andre C, et al. Diagnostic value of anti-F-actin antibodies in a French multicenter study. Ann N Y Acad Sci 2005;1050:266–73.
41. Farias AQ, Gonçalves LL, Bittencourt PL, et al. Applicability of the IAIHG scoring system to the diagnosis of antimitochondrial/anti-M2 seropositive variant form of autoimmune hepatitis. J Gastroenterol Hepatol 2006;21(5):887–93.
42. Balitzer D, Shafizadeh N, Peters M, et al. Autoimmune hepatitis: review of histologic features included in the simplified criteria proposed by the international autoimmune hepatitis group and proposal for new histologic criteria. Mod Pathol 2017;30:773–83.
43. Burt AD, Ferrell LD, Hübscher SG. MacSween's pathology of the liver, E-book. Elsevier Health Sciences; 2022.
44. Covelli C, Sacchi D, Sarcognato S, et al. Pathology of autoimmune hepatitis. Pathologica 2021;113(3):185–93.
45. Czaja AJ, Carpenter HA. Sensitivity, specificity, and predictability of biopsy interpretations in chronic hepatitis. Gastroenterology 1993;105(6):1824–32.
46. Kessler WR, Cummings OW, Eckert G, et al. Fulminant hepatic failure as the initial presentation of acute autoimmune hepatitis. Clin Gastroenterol Hepatol 2004; 2(7):625–31.

47. Gurung A, Assis DN, McCarty TR, et al. Histologic features of autoimmune hepatitis: a critical appraisal. Hum Pathol 2018;82:51–60.
48. Rubio CA, Truskaite K, Rajani R, et al. A method to assess the distribution and frequency of plasma cells and plasma cell precursors in autoimmune hepatitis. Anticancer Res 2013;33(2):665–9. PMID: 23393365.
49. Shen Y, Lu C, Men R, et al. Clinical and pathological characteristics of autoimmune hepatitis with acute presentation. Chin J Gastroenterol Hepatol 2018; 2018:3513206.
50. de Boer YS, van Nieuwkerk CM, Witte BI, et al. Assessment of the histopathological key features in autoimmune hepatitis. Histopathology 2015;66(3):351–62.
51. Stravitz RT, et al. Autoimmune acute liver failure: proposed clinical and histological criteria. Hepatology 2011;53(2):517–26.
52. Mohamadnejad M, Tavangar SM, Sotoudeh M, et al. Histopathological study of chronic hepatitis B: a comparative study of Ishak and METAVIR scoring systems. Int J Organ Transplant Med 2010;1(4):171–6.
53. Borssén ÅD, Palmqvist R, Kechagias S, et al. Histological improvement of liver fibrosis in well-treated patients with autoimmune hepatitis: a cohort study. Medicine (Baltim) 2017;96(34):e7708.
54. Colombato LA, Alvarez F, Côté J, et al. Autoimmune cholangiopathy: the result of consecutive primary biliary cirrhosis and autoimmune hepatitis? Gastroenterology 1994;107(6):1839–43.
55. Czaja AJ. Diagnosis and management of the overlap syndromes of autoimmune hepatitis. Can J Gastroenterol 2013;27(7):417–23.
56. Bairy I, Berwal A, Seshadri S. Autoimmune hepatitis - primary biliary cirrhosis overlap syndrome. J Clin Diagn Res 2017;11(7):OD07–9.
57. Chazouillères O, Wendum D, Serfaty L, et al. Long term outcome and response to therapy of primary biliary cirrhosis-autoimmune hepatitis overlap syndrome. J Hepatol 2006;44(2):400–6. Epub 2005 Nov 15. PMID: 16356577.
58. Chazouillères O, et al. Primary biliary cirrhosis–autoimmune hepatitis overlap syndrome: clinical features and response to therapy. Hepatology 1998;28(2):296–301.
59. Kuiper EM, Zondervan PE, van Buuren HR. Paris criteria are effective in diagnosis of primary biliary cirrhosis and autoimmune hepatitis overlap syndrome. Clin Gastroenterol Hepatol 2010;8(6):530–4.
60. Boberg KM, et al. Overlap syndromes: the International Autoimmune Hepatitis Group (IAIHG) position statement on a controversial issue. J Hepatol 2011; 54(2):374–85.
61. Li CP, Tong MJ, Hwang SJ, et al. Autoimmune cholangitis with features of autoimmune hepatitis: successful treatment with immunosuppressive agents and ursodeoxycholic acid. J Gastroenterol Hepatol 2000;15(1):95–8.
62. Boberg KM, Fausa O, Haaland T, et al. Features of autoimmune hepatitis in primary sclerosing cholangitis: an evaluation of 114 primary sclerosing cholangitis patients according to a scoring system for the diagnosis of autoimmune hepatitis. Hepatology 1996;23(6):1369–76.
63. Czaja AJ. Cholestatic phenotypes of autoimmune hepatitis. Clin Gastroenterol Hepatol 2014;12(9):1430–8.
64. Perdigoto R, Carpenter HA, Czaja AJ. Frequency and significance of chronic ulcerative colitis in severe corticosteroid-treated autoimmune hepatitis. J Hepatol 1992;14:325–31, 2-3.

65. Gregorio GV, Portmann B, Karani J, et al. Autoimmune hepatitis/sclerosing cholangitis overlap syndrome in childhood: a 16-year prospective study. Hepatology 2001;33(3):544–53.
66. Kaya M, Angulo P, Lindor KD. Overlap of autoimmune hepatitis and primary sclerosing cholangitis: an evaluation of a modified scoring system. J Hepatol 2000; 33(4):537–42.
67. Floreani A, Rizzotto ER, Ferrara F, et al. Clinical course and outcome of autoimmune hepatitis/primary sclerosing cholangitis overlap syndrome. Am J Gastroenterol 2005;100(7):1516–22.

Treatment of Autoimmune Hepatitis

Aparna Goel, MD*, Paul Kwo, MD[1]

KEYWORDS

- Autoimmune hepatitis • Treatment failure • Biochemical remission
- Immunosuppression • Liver transplant • Recurrent autoimmune hepatitis

KEY POINTS

- Treatment of autoimmune hepatitis should be considered in 2 phases: induction and maintenance. The goal of treatment is clinical and biochemical remission, defined as normal ALT and serum IgG levels.
- First-line therapy for autoimmune hepatitis is corticosteroids with subsequent initiation of azathioprine. Budesonide can be considered in patients without a severe acute presentation or cirrhosis.
- Side effects of corticosteroids and immunosuppressive regimen need to be considered before treatment and should be carefully monitored while on therapy.
- Alternative treatment options include mycophenolate mofetil, calcineurin inhibitors, mammalian target of rapamycin (mTOR) inhibitors, and rituximab.

INTRODUCTION

Autoimmune hepatitis (AIH) is a chronic immune-mediated inflammatory liver disease that presents across the demographic spectrum. The clinical presentation can range from asymptomatic disease and mild-to-moderate symptoms to acute liver failure. Without adequate control of autoimmune activity, the liver disease can progress to advanced fibrosis, cirrhosis, and liver failure. Treatment of AIH with immunosuppressive agents can significantly improve outcomes, but the efficacy of treatment regimens is variable and associated with long-term toxicity. In those with progressive liver disease, liver transplantation (LT) is considered an acceptable treatment option.

GOALS OF TREATMENT

There are several goals of AIH therapy including symptom control, biochemical remission, histologic remission, prevention of disease progression to decompensated cirrhosis or hepatocellular cancer, and regression of fibrosis. Biochemical remission

Division of Gastroenterology and Hepatology, Stanford University, Palo Alto, CA 94043, USA
[1] Present address: 430 Broadway Street, Pavilion C, 3rd Floor, Redwood City, CA 94043.
* Corresponding author. 430 Broadway Street, Pavilion C, 3rd Floor, Redwood City, CA 94043.
E-mail address: goela21@stanford.edu

Clin Liver Dis 28 (2024) 51–61
https://doi.org/10.1016/j.cld.2023.07.001
1089-3261/24/© 2023 Elsevier Inc. All rights reserved.

is defined as normalization of serum aspartate transferase (AST), alanine transferase (ALT), and immunoglobulin G (IgG) levels.[1] Histologic remission is the absence of inflammation in liver tissue after treatment.[2] In those that are able to achieve biochemical and histologic remission, it is possible to prevent disease progression and even reverse fibrosis.[3] Treatment should be considered in all patients with AIH except those with inactive disease based on clinical, laboratory, and histologic evaluation.

CONSIDERATIONS BEFORE TREATMENT

Treatment of AIH relies on potent immunosuppressive medications, hence baseline clinical and safety parameters need to be considered to guide the selection of therapy. Updated guidance from the American Association for the Study of Liver Diseases suggests the following list should be reviewed with patients in anticipation of treatment (**Table 1**).[2]

FIRST-LINE TREATMENT FOR AUTOIMMUNE HEPATITIS

The choice of first-line therapy depends on the clinical presentation of AIH including the presence of cirrhosis or acute severe AIH. There are 2 phases of therapy—

Table 1 Pre-treatment considerations for autoimmune hepatitis	
Vaccinations	• Follow age-specific guidelines of the Centers of Disease Control and Prevention • Complete vaccination series for hepatitis A and B infections, ideally before starting immunosuppressive therapy
Assessment of azathioprine safety	• Test thiopurine methyltransferase activity
Hepatitis B reactivation risk	• HBsAg-negative/anti-HBc-positive patients receiving high-dose predniso(lo)ne with azathioprine should have serial HBsAg and HBV DNA monitored • Preemptive antiviral therapy should be considered in those with prior HBV infection treated with high-dose predniso(lo)ne or potent immunomodulators, including B-cell depleting therapy
Bone health	• Assess serum 25-hydroxyvitamin D levels at diagnosis and replete appropriately • Bone density scan should be performed at the time of diagnosis in those with risk factors for osteoporosis
Metabolic syndrome	• Assess for the presence of metabolic syndrome, which may be exacerbated by immunosuppressive therapy, especially predniso(lo)ne
Family planning	• Women of reproductive potential should ideally be in remission for 1 y before conception • Risk of prematurity primarily in instances of active AIH or flare during pregnancy • Risk of flare after pregnancy is highest during the first 6 mo postpartum • Predniso(lo)ne and azathioprine should be continued during pregnancy • Mycophenolate mofetil is contraindicated in pregnancy

induction and maintenance. During the induction phase, higher doses of immunosuppression are used to control inflammatory activity rapidly and frequently laboratory testing is required. When there is an adequate biochemical response, the minimal immunosuppression dose should be continued to maintain remission (**Table 2**).[2]

Induction of Remission

First-line therapy to induce remission is usually monotherapy with a glucocorticoid and subsequent initiation of azathioprine (AZA). Several historical studies evaluating AZA monotherapy for induction noted higher mortality compared with prednisone, hence this is not a recommended strategy to induce remission.[4,5] Options for glucocorticoid therapy include budesonide, prednisone, or prednisolone. In patients with cirrhosis or acute severe AIH, budesonide should not be used as the presence of portal hypertensive shunts reduces efficacy.

Treatment is usually initiated with prednisone alone at a dose of 40 to 60 mg daily in adults. In Europe, the same dose or weight-based dose (0.5–1 mg/kg daily) of prednisolone is preferred over prednisone. Higher doses of predniso(lo)ne do not necessarily result in higher rates of biochemical remission in AIH.[6] Once biochemical improvement is demonstrated, AZA can be added, usually after 2 weeks. The rationale to delay the initiation of AZA is to assess treatment response to steroids, confirm thiopurine methyltransferase activity status and exclude the rare possibility of AZA-induced cholestatic hepatitis. Standard dosing of AZA varies based on region: 50 to 150 mg daily in the United States and 1 to 2 mg/kg daily in Europe. If combination therapy with AZA is preferred initially, the dose of prednisone can be reduced to 20 to 40 mg daily. Importantly, AZA should not be used in patients with decompensated cirrhosis or acute severe AIH until cholestasis has resolved due to risk of hepatotoxicity. In patients with acute severe AIH, high-dose predniso(lo)ne (60 mg daily) or intravenous (IV) methylprednisolone should be used for induction.

Budesonide is an acceptable induction agent in combination with AZA in patients without cirrhosis or acute severe AIH. Budesonide is initially started at 3 mg 3 times/day with weight-based AZA (1–2 mg/kg daily). The dose of budesonide is reduced to twice daily following remission. Studies comparing the efficacy of budesonide with AZA to prednisone have shown high rates of achieving biochemical remission at 6 months with fewer steroid-specific side effects, especially bone mineral density loss.[7] Patients with cirrhosis should not receive budesonide as the presence of portosystemic shunting reduces the efficacy of the drug and there is a risk of portal vein thrombosis.

During the induction phase, laboratory parameters are initially monitored every 1 to 2 weeks to determine whether there is a response to steroids ± AZA. If there is an

Table 2
Autoimmune hepatitis treatment regimens for both induction and maintenance phases using combination therapy

	Options for Combination Therapy	
Induction	Budesonide 9 mg daily AND Azathioprine 50–150 mg (or 1–2 mg/kg in Europe)	Prednisone 20–40 mg (or 0.5–1 mg/kg in Europe) AND Azathioprine 50–150 mg (or 1–2 mg/kg in Europe)
Maintenance	[a]Budesonide 3–6 mg daily AND Azathioprine 50–150 mg (or 1–2 mg/kg in Europe)	[a]Prednisone: 0–10 mg AND Azathioprine 50–150 mg (or 1–2 mg/kg in Europe)

[a] Lowest possible dose should be used.

appropriate biochemical response with normalization of transaminases and serum IgG levels after 4 to 8 weeks, a strategy of response-guided therapy is recommended to taper steroids. Predniso(lo)ne should be gradually reduced to 20 mg daily or the lowest dose required to maintain remission while monitoring laboratory tests every 2 weeks. The reduction of predniso(lo)ne from 20 mg to lower doses should be slow and gradual, usually no more than 2.5 to 5 mg every 2 to 4 weeks until the lowest possible dose or discontinuation of steroid while maintaining AZA or steroid-sparing agent.

Side effects of steroids are well documented and include diabetes, hypertension, cosmetic changes, osteoporosis, cataracts, opportunistic infections, depression, anxiety, psychosis, and ischemic necrosis of the hips. The intensity of these side effects is reduced with budesonide compared with prednisone due to first-pass metabolism in the liver.[7] AZA can cause bone marrow suppression resulting in mild cytopenias or bone marrow failure. AZA dose should be reduced or discontinued if cytopenias progress after 1 to 2 weeks after dose reduction. AZA dosage should also be adjusted to reduce hepatotoxicity and achieve therapeutic levels of 6 TGN. Routine 6 TGN levels are not recommended in adults, but 6-TGN levels of 100 to 300 pmol/8 $\times$ 10^6 are recommended in children. Thiopurine metabolites should be evaluated in adults who have an incomplete response to AZA to consider increasing the dose or adding allopurinol to alter AZA metabolism to form less 6 MMP and more 6 TGN.[8] GI intolerance with nausea and vomiting is also noted in ~10% of patients.[9] AZA should not be used in patients with active malignancy.

Maintenance of Remission

Once biochemical remission is achieved, laboratory tests should be monitored every 3 to 4 months. Withdrawal of steroids can be attempted while maintaining a steroid-sparing agent, such as AZA, mycophenolate mofetil, or calcineurin inhibitor (see *Alternative first-line therapies*). Complete clinical, biochemical, and histologic remission with a sustained response off immunosuppressant therapy is the most desirable endpoint; however, this does not occur in greater than 80% of patients.[10] Hence, a more practical goal is the maintenance of remission with the lowest possible immunosuppressive medication. Laboratory testing may be spaced out to every 4 to 6 months after prolonged remission of more than 2 years.

Follow-up biopsy is only recommended if histologic findings will result in a change in management. This is most often pursued in patients with an incomplete response to standard immunosuppression or for those hoping to withdraw immunosuppression after an extended period of biochemical remission. Transient elastography may be a reasonable noninvasive tool to follow changes in fibrosis as there is a good correlation with histology. However, increased liver stiffness may be due to inflammatory activity or fibrosis.[11,12] Hence, transient elastography should ideally be performed at least 6 months after biochemical remission to accurately identify the stage of fibrosis. With longitudinal follow-up, improvement in liver stiffness on transient elastography correlates with regression of fibrosis and favorable prognosis.[13]

Alternative First-Line Therapy

If there are contraindications to first-line therapy, alternative treatments should be considered. Corticosteroids are difficult to avoid in the treatment of AIH. However, if there are significant pre-existing conditions (eg, brittle diabetes, osteoporotic fractures) of which an exacerbation could be particularly harmful to the patient, it is prudent to minimize the dose of steroids and consider transitioning predniso(lo)ne to budesonide, if possible. Steroid-free induction with AZA monotherapy resulted in high mortality (30% during induction) in the 1970s and hence is not recommended in adults.[14] However, a recent small series suggests AZA monotherapy is a safe induction regimen in some children with mild AIH.[15] There are limited data on cyclosporine monotherapy as first-line therapy in children with subsequent use of low-dose steroids with AZA. This strategy prioritizes minimizing steroid exposure and seems to be effective in longer-term follow-up.[16] Similarly, there are sparse data on tacrolimus monotherapy for induction of remission in adults indicating limited success without the use of steroids or AZA.[17]

Induction treatment with MMF alone is not recommended at this time. However, the combination of MMF and predniso(lo)ne as first-line therapy seems to be at least as effective as AZA and predniso(lo)ne in achieving biochemical remission.[18–21] In a single observational study comparing MMF and prednisolone with prednisolone ± AZA as first-line treatment, the MMF group was more likely to achieve biochemical remission (72% vs 46%).[19] Data remain limited to case series or single-center studies and histologic outcomes are unknown. Importantly, MMF is contraindicated in pregnancy.

Second-Line Therapy

Second-line therapy should be considered in patients with intolerance or nonresponse to first-line therapy. Nonresponse to first-line therapy is reported in up to 20% of patients with AIH and is associated with an increased incidence of cirrhosis and LT.[22] It is critical to evaluate medication compliance with thiopurine metabolites in those with nonresponse to first-line therapy. Factors associated with nonresponse include age less than 40 years, less than 80% reduction in ALT after 8 weeks of therapy, serum IgG greater than $1.9\times$ upper limit normal (ULN), ferritin less than $2.1\times$ ULN, and vitamin D deficiency.[23–26] Nonresponse is further categorized into incomplete response and treatment failure.[2]

- Incomplete response is defined as an improvement of laboratory and histologic findings that are insufficient to satisfy the criteria for remission.
- Treatment failure is defined as worsening laboratory or histologic findings despite compliance with standard therapy.

In these instances, second-line therapy can serve as an alternative treatment option or an adjunct to first-line therapy. Second-line therapy options include MMF, calcineurin inhibitors, sirolimus, and biologics.

In patients treated with budesonide 9 mg/day to induce or maintain remission, replacement with predniso(lo)ne at a dose ≥20 mg/day should be considered. In patients treated with a predniso(lo)ne-based regimen, there are 3 possible options:

1. Increase the dose of predniso(lo)ne, although doses greater than 10 mg/day are not recommended in the long term due to side effects.
2. Increase AZA dose to 2 mg/kg/day along with low-dose predniso(lo)ne (5–10 mg/day). Targeting specific 6-TGN levels is not validated in adults.
3. Change AZA to another agent.

MMF is the most common second-line therapy for AIH. In several large case series and meta-analyses, MMF results in biochemical remission of varying degrees depending on the indication. In those started on MMF due to nonresponse to AZA, approximately one-third achieve biochemical remission compared with 60% to 90% when MMF is used due to AZA intolerance.[27–29] MMF tends to be well tolerated with the most common adverse effects leading to drug discontinuation being cytopenias and GI intolerance.

Tacrolimus has demonstrated efficacy as an alternative to AZA in those with intolerance or as a second-line agent. It has been studied in combination with other agents such as predniso(lo)ne, MMF, AZA, or as an alternative to AZA with serum trough levels ranging from 1 to 10 ng/mL.[30] The efficacy of tacrolimus in achieving biochemical remission is higher in those with AZA intolerance (94%) compared with nonresponse (57%).[29] Side effects of tacrolimus include neurotoxicity (tremors, headache), nephrotoxicity, and hair loss.

Cyclosporin can be considered as an alternative to tacrolimus in those with concurrent diabetes, although it has not been rigorously studied in AIH, so dosing and monitoring as not as well established. Data in adults with AIH are primarily limited to case series from the 1980s/1990s, indicating a positive response.[31] There are more data in the pediatric population suggesting efficacy in achieving biochemical remission.[16]

There are limited data on the efficacy of sirolimus for managing AIH that is refractory to first-line therapy. A small case series of 5 patients treated with sirolimus noted improvement in ALT in 80% of patients when targeting a median trough level of 12.5 ng/mL.[32] The main side effects of sirolimus include metabolic syndrome (weight gain, hyperlipidemia), proteinuria, and edema. Although the use of sirolimus as an initial second-line agent is not standard, it may be considered an alternative or adjunctive therapy in challenging cases.

Rituximab, an anti-CD-20 receptor monoclonal antibody, has been used to treat both children and adults with AIH. In a series of 22 adults who were given 2 doses of 1000 mg rituximab, administered 2 weeks apart, there was a notable improvement in transaminases within 1 month after the infusion, which sustained for approximately 24 months. Steroid dose was reduced in nearly two-thirds of the cohort.[33] However, given the extremely potent immunosuppressive effect with limited data in AIH, rituximab is not yet recommended as second-line therapy.

Common toxicity for the standard and alternative therapies for treatment of AIH along with strategies to manage common side effects are shown in **Table 3**.

Withdrawal of Immunosuppression

Immunosuppression withdrawal can be considered in patients with AIH that did not have an acute severe presentation. AST, ALT, and serum IgG levels should be normal for at least 2 years before attempting withdrawal. Although a liver biopsy is still recommended to evaluate for inflammation, an ALT level of less than 50% ULN and a normal serum IgG level of less than 1200 mg/dL (deep biochemical remission) may be more predictive of successful immunosuppression withdrawal. Approximately 50% of patients who met these parameters in a small study remained in remission for a median of 28 months after treatment withdrawal.[34] The utility of transient elastography in predicting outcome after immunosuppression withdrawal has not yet been validated. A recent report evaluated the utility of iron-corrected T1 (cT1) scores using multiparametric MR in patients with AIH, demonstrating that low cT1 scores could differentiate those in deep biochemical remission from those in normal biochemical remission, and this modality also deserves further study.[35] Liver enzymes should continue to be monitored indefinitely to ensure sustained remission.

Liver Transplantation

AIH is the indication for LT in approximately 5% of LT recipients in the United States. LT should be considered for patients with acute liver failure and complications from chronic liver disease including ascites, gastroesophageal variceal bleeding, hepatic encephalopathy, jaundice, and hepatocellular carcinoma. In those presenting with acute severe AIH, transplant candidacy should be assessed while initiating IV steroids as it is crucial not to delay the LT evaluation if hepatic encephalopathy develops.

Table 3
Side effects of standard immunosuppressive treatment options in autoimmune hepatitis and strategies to improve tolerability

	Standard Dose	Side Effects	Management Options
Predniso(lo)ne	40–60 mg/day 0.5–1 mg/kg/day	Metabolic—diabetes, weight gain, hypertension, osteoporosis, cataracts, glaucoma Cosmetic—moon facies, hirsutism, alopecia, striae Emotional lability, depression, anxiety, psychosis Ischemic necrosis of the hips	Use the lowest effective dose Lifestyle interventions for metabolic syndrome Calcium/vitamin D supplementation, bone density monitoring Eye examinations Discontinue treatment
Budesonide	3 mg TID	Reduced intensity of systemic steroids Portal vein thrombosis in cirrhosis—avoid in severe AIH	Use the lowest effective dose Do not use in cirrhosis or acute severe AIH
Azathioprine	50–150 mg/day 1–2 mg/kg/day	Bone marrow—cytopenia, leukopenia, bone marrow failure GI—nausea, vomiting, pancreatitis, cholestasis Non-melanoma skin cancer	Check test thiopurine methyltransferase status Lower dose if developing cytopenia Check thiopurine metabolites; consider allopurinol Discontinue if severe cytopenia Discontinue if severe GI intolerance Annual full-body skin examination Do not use in decompensated cirrhosis or acute severe AIH
MMF	1–3 g/day	Cytopenias GI intolerance	Reduce dose to minimize side effects
Tacrolimus	Target trough 1–10 ng/mL	Neurotoxicity—headache, tremor Nephrotoxicity—hypertension, insufficiency Hyperglycemia Hair loss Nausea	Reduce dose to minimize side effects
Cyclosporine	Unclear trough target	Nephrotoxicity—hypertension, insufficiency Gingival hyperplasia Hypertrichosis	Reduce dose to minimize side effects
Sirolimus	Unclear trough target	Metabolic syndrome—weight gain, hyperlipidemia Proteinuria Edema	Reduce dose to minimize side effects

Adapted from AASLD Guidelines in AIH.

AIH recurs in approximately 10% of patients within the first year of LT and 36% to 68% after 5 years. The diagnostic criteria for recurrent AIH (rAIH) are the same as for the original disease, although certain features may be less pronounced due to concurrent immunosuppressive therapy. The main histologic aspects are prominent lymphocytic interface activity, pseudo-rosetting of hepatocytes, and perivenular lymphoplasmacytic inflammation.[36] Clinical features range from asymptomatic presentation to graft failure. Serologic features of AIH such as hypergammaglobulinemia, positive smooth muscle, and antinuclear antibodies, should support the diagnosis. The severity of histologic inflammatory activity, elevated aminotransferases, and elevated serum IgG levels have been associated with a higher risk of rAIH possibly suggesting a more aggressive disease variant. Human leukocyte antigen (HLA) status of the donor and recipient remains a contro-versial risk factor with some studies reporting a higher risk of rAIH in HLA donor–recipient mismatches. Following LT, corticosteroid withdrawal, episodes of acute cellular rejection, and paradoxic stimulatory immune response induced by calci-neurin inhibitors have been proposed as risk factors for rAIH.[36,37] A long-term study from Birmingham demonstrated a reduced incidence of rAIH to 11% at 10 years with the maintenance of low-dose corticosteroid treatment (prednisolone 5–10 mg daily) following LT without significant adverse events.[38] However, data are limited to support long-term corticosteroids for all patients.[2] In general, maintaining corticosteroids and anti-metabolite therapy within the first year of transplant is recommended.

Management of rAIH depends on the presentation. Mild disease activity with minimal histologic or serologic changes can be treated with an increase in immunosuppression. However, in patients with moderate-to-severe rAIH, treatment with corticosteroids (predniso(lo)ne 30 mg daily), in combination with AZA (1–2 mg/kg daily) is recommen-ded. Failure of first-line therapy should prompt consideration of alternative treatment options including substituting MMF for AZA, changing calcineurin inhibitor, or starting sirolimus.[2] Progression to cirrhosis and graft failure has been reported in up to 50% of patients with rAIH, with a relatively short time between rAIH and graft loss compared with other disease states.[39]

CLINICS CARE POINTS

- Budesonide should only be used for treatment of AIH in patients without cirrhosis.
- Hepatic fibrosis is reversible in patients with AIH that achieve longterm biochemical remission.
- Biochemical remission is defined as normal liver tests and serum IgG level.

DISCLOSURES

No relevant financial disclosures.

REFERENCES

1. Manns MP, Czaja AJ, Gorham JD, et al. Diagnosis and management of autoim-mune hepatitis. Hepatology 2010;51(6):2193–213.
2. Mack CL, Adams D, Assis DN, et al. Diagnosis and management of autoimmune hepatitis in adults and children: 2019 practice guidance and Guidelines from the

American association for the study of liver diseases. Hepatology 2020;72(2): 671–722.

3. Czaja AJ. Review article: the prevention and reversal of hepatic fibrosis in auto-immune hepatitis. Aliment Pharmacol Ther 2014;39(4):385–406.

4. Early treatment response predicts the need for liver transplantation in autoimmune hepatitis - Tan - 2005 - Liver International - Wiley Online Library. https://onlinelibrary.wiley.com/doi/abs/10.1111/j.1478-3231.2005.01121.x. Accessed April 20, 2023.

5. Murray-Lyon I, Stern RB, Williams R. Controlled trial of prednisone and azathio-prine in active chronic hepatitis. Lancet 1973;301(7806):735–7.

6. Pape S, Gevers TJG, Belias M, et al. Predniso(lo)ne dosage and chance of remis-sion in patients with autoimmune hepatitis. Clin Gastroenterol Hepatol Off Clin Pract J Am Gastroenterol Assoc 2019;17(10):2068–75.e2.

7. Manns MP, Woynarowski M, Kreisel W, et al. Budesonide induces remission more effectively than prednisone in a controlled trial of patients with autoimmune hep-atitis. Gastroenterology 2010;139(4):1198–206.

8. Hindorf U, Jahed K, Bergquist A, et al. Characterisation and utility of thiopurine methyltransferase and thiopurine metabolite measurements in autoimmune hep-atitis. J Hepatol 2010;52(1):106–11.

9. Czaja AJ, Carpenter HA. Thiopurine methyltransferase deficiency and azathio-prine intolerance in autoimmune hepatitis. Dig Dis Sci 2006;51(5):968–75.

10. Czaja AJ, Menon KVN, Carpenter HA. Sustained remission after corticosteroid therapy for type 1 autoimmune hepatitis: a retrospective analysis. Hepatology 2002;35(4):890–7.

11. Hartl J, Denzer U, Ehlken H, et al. Transient elastography in autoimmune hepati-tis: timing determines the impact of inflammation and fibrosis. J Hepatol 2016; 65(4):769–75.

12. Xu Q, Sheng L, Bao H, et al. Evaluation of transient elastography in assessing liver fibrosis in patients with autoimmune hepatitis. J Gastroenterol Hepatol 2017;32(3):639–44.

13. Hartl J, Ehlken H, Sebode M, et al. Usefulness of biochemical remission and tran-sient elastography in monitoring disease course in autoimmune hepatitis. J Hepatol 2018;68(4):754–63.

14. Lamers MMH, van Oijen MGH, Pronk M, et al. Treatment options for autoimmune hepatitis: a systematic review of randomized controlled trials. J Hepatol 2010; 53(1):191–8.

15. Wehrman A, Waisbourd-Zinman O, Shah A, et al. Steroid free treatment of auto-immune hepatitis in selected children. J Pediatr 2019;207:244–7.

16. Nastasio S, Sciveres M, Matarazzo L, et al. Long-term follow-up of children and young adults with autoimmune hepatitis treated with cyclosporine. Dig Liver Dis Off J Ital Soc Gastroenterol Ital Assoc Study Liver 2019;51(5):712–8.

17. Marlaka JR, Papadogiannakis N, Fischler B, et al. Tacrolimus without or with the addition of conventional immunosuppressive treatment in juvenile autoimmune hepatitis. Acta Paediatr Oslo Nor 1992 2012;101(9):993–9.

18. Zachou K, Gatselis N, Papadamou G, et al. Mycophenolate for the treatment of autoimmune hepatitis: prospective assessment of its efficacy and safety for in-duction and maintenance of remission in a large cohort of treatment-naïve pa-tients. J Hepatol 2011;55(3):636–46.

19. Zachou K, Gatselis NK, Arvaniti P, et al. A real-world study focused on the long-term efficacy of mycophenolate mofetil as first-line treatment of autoimmune hep-atitis. Aliment Pharmacol Ther 2016;43(10):1035–47.

20. Hlivko JT, Shiffman ML, Stravitz RT, et al. A single center review of the use of mycophenolate mofetil in the treatment of autoimmune hepatitis. Clin Gastroenterol Hepatol Off Clin Pract J Am Gastroenterol Assoc 2008;6(9):1036–40.

21. Dalekos GN, Arvaniti P, Gatselis NK, et al. First results from a propensity matching trial of mycophenolate mofetil vs. Azathioprine in treatment-naive AIH patients. Front Immunol 2021;12:798602.

22. Muratori L, Muratori P, Lanzoni G, et al. Application of the 2010 American Association for the study of liver diseases criteria of remission to a cohort of Italian patients with autoimmune hepatitis. Hepatol Baltim Md 2010;52(5):1857 [author reply: 1857-1858].

23. Czaja AJ. Rapidity of treatment response and outcome in type 1 autoimmune hepatitis. J Hepatol 2009;51(1):161–7.

24. Pape S, Gevers TJG, Vrolijk JM, et al. Rapid response to treatment of autoimmune hepatitis associated with remission at 6 and 12 months. Clin Gastroenterol Hepatol Off Clin Pract J Am Gastroenterol Assoc 2020;18(7):1609–17.e4.

25. Kirstein MM, Metzler F, Geiger E, et al. Prediction of short- and long-term outcome in patients with autoimmune hepatitis. Hepatol Baltim Md 2015;62(5):1524–35.

26. Taubert R, Hardtke-Wolenski M, Noyan F, et al. Hyperferritinemia and hypergammaglobulinemia predict the treatment response to standard therapy in autoimmune hepatitis. PLoS One 2017;12(6):e0179074.

27. Santiago P, Schwartz I, Tamariz L, et al. Systematic review with meta-analysis: mycophenolate mofetil as a second-line therapy for autoimmune hepatitis. Aliment Pharmacol Ther 2019;49(7):830–9.

28. De Lemos-Bonotto M, Valle-Tovo C, Costabeber AM, et al. A systematic review and meta-analysis of second-line immunosuppressants for autoimmune hepatitis treatment. Eur J Gastroenterol Hepatol 2018;30(2):212–6.

29. Efe C, Hagström H, Ytting H, et al. Efficacy and safety of mycophenolate mofetil and tacrolimus as second-line therapy for patients with autoimmune hepatitis. Clin Gastroenterol Hepatol Off Clin Pract J Am Gastroenterol Assoc 2017; 15(12):1950–6.e1.

30. Hanouneh M, Ritchie MM, Ascha M, et al. A review of the utility of tacrolimus in the management of adults with autoimmune hepatitis. Scand J Gastroenterol 2019; 54(1):76–80.

31. Czaja AJ. Advances in the current treatment of autoimmune hepatitis. Dig Dis Sci 2012;57(8):1996–2010.

32. Chatrath H, Allen L, Boyer TD. Use of sirolimus in the treatment of refractory autoimmune hepatitis. Am J Med 2014;127(11):1128–31.

33. Than NN, Hodson J, Schmidt-Martin D, et al. Efficacy of rituximab in difficult-to-manage autoimmune hepatitis: results from the international autoimmune hepatitis group. JHEP Rep Innov Hepatol 2019;1(6):437–45.

34. Hartl J, Ehlken H, Weiler-Normann C, et al. Patient selection based on treatment duration and liver biochemistry increases success rates after treatment withdrawal in autoimmune hepatitis. J Hepatol 2015;62(3):642–6.

35. Heneghan MA, Shumbayawonda E, Dennis A, et al. Quantitative magnetic resonance imaging to aid clinical decision making in autoimmune hepatitis. EClinicalMedicine 2022;46:101325.

36. Stirnimann G, Ebadi M, Czaja AJ, et al. Recurrent and de novo autoimmune hepatitis. Liver Transplant 2019;25(1):152–66.

37. Visseren T, Darwish Murad S. Recurrence of primary sclerosing cholangitis, primary biliary cholangitis and auto-immune hepatitis after liver transplantation. Best Pract Res Clin Gastroenterol 2017;31(2):187–98.

38. Krishnamoorthy TL, Miezynska-Kurtycz J, Hodson J, et al. Longterm corticosteroid use after liver transplantation for autoimmune hepatitis is safe and associated with a lower incidence of recurrent disease. Liver Transplant 2016;22(1): 34–41.
39. Rowe IA, Webb K, Gunson BK, et al. The impact of disease recurrence on graft survival following liver transplantation: a single centre experience. Transpl Int 2008;21(5):459–65.

Primary Biliary Cholangitis
Epidemiology, Diagnosis, and Presentation

Muhammad Salman Faisal, MD[a], Humberto C. Gonzalez, MD[a,b],
Stuart C. Gordon, MD[a,b],*

KEYWORDS

- Primary biliary cholangitis • Epidemiology • Jaundice

KEY POINTS

- Primary biliary cholangitis (PBC) has an overall prevalence ranging from 1.9 to 40.2 cases per 100,000 with geographic variations.
- PBC generally presents in middle-aged women with a personal or family history of other autoimmune conditions.
- Autoimmune conditions associated with PBC are Sjögren syndrome; CREST (calcinosis, Raynaud, esophageal dysfunction, sclerodactyly, and telangiectasias)/scleroderma, and hypothyroidism.
- Persistant unexplained elevation of alkaline phosphatase and a positive anti-mitochondrial antibody secure the dignosis of PBC and liver biopsy is not required.
- Typical histopathological features include "florid duct lesions" with inflammation of the interlobular and septal bile ducts.

INTRODUCTION

Primary biliary cholangitis (PBC) is an uncommon cholestatic autoimmune disease of the liver. First described in western medical literature in 1949,[1] it was originally known as primary biliary cirrhosis. With the use of ursodeoxycholic acid (UDCA) as a standard treatment and the availibility of tests for antimitochondrial antibody (AMA) to accelerate diagnosis, survival of PBC patients has approached that of the general population. This led to a change in nomenclature from primary biliary cirrhosis to cholangitis to more accurately describe the disease.[2]

EPIDEMIOLOGY
Prevalence, Incidence, and Geographic Distribution

PBC is a rare disease, and prevalence estimates also range widely, from 1.9 to 40.2 cases per 100,000.[3] The highest prevalence in the literature—40.2 per

[a] Department of Gastroenterology and Hepatology, Henry Ford Health, 2799 West Grand Boulevard, Detroit, MI 48202, USA; [b] Wayne State University School of Medicine, 540 East Canfield Street, Detroit, MI 48201, USA
* Corresponding author. 2799 West Grand Boulevard, Detroit, MI 48202.
E-mail address: sgordon3@hfhs.org

Clin Liver Dis 28 (2024) 63–77
https://doi.org/10.1016/j.cld.2023.06.005
1089-3261/23/© 2023 Elsevier Inc. All rights reserved.

100,000—was reported in Minnesota (USA),[4] but it is possible this is not generalizable because of familial clustering and migration patterns to the area from mostly Scandinavian countries. A more recent multicenter US study estimated overall prevalence of 29.3 per 100,000 in a large health system-based population.[5] This estimate is similar to those from several Western countries: 22.7 per 100,000 from Canada,[6] 16.0 per 100,000 from Italy,[7] and 36.5 per 100,000 from Greece.[8] Notably, prevalence in Australia is estimated to be much lower, roughly 1.9 per 100,000, despite being a primarily European population; this suggests the possibility of interacting genetic and environmental factors.[9] However, there has historically been a lack of data from southeast Asian and African countries, but emerging data from Asian countries were recently summarized by Tanaka.[10] Reported prevalence in Hong Kong was 5.6 per 100,000,[11] South Korea 4.7 per 100,000,[12] and Japan 7.8 per 100,000.[13] Noting these patterns, Zhang and colleagues observed a latitudinal pattern of the disease, with higher prevalence in northern latitudes.[14]

Overall prevalence has increased in recent years. A Canadian study estimated that prevalence increased from 10.0 to 22.7 per 100,000[15] and an Australian study reported an increase from 1.0 to 5.1 per 100,000 from 1991 to 2004.[16] More recently, a US-based study found that prevalence increased from 21.7 to 39.4 per 100,000 from 2006 to 2014.[5] This is possibly due to better diagnostic tools and disease awareness in the medical community. Improved overall survival could also account for this increased prevalence.

A systematic review estimated the overall annual incidence of PBC to be 0.33 to 0.58 per 100,000 inhabitants.[17] Other authors have reported considerably higher estimates; an evaluation of Swedish health registry data estimated an annual incidence of 2.6 per 100,000, and a US health system-based study found steady annual incidence of roughly 4.3 per 100,000 from 2006 to 2014.[18] PBC has infrequently been reported in children.[19]

Sex Ratio

PBC has historically been described as a disease of white women in middle age. Older reports estimated a female to male incidence ratio as high as 10:1,[20] but more recent population-based studies indicate that this may be an overestimation. Population-based studies from Denmark and Italy show the ratios of 2:1 and 4:1[21]; a US-based study reported a similar 4:1 ratio.[17] Studies from Asian countries also report ratios of roughly 4:1. Notably, the female-to-male ratio for AMA-positivity in the general population is 2:1.[22]

Despite lower prevalence among men, their rates of mortality are higher. The population-based studies from Italy and Denmark report hazard ratios (HRs) for all-cause mortality of 2.36 and 3.04 for men versus women[21]; differences were similar but lower in the US health system–based study (HR = 1.47). Men are also less likely to respond to UDCA than female counterparts with PBC, as shown in a landmark study by Carbone and colleagues.[23]

Familial Clustering

Several genetic factors have been implicated in PBC pathogenesis; this is reflected in epidemiologic studies that show family clustering. PBC prevalence among first-degree relatives of known cases is estimated to be between 1.1% and 6.4% in case-based studies,[7,24] much higher than that in the general population. Prevalence in families with just one PBC-positive relative was 4.3%. Offspring of PBC patients have been reported to have higher risk of developing PBC than the general population (1.2%), with daughters at even higher risk (2.3%)[24]; this has been described as mother-daughter clustering.[25] AMA-positivity is also high among first-degree female relatives: 20.7% (sisters), 15.1% (mothers), and 9.8% (daughters).[26] The strongest evidence for a significant genetic component was reported by Selmi and colleagues, in a study of eight sets of monozygotic twins versus eight sets of dizygotic twins.[27] There was a 63% concordance rate among monozygotic twins (5 of 8 pairs) with no concordance among dizygotic pairs.[27] To distinguish between genetic and environmental factors, Mantaka and colleagues compared 111 PBC patients and 115 first-degree relatives. They found dyslipidemia and non-PBC autoimmune conditions were more common among first-degree relatives than in the general population, indicating an interaction between genetic and environmental factors.[28]

Genetic Associations

Genome-wide association studies and immunochip data suggest that most genetic linkages are associated with human leukocyte antigens (HLAs)[29]; non-HLA loci involved in regulation of different components of the immune system have also been identified.[30] Hirchfield and colleagues found that IL12RB2 and IL12 A increased the odds of PBC (odds ratios 1.51 and 1.54, respectively).[31] Genetic analysis conducted in European, Japanese, and Chinese cohorts demonstrates that PBC patients share some genetic susceptibility but also have a distinct profile.[32]

The strongest evidence for the underlying immune mechanism for PBC comes from the association with positive AMA. AMA targets a family of inner mitochondrial membrane enzymes within the biliary epithelial cells. These enzymes are known as 2-oxo-acid dehydrogenase complexes which are responsible for catalyzing oxidative decarboxylation of ketoacid substrates.[33,34] Pyruvate dehydrogenase (PDC2-E2) is the main enzyme implicated in PBC; however, branched-chain 2-oxo-dehydrogenase and 2-oxo glutaric acid dehydrogenase are also responsible for the immune-mediated injury which results in autolysis, apoptosis, and senescence of biliary epithelial cells.[35,36]

Environmental Associations

The autoantigen PDC-E2 is susceptible to environmental modification, particularly after certain infections and exposure to some chemicals found in cosmetics, perfumes, and food colors.[37] Several case-control studies of varied patient populations have identified specific environmental associations with PBC.[38] Most consistently, PBC has been associated with smoking and urinary tract infections—an association that may in part explain the female predominance of the disease. PDC is vital for cell survival; hence, it is reasonable that PDC-E2 is a well-preserved molecule among various species. The human PDC-E2 is similar to the *Escherichia coli* PCD-E2, especially in the AMA immunodominant epitope region.[39] This molecular mimicry has been implicated in the breakdown of tolerance and pathogenesis of the disease.[37,40] *Novosphingobium aromaticivorans*, betaviruses, and *Lactobacillus delbrueckii* have been suggested as potential contributors to PBC under the PDC-E2 tolerance breaking mechanism.[39]

Disease Associations

A study by Floreani and colleagues showed that Sjögren syndrome, CREST (calcinosis, Raynaud, esophageal dysfunction, sclerodactyly, and telangiectasias), scleroderma, and Raynaud disease are more likely to be present in patients with PBC than in the general population.[41] Celiac disease and autoimmune thyroid disease have also been associated with PBC.[42,43]

CLINICAL PRESENTATION
Signs and Symptoms

Fatigue
Most PBC patients—61% according to one study—are asymptomatic at the time of presentation.[44] When symptomatic, fatigue is the most reported complaint (50–78% of patients).[45] Positive AMA is a hallmark of the disease and is also believed to play a significant role in PBC pathogenesis. Given that autoantibodies against mitochondria lead to fatigue,[46] it is not surprising that it is the most common and earliest manifestation of presentation. Fatigue in PBC is associated with excessive day time somnolence. The degree of somnolence strongly correlates with fatigue severity.[47] Analysis of mitochondrial function (adenosine diphosphate and phosphocreatine) by magnetic resonance spectroscopy and muscle pH demonstrated mitochondrial dysfunction characterized by acidosis and delayed recovery of muscles markers, correlating with fatigue.[48] Fatigue also presents the biggest clinical challenge in early-stage disease and leads to poor quality of life.[49] It may also have prognostic implications, as severe fatigue has been associated with higher mortality in at least one study. Fatigue usually remains constant over time.[50]

Pruritus
Itching associated with PBC generally follows a circadian rhythm and is worse at night.[44] In older studies, prevalence of itching was reported to be 20% to 70%.[51] The etiology of pruritus in PBC remained to be fully elucidated. Bile salts that accumulate in excess in the skin and blood stream bind to the FXR and TGR5 (G-protein-coupled bile acid receptor) receptors, generating pruritus.[52] The reduction of bile acid levels by nasobiliary drainage and/or cholestyramine therapy has been shown to provide relief.[53] Ultraviolet B light therapy increases urinary excretion of bile acids and was found to provide symptomatic benefits.[54] The enzyme autotaxin and its by product lysophosphatidic acid have shown to be elevated in cases of cholestatic pruritus.[55] Other commonly implicated mechanisms include overproduction of endogenous opioids, which are elevated in PBC patients.[56,57]

Other symptoms
Inflammatory arthropathy leading to musculoskeletal complaints occurs in approximately 40% of PBC and can indicate coexistence of other autoimmune conditions. Common coexisting autoimmune conditions include thyroid disorders, rheumatoid arthritis, and CREST.[58,59] Less commonly, PBC patients may present with abdominal pain. One study reported rates as high as 8% to 17%. There was no correlation with disease stage or hepatomegaly; the pain may be self-resolving.[60] Another study found that more than half of the PBC patients demonstrated impairments in memory and concentration that were associated with autonomic dysfunction but not with severity of liver disease.[61] Disease progression may also be associated with fat-soluble vitamin deficiencies, although rare in the recent past. Vitamin A deficiencies may manifest with ocular symptoms (night blindness) and follicular hyperkeratosis. Vitamin D deficiency may lead to osteoporosis and osteomalacia, secondary to calcium deficiency, which may manifest as paresthesia and tetany in extreme circumstances. Vitamin K deficiency may lead to hematoma and increased risk of bleeding.[62] Patients may also develop steatorrhea manifested by pale and voluminous stool.[63]

Physical Examination

Most commonly, physical examination is normal in patients with PBC, especially in the early stages.[64] Late stages cases are now less common due to treatment, but characterized by manifestations of cirrhosis and portal hypertension, such as ascites, muscle wasting, spider nevi, and splenomegaly. Hepatomegaly may be detected earlier in the course of the disease.[65]

Dermatologic complaints associated with PBC have been described in literature but are less commonly seen with the advent of therapy.[66] Excoriations from itching may be present. PBC-related hyperlipidemia may manifest as xanthomas (5% of patients) and xanthelasmas (10%). Xanthomas are clusters of foam cells formed from excess cholesterol within macrophages that are deposited in skin, tendons, and occasionally in the periosteum. They most commonly present as yellow, small, flat, or minimally elevated plaques on the upper and/or lower eyelids known as xanthelasmas.[67] Hyper-pigmentation from an unknown mechanism may also be present (25%–50% of patients). Fungal infections of feet and nails are also reported.

Laboratories

Liver biochemistries
Elevated alkaline phosphatase (ALP) is a hallmark of PBC. ALP and higher bilirubin elevation both indicate severity of ductopenia and inflammation.[67] Higher bilirubin is associated with poor disease outcomes and biliary necrosis.[68] Alanine and aspartate aminotransferases (ALT and AST) may be normal or slightly elevated. Elevation of AST or ALT to more than five times the upper limit of normal (ULN) should indicate evaluation for an alternate diagnosis or overlap of PBC with autoimmune hepatitis.[69]

Serology
More than 95% of PBC patients have antimitochondrial antibodies.[70] AMA can be detected using indirect immunofluorescence, immunoblotting, enzyme immunoassay, Luminex beads assay, and enzyme inhibition assay. However, 5% to 15% of PBC patients are AMA-negative, depending on the modality of antibody testing.[71] AMA-positivity is also present in the general population; rates of 0.5% were found in Italy[72] and 0.64% in a study of 1714 healthy subjects in Japan.[73] The 5-year incidence of PBC development among individuals with AMA was 16% in one study.[74]

Addtional serologic tests often positive in PBC patients include antinuclear antibody (ANA), which is present in 70% of PBC patients. ANA patterns associated with PBC include multiple nuclear dots pattern (target antigen, Sp100) and the rim-like/membranous pattern (target antigens, glycoprotein gp210, nucleoporin p62, and the lamin B receptor). In a study of 80 patients with long-term follow-up, higher levels of gp210 were associated with higher risk of progression than negative or lower levels.[75] Other studies have also suggested that ANA presence may be associated with worse disease outcomes.[76] A polyclonal elevation in IgM is also seen in PBC. In one study, the mean IgM concentration was 2.4 times the ULN in all 25 PBC patients in the study.[77] Reductions in IgM have been observed with UDCA treatment, but the role of IgM in disease pathogenesis and prognosis is unclear.[78]

Other laboratory tests
With progression of disease and development of cirrhosis, additional lab abnormalities such as low platelets, hypoalbuminemia, elevated prothrombin time, and international normalized ratio will manifest.[65] A systematic review showed that PBC is associated with markedly elevated lipid levels—cholesterol may reach 1000 mg/dL, but with significant elevation of high-density lipoprotein and milder elevation of low-density lipoprotein and very-low-density lipoprotein.[79]

Imaging

The American Association for the Study of Liver Diseases guidelines recommend noninvasive imaging of the liver and biliary tree in all patients with evidence of cholestasis. Magnetic resonance cholangiography is the preferred modality to exclude other causes of biliary obstruction, such as choledocholithiasis and primary sclerosing

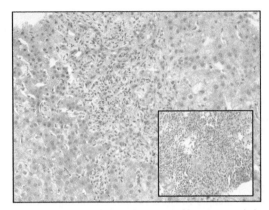

Fig. 1. Portal bile ductular injury with lymphocytic infiltration and degenerative changes characterized by dense eosinophilic cytoplasm or cytoplasmic vacuolization, shrunken and irregular nuclei, and stratification. Non-necrotizing epithelioid granulomatous inflammation may be seen (*inset*). Granulomata may be centered on bile ducts (florid duct lesions; not pictured). Image credit: *Brian Thiesen MD, Senior Staff Pathologist, Henry Ford Health*

cholangitis (PSC),[80] but is rarely needed unless there is a reason to suspect biliary tract obstruction. Transient elastography is increasingly being used as a noninvasive measure of liver stiffness. Successful medical therapy is associated with slowing the progression of liver stiffness, while advancing stiffness is associated with worse outcomes.[81] To date, there is no role of serial imaging in PBC.

Histology

Biopsies are not required to diagnose most cases of PBC,[80] except in cases of AMA-negative individuals or when concomitant autoimmune hepatitis and non-alcoholic steatohepatitis (NASH) are suspected. Given that PBC has a patchy distribution, at least 10 to 15 portal tracts are needed to observe cholangitis and rule the diagnosis in or out. Histology (**Figs. 1–4**) is characterized by inflammation of the

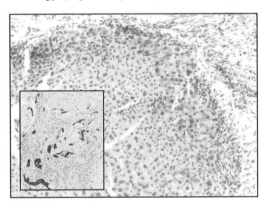

Fig. 2. Ancillary studies can highlight the characteristic features of a chronic cholestatic hepatitis. Rhodanine copper stain highlights periportal copper granules in swollen hepatocytes (*red-brown* granular staining). Only a few copper granules may be seen in some cases. (*Inset*) An immunohistochemical stain for Cytokeratin 7 highlights the ductular reaction which occurs secondary to ductular metaplasia (faint brown staining hepatocytes) or proliferation of preexisting portal ductules. Image credit: *Brian Thiesen MD, Senior Staff Pathologist, Henry Ford Health*

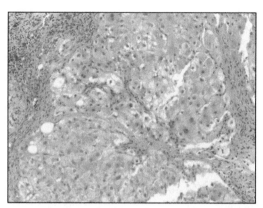

Fig. 3. Swollen periportal hepatocytes with cleared cytoplasm (feathery degeneration) characteristic of cholate stasis. Mallory's hyaline may be seen (not pictured). Image credit: *Brian Thiesen MD, Senior Staff Pathologist, Henry Ford Health*

interlobular and septal bile ducts that can form focal lesions with intense inflammatory changes and necrosis. These lesions are often referred to as "florid duct lesions." Epithelioid granulomas can be present in early stages of the disease. The inflammatory infiltrate is primarily composed of plasma cells but may also contain macrophages, eosinophils, and other polymorphonuclear cells.[70]

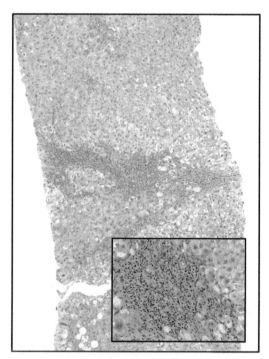

Fig. 4. Lower power magnification demonstrates moderate portal inflammation composed predominately of lymphocytes and plasma cells with occasional neutrophils and eosinophils (*inset*). Image credit: *Brian Thiesen MD, Senior Staff Pathologist, Henry Ford Health*

Nakanuma and colleagues developed a four-stage model for PBC histology in 2010.[82] Stage I is defined by inflammation confined to the portal triad with or without florid ductal lesions. Stage II is defined by interface hepatitis, which can be lymphocytic piecemeal necrosis-like autoimmune hepatitis or biliary piecemeal necrosis with periportal lesions spreading into the hepatic parenchyma. Stage III is characterized by distortion of the hepatic architecture with fibrous septa. Stage IV is defined by the presence of cirrhosis and regenerative nodules. Nodular regenerative hyperplasia can lead to portal hypertension without cirrhosis and is a known complication of PBC.[82]

Complications

Progression to cirrhosis

PBC can lead to cirrhosis and associated portal hypertension. It may also cause presinusoidal portal hypertension without advanced fibrosis, due to nodular regenerative hyperplasia.[83] Clinical manifestations after progression to cirrhosis from PBC are similar to those of other cirrhosis patients, with initial symptoms of anorexia, fatigue, and loss of muscle mass. Progression to decompensated cirrhosis can manifest with ascites, hepatic encephalopathy, and variceal bleeding.[84]

Hepatocellular carcinoma

PBC increases the risk of hepatocellular carcinoma (HCC); one study demonstrated an incidence rate of 3.9 per 1000 per year, with higher risk associated with suboptimal response to therapy.[85] Men are twice as likely to develop HCC than women.[86] Twice-yearly HCC screening is recommended for all men with PBC and for all patients with cirrhosis secondary to PBC; this has shown to be associated with better clinical outcomes.[87] Noninvasive measures of liver fibrosis (platelet levels and vibration controlled transient elastography [VCTE]) can be used to identify patients who need screening among patients without liver biopsy.[87]

Metabolic bone disease

PBC increases the risk of metabolic bone disease such as osteopenia and osteoporosis. Menon and colleagues estimated this risk to be 32.1 times higher than that in the general population, and 20% of PBC patients in their sample had osteoporosis.[88] Poor vitamin D absorption might play a role along with a possible inhibitory toxin acting on osteoblasts.[88]

DIAGNOSIS
Approach

PBC classically presents in middle age, with fatigue, pruritus, and elevated ALP. The disease runs a spectrum, however, and pruritus is not always present at the outset.

American Association for the Study of Liver Disease (AASLD) criteria for the diagnosis of PBC relies on meeting two of the following three criteria.[80]

- Elevated ALP
- Positive AMA
- Histologic evidence of nonsuppurative cholangitis with destruction of small- or medium-sized bile ducts.

We recommend a structured diagnostic approach. All patients should have imaging, starting with right-upper-quadrant ultrasound, ideally followed by a magnetic resonance (MR) scan of the liver and bile ducts to rule out extrahepatic biliary obstruction. Serology should include AMA along with other autoimmune liver markers such as ANA and antismooth muscle antibody. Biopsy is not required to confirm a diagnosis if ALP is >1.5 times the ULN, AMA is positive, and there is no sign of biliary obstruction on imaging. If ALP is elevated and AMA is positive but the patient is atypical for PBC (eg, male with comorbidities such as diabetes and hypertension that might increase the risk of nonalcoholic steatohepatitis), biopsy may help to confirm the diagnosis. Biopsy may also provide important diagnostic and staging information in situations where either ALP is elevated or AMA is positive but not both. If ALP is normal and AMA is negative, other disease etiologies should be considered, as PBC is unlikely in this scenario. Biopsy may also be helpful if a patient does not respond appropriately to therapy.

Differential Diagnosis

The diagnostic workup should rule out other etiologies of cholestasis. Imaging can assess for biliary obstruction secondary to choledocholithiasis or malignancy. Another common etiology of cholestasis in the absence of anatomic obstruction are drugs, such as anabolic steroids, trimethoprim sulfamethoxazole, ampicillin, oxacillin, and nonsteroidal anti-inflammatory drugs such as diclofenac; occasionally such acute drug reactions may lead to chronic cholestasis. Viral infections should also be ruled out, particularly if there are also concomitant transaminase elevations. Infiltrative diseases such as sarcoidosis, lymphoma, and solid-organ malignancies may also manifest with elevated ALP; congestive heart failure and total parenteral nutrition have also been shown to be associated with increased ALP levels. Differentiating PBC from PSC is also vitally important because of differences in treatment and prognostic implications. PSC should be suspected in cases of unexplained ALP elevation in the absence of AMA positivity, especially in men; it is often associated with inflammatory bowel disease. It has characteristic features on cholangiography, whether MR or endoscopic modality. Biopsy can help differentiate between small duct PSC and PBC.

Special Situations

Antimitochondrial antibody-negative primary biliary cholangitis
This describes a set of individuals whose clinical presentation and histology are consistent with PBC but test negative for AMA. In these situations, detection of other autoantibodies—such as sp100, gp210, anti-kelch-like 12, and anti-hexokinase-1— can aid in diagnosis.[89] Studies have shown faster rate of progression, later diagnosis, and worse social and emotional quality of life for these patients.[90,91]

Overlap syndrome
Autoimmune Hepatitis (AIH) and PBC overlap has been described in the literature but lacks a clear definition. AASLD guidelines recommend labeling PBC patients with ANA positivity and mild interface hepatitis as having overlap syndrome because these features are common in PBC. PBC/AIH overlap patients have shown to have similar response to treatment. It might also represent PBC patients who subsequently develop autoimmune hepatitis or vice versa.[92] Further studies are needed for better characterization of this syndrome. As noted by Levy and colleagues, overlap syndrome is more common in the Hispanic population in Miami.[93] They were also found to be more likely to present with decompensated disease than the general population.[93]

SUMMARY

PBC represents a rare clinical syndrome mostly presenting in middle age, either as asymptomatic ALP elevation or with associated fatigue and pruritus. Diagnosis can be made via serology showing positive AMA and confirmed by histology showing nonsuppurative bile duct inflammation.

CLINICS CARE POINTS

- The most common presentation is an incidental alkaline phosphatase elevation with a positive AMA; patients are usually asymptomatic but may have undisclosed pruritus and should be queried about its presence.
- Fatigue is the most common symptom of PBC and can be present in up to 50% of patients, negatively impacting quality of life.
- PBC is associated with a high incidence of osteopenia and osteoporosis, for which screening with DEXA scan is recommended every 2 years.
- PBC increases the risk for hepatocellular cancer (HCC) especially in men and UCDA non-responders; twice yearly HCC screening is recommended for patients at high risk.

DISCLOSURE

The authors have no disclosures for this article.

ACKNOWLEDGEMENTS

Dr. Brian Thiesen (Department of Pathology, Henry Ford Health, Detroit MI) provided biopsy images and descriptions. Sheri Trudeau MPH (Department of Public Health Sciences, Henry Ford Health, Detroit MI) provided writing assistance.

REFERENCES

1. Dauphinee JA, Sinclair JC. Primary biliary cirrhosis. Can Med Assoc J 1949; 61(1):1–6.
2. Beuers U, Gershwin ME, Gish RG, et al. Changing nomenclature for PBC: from 'cirrhosis' to 'cholangitis'. J Hepatol 2015;64(11):1671–2.
3. Lleo A, FJCild Colapietro. Changes in the epidemiology of primary biliary cholangitis. Clin Liver Dis 2018;22(3):429–41.
4. Kim WR, Lindor KD, Locke GR III, et al. Epidemiology and natural history of primary biliary cirrhosis in a US community. Gastroenterology 2000;119(6):1631–6.
5. Lu M, Li J, Haller IV, et al. Factors associated with prevalence and treatment of primary biliary cholangitis in United States health systems. Clin Gastroenterol Hepatol 2018;16(8):1333–41, e1336.
6. Witt-Sullivan H, Heathcote J, Cauch K, et al. The demography of primary biliary cirrhosis in Ontario, Canada. Hepatology 1990;12(1):98–105.
7. Floreani AJJH. Prevalence of familial disease in primary biliary cirrhosis in Italy. J Hepatol 1997;26:737–8.
8. Koulentaki M, Mantaka A, Sifaki-Pistolla D, et al. Geoepidemiology and space–time analysis of Primary biliary cirrhosis in Crete, Greece. Liver Int 2014;34(7): e200–7.
9. Watson R, Angus PW, Dewar M, et al. Low prevalence of primary biliary cirrhosis in Victoria, Australia. Melbourne Liver Group 1995;36(6):927–30.
10. Tanaka AJCLD. PBC: No longer a western disease? Clin Liver Dis 2020; 16(6):227.
11. Cheung K-S, Seto W-K, Fung J, et al. Epidemiology and natural history of primary biliary cholangitis in the Chinese: a territory-based study in Hong Kong between 2000 and 2015. Clin Transl Gastroenterol 2017;8(8):e116.

12. Kim KA, Ki M, Choi H, et al. Population-based epidemiology of primary biliary cirrhosis in South Korea. Aliment Pharmacol Ther 2016;43(1):154–62.
13. Sakauchi F, Mori M, Zeniya M, et al. A cross-sectional study of primary biliary cirrhosis in Japan: utilization of clinical data when patients applied to receive public financial aid. J Epidemiol 2005;15(1):24–8.
14. Zhang H, Carbone M, Lleo A, et al. Geoepidemiology, genetic and environmental risk factors for PBC. Dig Dis 2015;33(Suppl. 2):94–101.
15. Myers RP, Shaheen AAM, Fong A, et al. Epidemiology and natural history of primary biliary cirrhosis in a Canadian health region: a population-based study. Hepatology 2009;50(6):1884–92.
16. Sood S, Gow PJ, Christie JM, et al. Epidemiology of primary biliary cirrhosis in Victoria, Australia: high prevalence in migrant populations. Gastroenterology 2004;127(2):470–5.
17. Boonstra K, Beuers U, CYJJoh Ponsioen. Epidemiology of primary sclerosing cholangitis and primary biliary cirrhosis: a systematic review. J Hepatol 2012; 56(5):1181–8.
18. Lu M, Zhou Y, Haller IV, et al. Increasing prevalence of primary biliary cholangitis and reduced mortality with treatment. Clin Gastroenterol Hepatol 2018;16(8): 1342–50, e1341.
19. Lleo A, Wang G-Q, Gershwin ME, Hirschfield GMJTL. Primary biliary cholangitis. 2020;396(10266):1915-1926.
20. Metcalf J, Bhopal R, Gray J, et al. Incidence and prevalence of primary biliary cirrhosis in the city of Newcastle upon Tyne, England. Int J Epidemiol 1997; 26(4):830–6.
21. Lleo A, Jepsen P, Morenghi E, et al. Evolving trends in female to male incidence and male mortality of primary biliary cholangitis. Sci Rep 2016;6(1):1–8.
22. Turchany J, Uibo R, Kivik T, et al. A study of antimitochondrial antibodies in a random population in Estonia. Am J Gastroenterol 1997;92(1):124–6.
23. Carbone M, Mells GF, Pells G, et al. Sex and age are determinants of the clinical phenotype of primary biliary cirrhosis and response to ursodeoxycholic acid. Gastroenterology 2013;144(3):560–9, e567.
24. Jones DE, Watt FE, Metcalf JV, et al. Familial primary biliary cirrhosis reassessed: a geographically-based population study. J Hepatol 1999;30(3):402–7.
25. Smyk D, Cholongitas E, Kriese S, et al. Primary biliary cirrhosis: family stories. Autoimmune Dis 2011;2011:189585.
26. Lazaridis KN, Juran BD, Boe GM, et al. Increased prevalence of antimitochondrial antibodies in first-degree relatives of patients with primary biliary cirrhosis. Hepatology 2007;46(3):785–92.
27. Selmi C, Mayo MJ, Bach N, et al. Primary biliary cirrhosis in monozygotic and dizygotic twins: genetics, epigenetics, and environment. Gastroenterology 2004;127(2):485–92.
28. Mantaka A, Koulentaki M, Chlouverakis G, et al. Primary biliary cirrhosis in a genetically homogeneous population: disease associations and familial occurrence rates. BMC Gastroenterol 2012;12(1):1–8.
29. Invernizzi P, Ransom M, Raychaudhuri S, et al. Classical HLA-DRB1 and DPB1 alleles account for HLA associations with primary biliary cirrhosis. Genes Immun 2012;13(6):461–8.
30. Nakamura M, Nishida N, Kawashima M, et al. Genome-wide association study identifies TNFSF15 and POU2AF1 as susceptibility loci for primary biliary cirrhosis in the Japanese population. Am J Hum Genet 2012;91(4):721–8.

31. Hirschfield GM, Liu X, Xu C, et al. Primary biliary cirrhosis associated with HLA, IL12A, and IL12RB2 variants. N Engl J Med 2009;360(24):2544–55.
32. Qiu F, Tang R, Zuo X, et al. A genome-wide association study identifies six novel risk loci for primary biliary cholangitis. Nat Commun 2017;8(1):14828.
33. Kita H, Matsumura S, He X-S, et al. Quantitative and functional analysis of PDC-E2–specific autoreactive cytotoxic T lymphocytes in primary biliary cirrhosis. J Clin Invest 2002;109(9):1231–40.
34. Leung KK, Deeb M, GMJAP Hirschfield. Pathophysiology and management of primary biliary cholangitis. Aliment Pharmacol Ther 2020;52(7):1150–64.
35. Shimoda S, Van de Water J, Ansari A, et al. Identification and precursor frequency analysis of a common T cell epitope motif in mitochondrial autoantigens in primary biliary cirrhosis. J Clin Invest 1998;102(10):1831–40.
36. Kamihira T, Shimoda S, Harada K, et al. Distinct costimulation dependent and independent autoreactive T-cell clones in primary biliary cirrhosis. Gastroenterology 2003;125(5):1379–87.
37. Leung PS, Wang J, Naiyanetr P, et al. Environment and primary biliary cirrhosis: electrophilic drugs and the induction of AMA. J Autoimmun 2013;41:79–86.
38. Gershwin ME, Selmi C, Worman HJ, et al. Risk factors and comorbidities in primary biliary cirrhosis: a controlled interview-based study of 1032 patients. Hepatology 2005;42(5):1194–202.
39. Tanaka A, Leung P, Gershwin MJC, et al. Pathogen infections and primary biliary cholangitis. Clin Exp Immunol 2019;195(1):25–34.
40. Shimoda S, Nakamura M, Ishibashi H, et al. Molecular mimicry of mitochondrial and nuclear autoantigens in primary biliary cirrhosis. Gastroenterology 2003;124(7):1915–25.
41. Floreani A, Franceschet I, Cazzagon N, et al. Extrahepatic autoimmune conditions associated with primary biliary cirrhosis. Clin Rev Allergy Immunol 2015;48:192–7.
42. Bizzaro N, Tampoia M, Villalta D, et al. Low specificity of anti-tissue transglutaminase antibodies in patients with primary biliary cirrhosis. J Clin Lab Anal 2006;20(5):184–9.
43. Floreani A, Mangini C, Reig A, et al. Thyroid dysfunction in primary biliary cholangitis: a comparative study at two European centers. Am J Gastroenterol 2017;112(1):114–9.
44. Prince M, Chetwynd A, Craig W, et al. Asymptomatic primary biliary cirrhosis: clinical features, prognosis, and symptom progression in a large population based cohort. Gut 2004;53(6):865–70.
45. Poupon RE, Chrétien Y, Chazouillères O, et al. Quality of life in patients with primary biliary cirrhosis. Hepatology 2004;40(2):489–94.
46. Filler K, Lyon D, Bennett J, et al. Association of mitochondrial dysfunction and fatigue: a review of the literature. BBA Clin 2014;1:12–23.
47. Newton JL, Gibson GJ, Tomlinson M, et al. Fatigue in primary biliary cirrhosis is associated with excessive daytime somnolence. Hepatology 2006;44(1):91–8.
48. Hollingsworth KG, Newton JL, Taylor R, et al. Pilot study of peripheral muscle function in primary biliary cirrhosis: potential implications for fatigue pathogenesis. Clin Gastroenterol Hepatol 2008;6(9):1041–8.
49. Jopson L, Jones DE. Fatigue in primary biliary cirrhosis: prevalence, pathogenesis and management. Dig Dis 2015;33(Suppl 2):109–14.
50. Jones DE, Al-Rifai A, Frith J, et al. The independent effects of fatigue and UDCA therapy on mortality in primary biliary cirrhosis: results of a 9 year follow-up. J Hepatol 2010;53(5):911–7.

51. Talwalkar JA, Souto E, Jorgensen RA, et al. Natural history of pruritus in primary biliary cirrhosis. Clin Gastroenterol Hepatol 2003;1(4):297–302.
52. Hussain A, Samuel R, Hegade V, et al. Pruritus secondary to primary biliary cholangitis: a review of the pathophysiology and management with phototherapy. Br J Dermatol 2019;181(6):1138–45.
53. Danese S, Semeraro S, Papa A, et al. Extraintestinal manifestations in inflammatory bowel disease. 2005;11(46):7227.
54. Rosenthal E, Diamond E, Benderly A, et al. Cholestatic pruritus: effect of phototherapy on pruritus and excretion of bile acids in urine. Acta Paediatr 1994;83(8): 888–91.
55. Kremer AE, van Dijk R, Leckie P, et al. Serum autotaxin is increased in pruritus of cholestasis, but not of other origin, and responds to therapeutic interventions. Hepatology 2012;56(4):1391–400.
56. Jones EA, Bergasa NV. The pruritus of cholestasis: from bile acids to opiate agonists. Hepatology 1990;11(5):884–7.
57. Abboud TK, Lee K, Zhu J, et al. Prophylactic oral naltrexone with intrathecal morphine for cesarean section: effects on adverse reactions and analgesia. Anesth Analg 1990;71(4):367–70.
58. Siegel JL, Luthra H, Donlinger J, et al. Association of primary biliary cirrhosis and rheumatoid arthritis. J Clin Rheumatol 2003;9(6):340–3.
59. Tojo J, Ohira H, Suzuki T, et al. Clinicolaboratory characteristics of patients with primary biliary cirrhosis associated with CREST symptoms. Hepatol Res 2002; 22(3):187–95.
60. Laurin JM, DeSotel CK, Jorgensen RA, et al. The natural history of abdominal pain associated with primary biliary cirrhosis. Am J Gastroenterol 1994;89(10):1840–3.
61. Newton JL, Hollingsworth KG, Taylor R, et al. Cognitive impairment in primary biliary cirrhosis: symptom impact and potential etiology. Hepatology 2008; 48(2):541–9.
62. Phillips JR, Angulo P, Petterson T, et al. Fat-soluble vitamin levels in patients with primary biliary cirrhosis. Am J Gastroenterol 2001;96(9):2745–50.
63. Selmi C, Bowlus CL, Gershwin ME, et al. Primary biliary cirrhosis. Lancet (London, England) 2011;377(9777):1600–9.
64. Long RG, Scheuer PJ, Sherlock S. Presentation and course of asymptomatic primary biliary cirrhosis. Gastroenterology 1977;72(6):1204–7.
65. Garcia-Pagan JC, Francoz C, Montagnese S, et al. Management of the major complications of cirrhosis: beyond guidelines. Journal of hepatology 2021; 75(Suppl 1):S135–s146.
66. Koulentaki M, Ioannidou D, Stefanidou M, et al. Dermatological manifestations in primary biliary cirrhosis patients: a case control study. Am J Gastroenterol 2006; 101(3):541–6.
67. Zak A, Zeman M, Slaby A, Vecka MJBPotMFoPUiO. Xanthomas: clinical and pathophysiological relations. 2014;158(2).
68. Poupon R, Chazouillères O, Balkau B, et al. Clinical and biochemical expression of the histopathological lesions of primary biliary cirrhosis. UDCA-PBC Group. Journal of hepatology 1999;30(3):408–12.
69. Corpechot C, Poujol-Robert A, Wendum D, et al. Biochemical markers of liver fibrosis and lymphocytic piecemeal necrosis in UDCA-treated patients with primary biliary cirrhosis. Liver Int 2004;24(3):187–93.
70. Kaplan MM, Gershwin ME. Primary biliary cirrhosis. N Engl J Med 2005;353(12): 1261–73.

71. Bizzaro N, Covini G, Rosina F, et al. Overcoming a "probable" diagnosis in anti-mitochondrial antibody negative primary biliary cirrhosis: study of 100 sera and review of the literature. Clin Rev Allergy Immunol 2012;42(3):288–97.

72. Mattalia A, Quaranta S, Leung PS, et al. Characterization of antimitochondrial antibodies in healthy adults. 1998;27(3):656-661.

73. Shibata M, Onozuka Y, Morizane T, et al. Prevalence of antimitochondrial antibody in Japanese corporate workers in Kanagawa prefecture. J Gastroenterol 2004;39: 255–9.

74. Dahlqvist G, Gaouar F, Carrat F, et al. Large-scale characterization study of patients with antimitochondrial antibodies but nonestablished primary biliary cholangitis. Hepatology 2017;65(1):152–63.

75. Nakamura M, Shimizu-Yoshida Y, Takii Y, et al. Antibody titer to gp210-C terminal peptide as a clinical parameter for monitoring primary biliary cirrhosis. J Hepatol 2005;42(3):386–92.

76. Nakamura M, Kondo H, Mori T, et al. Anti-gp210 and anti-centromere antibodies are different risk factors for the progression of primary biliary cirrhosis. Hepatology 2007;45(1):118–27.

77. Taal B, Schalm S, De Bruyn A, De Rooy F, Klein FJCCA. Serum IgM in primary biliary cirrhosis. 1980;108(3):457-463.

78. Poupon R, Chazouillères O, Balkau B, et al. Clinical and biochemical expression of the histopathological lesions of primary biliary cirrhosis. J Hepatol 1999;30(3): 408–12.

79. Sorokin A, Brown JL, Thompson PD. Primary biliary cirrhosis, hyperlipidemia, and atherosclerotic risk: a systematic review. Atherosclerosis 2007;194(2):293–9.

80. Lindor KD, Bowlus CL, Boyer J, et al. Primary biliary cholangitis: 2018 practice guidance from the American association for the study of liver diseases. Hepatology 2019;69(1):394–419.

81. Corpechot C, Carrat F, Poujol-Robert A, et al. Noninvasive elastography-based assessment of liver fibrosis progression and prognosis in primary biliary cirrhosis. Hepatology 2012;56(1):198–208.

82. Nakanuma Y, Zen Y, Harada K, et al. Application of a new histological staging and grading system for primary biliary cirrhosis to liver biopsy specimens: interobserver agreement. Pathol Int 2010;60(3):167–74.

83. Abraham SC, Kamath PS, Eghtesad B, et al. Liver transplantation in precirrhotic biliary tract disease: portal hypertension is frequently associated with nodular regenerative hyperplasia and obliterative portal venopathy. Am J Surg Pathol 2006;30(11):1454–61.

84. Garcia-Tsao G, Abraldes JG, Berzigotti A, et al. Portal hypertensive bleeding in cirrhosis: risk stratification, diagnosis, and management: 2016 practice guidance by the American Association for the study of liver diseases. Hepatology 2017; 65(1):310–35.

85. Trivedi PJ, Bruns T, Cheung A, et al. Optimising risk stratification in primary biliary cirrhosis: AST/platelet ratio index predicts outcome independent of ursodeoxycholic acid response. J Hepatol 2014;60(6):1249–58.

86. Rong G, Wang H, Bowlus CL, et al. Incidence and risk factors for hepatocellular carcinoma in primary biliary cirrhosis. Clin Rev Allergy Immunol 2015;48(2–3): 132–41.

87. Bruix J, Sherman M. Management of hepatocellular carcinoma. Hepatology 2005; 42(5):1208–36.

88. Menon KV, Angulo P, Weston S, et al. Bone disease in primary biliary cirrhosis: independent indicators and rate of progression. J Hepatol 2001;35(3):316–23.

89. Sakauchi F, Mori M, Zeniya M, et al. Antimitochondrial antibody negative primary biliary cirrhosis in Japan: utilization of clinical data when patients applied to receive public financial aid. J Epidemiol 2006;16(1):30–4.
90. Taylor SL, Dean PJ, Riely CA. Primary autoimmune cholangitis. An alternative to antimitochondrial antibody-negative primary biliary cirrhosis. Am J Surg Pathol 1994;18(1):91–9.
91. Juliusson G, Imam M, Björnsson ES, et al. Long-term outcomes in antimitochondrial antibody negative primary biliary cirrhosis. Scand J Gastroenterol 2016; 51(6):745–52.
92. Jin Q, Moritoki Y, Lleo A, et al. Comparative analysis of portal cell infiltrates in antimitochondrial autoantibody-positive versus antimitochondrial autoantibody-negative primary biliary cirrhosis. Hepatology 2012;55(5):1495–506.
93. Levy C, Naik J, Giordano C, et al. Hispanics with primary biliary cirrhosis are more likely to have features of autoimmune hepatitis and reduced response to ursodeoxycholic acid than non-Hispanics. Clin Gastroenterol Hepatol 2014;12(8): 1398–405.

Primary Biliary Cholangitis
Pathophysiology

Inbal Houri, MD, Gideon M. Hirschfield, MB BChir, PhD, FRCP*

KEYWORDS

- Autoimmune • Biliary epithelial cell • GWAS • Epigenetics

KEY POINTS

- Primary biliary cholangitis is initiated by an autoimmune response.
- Biliary epithelial cell damage follows and can progress to biliary-type fibrosis.
- Multiple immune pathways are involved, as demonstrated by genome-wide association studies.
- Potential triggers for the immune response may be environmental factors.

INTRODUCTION

Primary biliary cholangitis (PBC) is the most common of the autoimmune liver diseases, with a female predominance and prevalence that varies greatly geographically with reports of 19 to 402 cases per million persons. Classically it is considered an archetypal chronic autoimmune injury to the liver, with persistent cholestasis and secondary biliary fibrosis developing as a result of biliary epithelial cell (BEC) injury and loss. Autoimmunity is usually considered the primary initiating disease factor for several reasons, including female-predominant disease, the histologic appearance is of a lymphocytic cholangitis, a very high prevalence of specific autoreactivity with circulating anti-mitochondrial antibodies (AMAs), patients and their family members have increased rates of other autoimmune disease, and there is no known pathogenic agent identified (**Box 1**). The pathophysiological hallmark of PBC relates to a highly specific loss of tolerance to the E2 subunit of the mitochondrial pyruvate dehydrogenase complex (PDC-E2).

From a pathophysiologic perspective, evidence identifies three major themes of interest. First, there is a genetic predisposition, with common genetic variation in human leukocyte antigen (HLA) and non-HLA regions of the genome. The non-HLA genetic signatures have largely arisen in immunologically relevant genes and pathways.

Division of Gastroenterology and Hepatology, Toronto Centre for Liver Disease, University of Toronto, 9th Floor Eaton Building, North Wing 219-B, 200 Elizabeth Street, Toronto, Ontario M5G 2C4, Canada
* Corresponding author.
E-mail address: Gideon.hirschfield@uhn.ca

Clin Liver Dis 28 (2024) 79–92
https://doi.org/10.1016/j.cld.2023.06.006
1089-3261/24/© 2023 Elsevier Inc. All rights reserved.

Box 1
Considerations for autoimmunity in PBC

Female predominance

Lymphocytic cholangitis per histology

High prevalence of specific autoantibodies—AMA

Increased rate of other autoimmune diseases in patients and family members

Recurrence after transplant

No known pathogenic agent

Second, environmental factors are believed to be relevant on a background of this genetic predisposition to autoimmunity. Environmental factors proposed include smoking, exposure to toxins and xenobiotics, and infectious agents. Finally, as the disease is restricted to the small bile ducts, cellular responses to injury by BECs (eg, senescence, apoptosis, bicarbonate excretion) are thought relevant to disease expression and response to treatment. Given that disease is seen globally but with significant heterogeneity in presentation and outcome, it is assumed that in any individual, there can be variation in the relative contribution of the proposed risk factors.

When examining the pathophysiology of PBC, there are thus two main chronic processes involved—an immune dysregulation and injury to the BEC. Although it is clear that both these processes are crucial to the development of the disease phenotype, there is an ongoing debate as to the role of each of these processes at the different stages of disease development. Both processes are influenced by genetic, epigenetic, and environmental factors, suggesting "multiple hits" are required for disease to present (**Fig. 1**A).

Histopathology

PBC is defined by a chronic immune-driven injury to the small bile ducts with destructive lymphocytic cholangitis, granulomas, and cholestasis. This chronic injury leads with time to biliary fibrosis and later to cirrhosis. The histology of early-stage disease is macroscopically described as inflammation and/or abnormal connective tissue confined to the portal areas. In stage 2 disease, inflammation and/or fibrosis can be seen also in periportal areas, and stage 3 and 4 signify bridging fibrosis and cirrhosis, respectively. Florid bile duct lesions (**Fig. 2**) are considered a pathognomonic finding for PBC, although not commonly seen in biopsy specimens. Other features that may be seen are granulomas and duct loss (ductopenia). Immunophenotyping identifies mixed populations of cells (eg, T cells, B cells, macrophages, eosinophils, and so on).

Immune Dysregulation

There are many epidemiologic features of PBC that suggest an immune-mediated process is the driving factor in PBC development (see **Box 1**), mainly:

- Female predominance,[1] as has been described in most other autoimmune diseases.
- Association with other autoimmune conditions: PBC patients have more frequent comorbidity with other autoimmune conditions, including but not limited to thyroid disease, celiac disease, and more.[2]
- Extra-hepatic manifestations: Sicca symptoms are common in PBC patients, presenting as a spectrum between mild symptoms to severe that meet

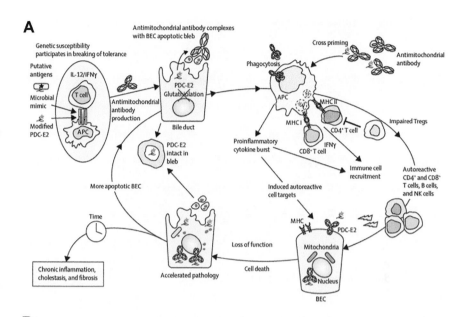

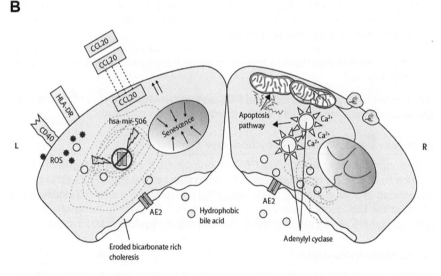

Fig. 1. Biological understanding of disease pathophysiology.[76] (*A*) Autoimmune susceptibility participates in breaking of tolerance, eventually producing antimitochondrial antibodies and a cycle of immune-mediated injury. (*B*) An active BEC bicarbonate-rich choleresis (which is membrane protective) is eroded because of low expression of AE2 solute transporter. Without the bicarbonate umbrella, hydrophobic bile acids permeate BEC membranes in an uncontrolled manner. APC, antigen-presenting cell; BEC, biliary epithelial cell; IL-12, interleukin-12; NK cells, natural killer cells; PDC-E2, E2 component of the pyruvate dehydrogenase complex; ROS, reactive oxygen species. Tregs, T-regulatory cells. Reprinted with permission from Elsevier. The Lancet, Dec 2020, 396 (10266), 1915-1926.

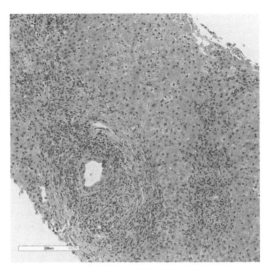

Fig. 2. Florid duct lesion: from a biopsy of a PBC patient.

diagnostic criteria for Sjogren syndrome. Salivary PDC-E2 has been shown to have aberrant expression in the salivary glands of patients with PBC, independent of Sjogren's syndrome diagnosis.[3]

- Recurrence after transplant: The frequent recurrence of PBC after liver transplantation indicates that disease activity includes both adaptive and innate immune mechanisms.[4]

While there are no animal models of PBC as such, multiple studies of murine autoimmune cholangitis support key involvement by immune pathways.[5,6]

Loss of Tolerance to Pyruvate Dehydrogenase Complex-E2

The E2 subunit of the mitochondrial PDC-E2 complex is the target of AMAs.[7,8] Loss of tolerance to PDC-E2 is associated with targeted injury of the BEC. PDC-E2 is present in mitochondria of all nucleated cells, raising the question of the specific localization of PBC to small bile ducts. Localization of unmodified PDC-E2 in apoptotic blebs of BECs may create an opportunity for immune reactivity by AMAs and T cells.[9-11]

Immune Microenvironment

As detailed previously, liver histology in PBC shows a progressive lymphocytic cholangitis, centered on small intrahepatic bile ducts, often associated with portal and parenchymal granulomata. There is infiltration of antigen-specific CD4+ T cells and CD8+ T cells within the portal tracts.[12] CD8+ T-cell subsets with an effector memory phenotype are resistant to apoptosis, and in PBC, they have been shown to accumulate around the portal area,[13] possibly promoted by CXCR3.[14]

Th17 cells and T-regulatory cells, and more specifically the balance between them, have been shown to correlate with disease severity.[15,16] The ratio between follicular helper T (Tfh) cells and follicular regulatory T (Tfr) cells is also changed in PBC due to a decrease in Tfr cells.[17] Tfh cells have been shown to be increased both in liver and in circulation of PBC patients and also differentiate between ursodeoxycholic acid (UDCA) responders and nonresponders.[18]

The innate immune system also plays a part in PBC pathogenesis, as demonstrated by the presence of granulomatous inflammation and polyclonal immunoglobulin (Ig) M production. There is an expansion of innate immune cells in patients with PBC, further emphasizing its role in disease pathogenesis.[19] This response may be mediated by Toll-like receptors (TLRs) that are expressed on BECs.[20,21] TLRs can be activated by various ligands, which may contribute to cellular injury by activating proinflammatory pathways and recruiting lymphoid cells.

The role of various liver mononuclear populations in PBC has been investigated. Peripheral blood myeloid-derived suppressor cells in PBC patients were elevated compared to controls, with significant correlation to biochemical disease markers and higher amounts in UDCA responders.[22] Macrophages react, together with circulating AMAs, to the presence of PDC-E2-containing apoptotic bodies from BECs, with upregulation of IL-12 and other proinflammatory cytokines.[23]

Another link to the innate immune system is by natural killer (NK) cells, which are increased both in the blood and liver of PBC patients and also show higher cytotoxic activity.[24] NK cells likely have a role both at initial phases of PBC inflammation and in facilitating chronic cytopathic effect of CD4+ cells via interferon gamma (IFNγ) secretion.[25]

Mucosal invariant T (MAIT) cells, a subset of innate-like T cells that produce proinflammatory cytokines, are predominantly localized to bile ducts in the portal tracts.[26] In a healthy liver, antigenic exposure causes activation of MAIT cells, initiating a localized immune response. In the liver of PBC patients as well as their systemic circulation, MAIT cells are reduced in number and furthermore express signs of exhaustion with a profibrogenic phenotype.[27] Interestingly, MAIT cells did not recover even after UDCA treatment response,[28] which may explain observations of progressive injury despite biochemical remission.

Despite the clear evidence of autoimmunity, PBC does not respond to immunosuppression but is rather treated by interventions aimed at the biliary component. The proposed explanation for this phenomenon lies in the timeline of disease process, assuming that the initial immune dysregulation occurs earlier than the actual presentation with symptoms or elevated liver enzymes, and treatment targeting the immune response at that point is therefore less effective.

BILIARY EPITHELIAL CELLS CHANGES
The Biliary Bicarbonate Umbrella

As bile is an acidic substance, BEC normally produce bicarbonate which is secreted to the epithelial surface, creating a "bicarbonate umbrella" and protecting cellular integrity. Anion exchanger 2 (AE2) is the major Cl-/HCO3- exchanger expressed by BECs and is key in creating a bicarbonate-rich umbrella on the apical surface of cholangiocytes, thus protecting BECs. AE2 is downregulated in PBC patients, leading to exposure of BECs to the acidic environment. In addition, there is increased bicarbonate in the intracellular compartment, affecting soluble intracellular adenylyl cyclase that sensitizes BECs to bile salt-induced apoptosis.[29,30] In support of this theory, an Ae2a,b-deficient mouse model developed features of PBC, including positive AMAs, high IgM and IgG, and elevated ALP. One-third of the mice had extensive portal inflammation with lymphocytic infiltrate. The regulation of AE2 levels may be via an epigenetic mechanism.

Biliary Epithelial Cells Senescence

An additional process contributing to ongoing injury is cholangiocyte senescence. BECs in PBC show senescent features, and telomere shortening may play a role.[31]

These senescent cells express a higher level of chemokines including CCL-2 and CX3CL1, thus modulating the bile duct microenvironment and promoting a proinflammatory reaction[32,33] (**Fig. 1**B).

Bile Acid Metabolism and Treatment Mechanisms

Bile acids are synthesized in the liver through the classical and alternative pathways, resulting in formation of the primary bile acids cholic acid and chenodeoxycholic acid (CDCA) that are subsequently conjugated to enhance solubility.[34] The bile salt export pump (BSEP) is an active transporter through which most conjugated bile acids are secreted, whereas the multidrug resistance proteins (MDRs) ABCB1 and ABCC2 facilitate secretion of less-common bile acids.

Cholestatic disease develops when there is impairment of bile formation or flow,[35] and the current treatment paradigm in PBC is aimed at influencing cholestasis.

UDCA, which is the first-line treatment for PBC, is a hydrophilic dihydroxy bile acid. Pharmacologically, UDCA increases metabolic conversion of cholesterol to bile acids. Several mechanisms of action have been suggested, including replacement of endogenous hydrophobic toxic bile acids by UDCA, thus preventing their accumulation; upregulation of AE2 expression on the surface of BECs; immune modulation; and possible activation of antiapoptotic pathways.

Bile acids are natural ligands of various intracellular and membrane receptors, effecting downstream signaling pathways.

Farnesoid X receptor (FXR) is a nuclear receptor that regulates absorption, transport, and synthesis of bile acids. Cholic acid and CDCA, both primary bile acids, bind FXR, which then together with retinoid X receptor binds to the promotor region of relevant target genes, including small heterodimer partner (SHP), FGF19, bile transporter BSEP, and more. SHP represses transcription of CYP7A1, resulting in suppression of bile acid synthesis. FXR receptors are also present in ileal enterocytes, and when activated by reabsorbed bile acids, they lead to expression of FGF19, which then enters the portal circulation. It binds to receptors on hepatocytes leading to CYP7A1 suppression via a different pathway. Beyond this effect on bile acid synthesis, FXR induces expression of bile acid transporters including BSEP, promoting export of bile acids from hepatocytes.[36] Highlighting the importance of this pathway in PBC, obeticholic acid, a semi-synthetic FXR agonist, is used as a therapy in PBC, promoting cholestasis and reducing liver injury.

Peroxisome proliferator-activated receptors (PPARs) are an additional group of nuclear receptors that are activated by fatty acids and their metabolites. They appear important in cholestatic liver injuries including PBC, and when activated, they improve markers of cholestasis significantly as well as helping pruritus, an important patient-reported symptom.

Three PPAR isoforms have been described, PPARα, PPARβ/δ, and PPARγ, with PPARα predominantly expressed in hepatocytes and PPARβ/δ and PPARγ in various tissues. PPARδ are active in the liver also in cholangiocytes, Kupffer cells, and hepatic stellate cells.

These receptors induce regulation of bile acid synthesis, transport, and detoxification, as well as energy metabolism and fatty acid transport and oxidation. PPAR agonism suppresses expression of CYP7A1 and CYP27A1,[37,38] leading to reduced bile acid synthesis. PPARα-mediated upregulation enzymes including CYP3A4, the UDP-glucuronosyltransferase (UGT)[39] enzyme family, and sulfotransferase 2A1 (SULT2A1)[40] result in detoxification of bile acids via conjugation of toxic hydrophobic bile acids. Phosphatidylcholine translocator ABCB4 (also known as MDR3), which translocates phosphatidylcholine across the inner canalicular membrane,[41] is also induced by PPARα. Phosphatidylcholine is an essential component of biliary micelles that protect BECs from bile salt irritation and subsequent cholestatic injury. Anti-inflammatory actions of PPARs have also been reported.[42]

There are several drugs targeting PPARs. Fibrates, initially developed for treatment of hypertriglyceridemia, are commercially available in some countries although not licensed for treatment of PBC. The fibrates differ in their specificity for PPAR sub-types—bezafibrate activates all three isoforms, whereas fenofibrate is more selective for PPARα, although the clinical relevance of this is not clearly defined.[43]

Seladelpar is a drug currently in phase-3 studies, with highly selective PPARδ activity, and has shown promising results for treating PBC.[44] Elafibranor, also in development, has dual PPARα/δ agonist properties and has also shown promising results.[45]

Pregnane X receptor (PXR) is another nuclear receptor that heterodimerizes with the retinoid X receptor when activated and regulates drug and bile acid metabolism.[46] PXR is highly expressed in the liver and induces molecules involved in metabolism such as the CYP450 family of enzymes.[47] PXR plays a role in detoxification and solubilization of bile acids. Rifampicin, which is currently used as an antipruritic agent in cholestatic liver diseases, is a potent PXR agonist and was shown to enhance bile acid detoxification as well as bilirubin conjugation and excretion as reflected by enhanced expression of CYP3A4, UGT1A1, and MRP2.[48] However, unlike other nuclear receptors discussed previously, PXR agonism with rifampicin has not been shown to modify disease progression.

INFLUENCING FACTORS
Genetic Factors

There is increased risk of PBC development in relatives of diagnosed patients,[49] including a high concordance of 63% in monozygotic twins.[50] Genome-wide association studies (GWAS) in PBC patients have shown significant associations to both HLA and non-HLA loci. A large, multi-ethnic GWAS combining the various cohorts identified additional loci, and as of 2022, 70 susceptibility loci have been identified.[51]

HLA loci have particularly strong associations with PBC; however, the specific associations differ between populations.[52,53]

Several non-HLA loci are also associated with PBC, all of which are associated with different components of the immune system. Over 80% of these overlap with loci implicated in other autoimmune diseases, while the few others are seemingly specific for PBC.[51]

The IL-12 signaling pathway is key in immune regulation, both by activating proinflammatory T helper 1 cells and by inhibiting Th17 cells via stimulation of IFNγ.

Other pathways involved are cellular responses to tumor necrosis factor and B-cell activation pathways.

Initial GWAS published did not find any potential loci on the X-chromosome. A recent study using 5 cohorts from previous GWAS examined X-chromosome loci and identified a novel locus, characterized by the presence of different genes and of a superenhancer possibly involved in their coregulation, as well as in the regulation of FOXP3, a major factor in T-cell regulation.[54]

Environmental Factors

Environmental factors are either chemical or infectious and are thought to trigger disease processes through molecular mimicry. As mentioned previously, a "multiple-hit" process is probably required, initiated by exposure to an external substance, leading to antigen-presentation, activation of co-stimulatory pathways, thus causing immune activation and biliary damage.

Data suggest geographic clustering of PBC cases,[55] with multiple studies failing to show a clear genetic association in those areas, suggesting a dominant role for environmental factors.

A large study mapping PBC cases in north-east of England and north Cumbria showed a distinct pattern, with a high prevalence of PBC found in urban, postindustrial areas with a strong coal-mining heritage and increased environmental cadmium levels.[56] Multiple studies have shown a significant association between smoking history and PBC.[57,58]

Urinary tract infections are more common in patients with PBC; however, it is unclear if this is through a shared mechanism of epithelial dysfunction or if this may be an environmental trigger causing autoreactivity. One proposed mechanism is via the significant similarity of the PDC-E2 between mammals and bacteria, including in *Escherichia coli*.[59]

Xenobiotics have also been implicated as environmental triggers, including some present in cosmetics and food additives such as 2-octynoic acid[60,61] and 2-nonynoic acid,[62] and have also been shown to induce immunologic and histologic features of human PBC in animal models.

The mechanism of these associations is presumably one of molecular mimicry, contributing to loss of self-tolerance.[63] However, direct toxicity to BECs has been suggested as an additional potential mechanism.

Epigenetics—microRNAs

Beyond genetic associations, posttranscriptional regulation of gene expression can be done via microRNAs.

Explanted livers of PBC patients have been shown to have different expression of 35 miRNAs compared to controls, with predicted targets known to affect cell proliferation, apoptosis, inflammation, oxidative stress, and metabolism.[64] Specifically, miR-506 is upregulated in PBC and has been shown to impact disease processes in various mechanisms including inducing de-differentiation by downregulating biliary and epithelial markers and upregulating proinflammatory and profibrotic markers. This is presumed to be via targeting the Cl-/HCO3- AE2 as mentioned previously. miR-506 Also regulates type III inositol 1,4,5-triphosphate receptor that is involved in maintaining the biliary bicarbonate umbrella via regulation of calcium release in cholangiocytes.

Gut–Liver Axis

After being absorbed, gut-derived products enter the portal circulation and reach the liver. These include bacterial components, nutrients, and all other orally introduced agents and create complex interactions in the gut–liver axis.[65] The liver in turn can influence absorptive processes in the intestinal system via the enterohepatic circulation. Bile duct ligation in a mouse model causes bacterial overgrowth and mucosal injury in the ileum, and FXR activation has been shown to induce genes involved in enteroprotection and prevent epithelial deterioration.[66]

Microbiome

Dysbiosis of the gut microbiome has been implicated in many disease processes, including a variety of autoimmune processes.[67] A growing body of evidence demonstrates changes in gut microbiota in PBC patients.[68,69] In particular, lower levels of *Oscillospira* correlated with anti-gp210 positivity.

Female predominance of autoimmune disease may be explained in part by gut microbiome influence, as was suggested by the nonobese diabetic model of type 1 diabetes mellitus.[70,71] This has been associated with hormonal effects, suggesting

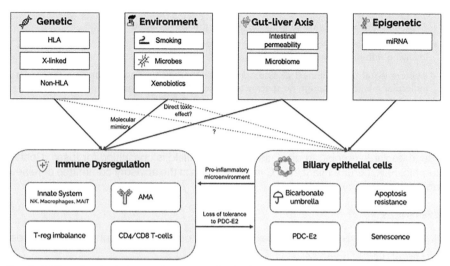

Fig. 3. PBC pathophysiology concepts. Multiple factors mutually interact and lead to a "multi-hit" process resulting in PBC development. The main processes are immune dysregulation and damage to biliary epithelial cells, with influences from genetic factors, epigenetics, the gut–liver axis, and environmental exposures. HLA, human leukocyte antigen; miRNA, microRNA; NK, natural killer cells; MAIT, mucosal invariant T cells; AMA, antimitochondrial antibodies; PDC-E2, E2 component of the pyruvate dehydrogenase complex.

cross-reaction between hormones and the microbiome. Interestingly, testosterone has been showed to suppress hepatic inflammation in a mouse model of acute cholangitis.[72]

Intestinal permeability
Changes along the liver–gut axis may influence intestinal permeability,[73] and this loss of barrier function can result in the increased delivery to the liver of potentially toxic substances, including free fatty acids, endotoxins, and gut microbial components.

IgA
Portal plasma cells produce secretory IgA, and this liver-derived immunoglobulin is secreted into the lumen via bile. In the intestinal lumen, IgA prevents bacterial translocation by contributing to biofilm formation.[74] Duodenal enterocytes in PBC patients show reduced secretory IgA compared with controls.[75]

SUMMARY

PBC is a heterogenous and multifaceted disease, with varying presentations and disease course. Phenotype arises from a biliary epithelial response to a complex, chronic, and evolving cascade of immunologic and bile acid interactions, leading to inflammatory and fibrotic changes (**Fig. 3**). The advances in treatment in recent years have stemmed from better biologic understanding of the underlying mechanisms although there is still much left to learn in the hope of achieving disease cure in the future.

CLINICS CARE POINTS

- Disease process in PBC involves both biliary epithelial cell damage and immune dysregulation.

- Autoimmunity is usually considered the primary disease-initiating factor.
- Genome-wide association studies have recognized multiple loci in association with PBC, involving different immune pathways.
- Environmental factors impact disease risk and are thought to trigger immune response via molecular mimicry, although no specific toxic agent has been identified to date.

DISCLOSURES

I. Houri declares nothing to disclose. G.M. Hirschfield is consulting for Ipsen, Roche, Morphic, Falk, Mirum, Pliant, and CymaBay and is in the advisory committee or review panel of Intercept and GSK.

REFERENCES

1. Schwinge D, Schramm C. Sex-related factors in autoimmune liver diseases. Semin Immunopathol 2019;41(2):165–75.
2. Efe C, Torgutalp M, Henriksson I, et al. Extrahepatic autoimmune diseases in primary biliary cholangitis: prevalence and significance for clinical presentation and disease outcome. J Gastroenterol Hepatol 2021;36(4):936–42.
3. Tsuneyama K, Water JVD, Yamazaki K, et al. Primary biliary cirrhosis an E pi thelitis: evidence of abnormal salivary gland Immunohistochemistry. Autoimmunity 1997;26(1):23–31.
4. Montano-Loza AJ, Hansen BE, Corpechot C, et al. Factors associated with recurrence of primary biliary cholangitis after liver transplantation and effects on graft and patient survival. Gastroenterology 2019;156(1):96–107.e1.
5. Bae HR, Leung PSC, Tsuneyama K, et al. Chronic expression of interferon-gamma leads to murine autoimmune cholangitis with a female predominance. Hepatology 2016;64(4):1189–201.
6. Bae HR, Hodge DL, Yang GX, et al. The interplay of type I and type II interferons in murine autoimmune cholangitis as a basis for sex-biased autoimmunity. Hepatology 2018;67(4):1408–19.
7. Yeaman SJ, Fussey SP, Danner DJ, et al. Primary biliary cirrhosis: identification of two major M2 mitochondrial autoantigens. Lancet 1988;1(8594):1067–70.
8. Invernizzi P, Lleo A, Podda M. Interpreting serological tests in diagnosing autoimmune liver diseases. Semin Liver Dis 2007;27(2):161–72.
9. Lleo A, Bowlus CL, Yang GX, et al. Biliary apotopes and anti-mitochondrial antibodies activate innate immune responses in primary biliary cirrhosis. Hepatology 2010;52(3):987–98.
10. Lleo A, Selmi C, Invernizzi P, et al. Apotopes and the biliary specificity of primary biliary cirrhosis. Hepatology 2009;49(3):871–9.
11. Shimoda S, Miyakawa H, Nakamura M, et al. CD4 T-cell autoreactivity to the mitochondrial autoantigen PDC-E2 in AMA-negative primary biliary cirrhosis. J Autoimmun 2008;31(2):110–5.
12. Kita H, Lian ZX, Van de Water J, et al. Identification of HLA-A2-restricted CD8(+) cytotoxic T cell responses in primary biliary cirrhosis: T cell activation is augmented by immune complexes cross-presented by dendritic cells. J Exp Med 2002;195(1):113–23.
13. Tsuda M, Ambrosini YM, Zhang W, et al. Fine phenotypic and functional characterization of effector cluster of differentiation 8 positive T cells in human patients with primary biliary cirrhosis. Hepatology 2011;54(4):1293–302.

14. Ma HD, Ma WT, Liu QZ, et al. Chemokine receptor CXCR3 deficiency exacerbates murine autoimmune cholangitis by promoting pathogenic CD8+ T cell activation. J Autoimmun 2017;78:19–28.
15. Rong G, Zhou Y, Xiong Y, et al. Imbalance between T helper type 17 and T regulatory cells in patients with primary biliary cirrhosis: the serum cytokine profile and peripheral cell population. Clin Exp Immunol 2009;156(2):217–25.
16. Yang CY, Ma X, Tsuneyama K, et al. IL-12/Th1 and IL-23/Th17 biliary microenvironment in primary biliary cirrhosis: implications for therapy. Hepatology 2014; 59(5):1944–53.
17. Zheng J, Wang T, Zhang L, et al. Dysregulation of circulating Tfr/Tfh ratio in primary biliary cholangitis. Scand J Immunol 2017;86(6):452–61.
18. Wang L, Sun Y, Zhang Z, et al. CXCR5+ CD4+ T follicular helper cells participate in the pathogenesis of primary biliary cirrhosis. Hepatology 2015;61(2):627–38.
19. Selmi C, Lleo A, Pasini S, et al. Innate immunity and primary biliary cirrhosis. Curr Mol Med 2009;9(1):45–51.
20. Yokoyama T, Komori A, Nakamura M, et al. Human intrahepatic biliary epithelial cells function in innate immunity by producing IL-6 and IL-8 via the TLR4-NF-kappaB and -MAPK signaling pathways. Liver Int 2006;26(4):467–76.
21. Harada K, Isse K, Nakanuma Y. Interferon gamma accelerates NF-kappaB activation of biliary epithelial cells induced by Toll-like receptor and ligand interaction. J Clin Pathol 2006;59(2):184–90.
22. Zhang H, Lian M, Zhang J, et al. A functional characteristic of cysteine-rich protein 61: modulation of myeloid-derived suppressor cells in liver inflammation. Hepatology 2018;67(1):232–46.
23. Lleo A, Invernizzi P. Apotopes and innate immune system: novel players in the primary biliary cirrhosis scenario. Dig Liver Dis 2013;45(8):630–6.
24. Chuang YH, Lian ZX, Tsuneyama K, et al. Increased killing activity and decreased cytokine production in NK cells in patients with primary biliary cirrhosis. J Autoimmun 2006;26(4):232–40.
25. Shimoda S, Hisamoto S, Harada K, et al. Natural killer cells regulate T cell immune responses in primary biliary cirrhosis. Hepatology 2015;62(6):1817–27.
26. Jeffery HC, van Wilgenburg B, Kurioka A, et al. Biliary epithelium and liver B cells exposed to bacteria activate intrahepatic MAIT cells through MR1. J Hepatol 2016;64(5):1118–27.
27. Böttcher K, Rombouts K, Saffioti F, et al. MAIT cells are chronically activated in patients with autoimmune liver disease and promote profibrogenic hepatic stellate cell activation. Hepatology 2018;68(1):172–86.
28. Setsu T, Yamagiwa S, Tominaga K, et al. Persistent reduction of mucosal-associated invariant T cells in primary biliary cholangitis. J Gastroenterol Hepatol 2018;33(6):1286–94.
29. Kleinboelting S, Diaz A, Moniot S, et al. Crystal structures of human soluble adenylyl cyclase reveal mechanisms of catalysis and of its activation through bicarbonate. Proc Natl Acad Sci U S A 2014;111(10):3727–32.
30. Chang JC, Go S, de Waart DR, et al. Soluble adenylyl cyclase regulates bile salt-induced apoptosis in human cholangiocytes. Hepatology 2016;64(2):522–34.
31. Sasaki M, Ikeda H, Yamaguchi J, et al. Telomere shortening in the damaged small bile ducts in primary biliary cirrhosis reflects ongoing cellular senescence. Hepatology 2008;48(1):186–95.
32. Sasaki M, Miyakoshi M, Sato Y, et al. Chemokine-chemokine receptor CCL2-CCR2 and CX3CL1-CX3CR1 axis may play a role in the aggravated inflammation in primary biliary cirrhosis. Dig Dis Sci 2014;59(2):358–64.

33. Sasaki M, Miyakoshi M, Sato Y, et al. Modulation of the microenvironment by se-nescent biliary epithelial cells may be involved in the pathogenesis of primary biliary cirrhosis. J Hepatol 2010;53(2):318–25.

34. Chiang JYL. Regulation of bile acid synthesis: pathways, nuclear receptors, and mechanisms. J Hepatol 2004;40(3):539–51.

35. Beuers U, Trauner M, Jansen P, et al. New paradigms in the treatment of hepatic cholestasis: from UDCA to FXR, PXR and beyond. J Hepatol 2015;62(1 Suppl): S25–37.

36. Ananthanarayanan M, Balasubramanian N, Makishima M, et al. Human bile salt export pump promoter is transactivated by the farnesoid X receptor/bile acid re-ceptor. J Biol Chem 2001;276(31):28857–65.

37. Marrapodi M, Chiang JY. Peroxisome proliferator-activated receptor alpha (PPAR-alpha) and agonist inhibit cholesterol 7alpha-hydroxylase gene (CYP7A1) tran-scription. J Lipid Res 2000;41(4):514–20.

38. Post SM, Duez H, Gervois PP, et al. Fibrates suppress bile acid synthesis via peroxisome proliferator-activated receptor-alpha-mediated downregulation of cholesterol 7alpha-hydroxylase and sterol 27-hydroxylase expression. Arterios-cler Thromb Vasc Biol 2001;21(11):1840–5.

39. Barbier O, Duran-Sandoval D, Pineda-Torra I, et al. Peroxisome proliferator-activated receptor alpha induces hepatic expression of the human bile acid glu-curonidating UDP-glucuronosyltransferase 2B4 enzyme. J Biol Chem 2003; 278(35):32852–60.

40. Kitada H, Miyata M, Nakamura T, et al. Protective role of hydroxysteroid sulfo-transferase in lithocholic acid-induced liver toxicity. J Biol Chem 2003;278(20): 17838–44.

41. Ghonem NS, Ananthanarayanan M, Soroka CJ, et al. Peroxisome proliferator-activated receptor α activates human multidrug resistance transporter 3/ATP-binding cassette protein subfamily B4 transcription and increases rat biliary phosphatidylcholine secretion. Hepatology 2014;59(3):1030–42.

42. Lee MY, Choi R, Kim HM, et al. Peroxisome proliferator-activated receptor δ agonist attenuates hepatic steatosis by anti-inflammatory mechanism. Exp Mol Med 2012;44(10):578–85.

43. Willson TM, Brown PJ, Sternbach DD, et al. The PPARs: from orphan receptors to drug discovery. J Med Chem 2000;43(4):527–50.

44. Wetten A, Jones DEJ, Dyson JK. Seladelpar: an investigational drug for the treat-ment of early-stage primary biliary cholangitis (PBC). Expert Opin Investig Drugs 2022;31(10):1101–7.

45. Schattenberg JM, Pares A, Kowdley KV, et al. A randomized placebo-controlled trial of elafibranor in patients with primary biliary cholangitis and incomplete response to UDCA. J Hepatol 2021;74(6):1344–54.

46. Staudinger JL, Goodwin B, Jones SA, et al. The nuclear receptor PXR is a litho-cholic acid sensor that protects against liver toxicity. Proc Natl Acad Sci U S A 2001;98(6):3369–74.

47. Ihunnah CA, Jiang M, Xie W. Nuclear receptor PXR, transcriptional circuits and metabolic relevance. Biochim Biophys Acta 2011;1812(8):956–63.

48. Marschall HU, Wagner M, Zollner G, et al. Complementary stimulation of hepato-biliary transport and detoxification systems by rifampicin and ursodeoxycholic acid in humans. Gastroenterology 2005;129(2):476–85.

49. Tsuji K, Watanabe Y, Van De Water J, et al. Familial primary biliary cirrhosis in Hir-oshima. J Autoimmun 1999;13(1):171–8.

50. Selmi C, Mayo MJ, Bach N, et al. Primary biliary cirrhosis in monozygotic and dizygotic twins: genetics, epigenetics, and environment. Gastroenterology 2004;127(2):485–92.
51. Hitomi Y, Nakamura M. The genetics of primary biliary cholangitis: a GWAS and post-GWAS update. Genes (Basel) 2023;14(2):405.
52. Begovich AB, Klitz W, Moonsamy PV, et al. Genes within the HLA class II region confer both predisposition and resistance to primary biliary cirrhosis. Tissue Antigens 1994;43(2):71–7.
53. Yasunami M, Nakamura H, Tokunaga K, et al. Principal contribution of HLA-DQ alleles, DQB1*06:04 and DQB1*03:01, to disease resistance against primary biliary cholangitis in a Japanese population. Sci Rep 2017;7(1):11093.
54. Asselta R, Paraboschi EM, Gerussi A, et al. X chromosome contribution to the genetic architecture of primary biliary cholangitis. Gastroenterology 2021;160(7): 2483–95.e26.
55. Hamlyn AN, Macklon AF, James O. Primary biliary cirrhosis: geographical clustering and symptomatic onset seasonality. Gut 1983;24(10):940–5.
56. Dyson JK, Blain A, Foster Shirley MD, et al. Geo-epidemiology and environmental co-variate mapping of primary biliary cholangitis and primary sclerosing cholangitis. JHEP Rep 2020;3(1):100202.
57. Corpechot C, Chrétien Y, Chazouillères O, et al. Demographic, lifestyle, medical and familial factors associated with primary biliary cirrhosis. J Hepatol 2010; 53(1):162–9.
58. Gershwin ME, Selmi C, Worman HJ, et al. Risk factors and comorbidities in primary biliary cirrhosis: a controlled Interview-based study of 1032 patients. Hepatology 2005;42(5):1194–202.
59. Wang JJ, Yang GX, Zhang WC, et al. Escherichia coli infection induces autoimmune cholangitis and anti-mitochondrial antibodies in non-obese diabetic (NOD).B6 (Idd10/Idd18) mice. Clin Exp Immunol 2014;175(2):192–201.
60. Amano K, Leung PSC, Rieger R, et al. Chemical xenobiotics and mitochondrial autoantigens in primary biliary cirrhosis: identification of antibodies against a common environmental, cosmetic, and food additive, 2-octynoic acid. J Immunol 2005;174(9):5874–83.
61. Wakabayashi K, Lian ZX, Leung PSC, et al. Loss of tolerance in C57BL/6 mice to the autoantigen E2 subunit of pyruvate dehydrogenase by a xenobiotic with ensuing biliary ductular disease. Hepatology 2008;48(2):531–40.
62. Rieger R, Leung PSC, Jeddeloh MR, et al. Identification of 2-nonynoic acid, a cosmetic component, as a potential trigger of primary biliary cirrhosis. J Autoimmun 2006;27(1):7–16.
63. Shimoda S, Nakamura M, Ishibashi H, et al. HLA DRB4 0101-restricted immunodominant T cell autoepitope of pyruvate dehydrogenase complex in primary biliary cirrhosis: evidence of molecular mimicry in human autoimmune diseases. J Exp Med 1995;181(5):1835–45.
64. Padgett KA, Lan RY, Leung PC, et al. Primary biliary cirrhosis is associated with altered hepatic microRNA expression. J Autoimmun 2009;32(3–4):246–53.
65. Acharya C, Sahingur SE, Bajaj JS. Microbiota, cirrhosis, and the emerging oral-gut-liver axis. JCI Insight 2017;2(19):e94416.
66. Inagaki T, Moschetta A, Lee YK, et al. Regulation of antibacterial defense in the small intestine by the nuclear bile acid receptor. Proc Natl Acad Sci U S A 2006;103(10):3920–5.
67. Li B, Selmi C, Tang R, et al. The microbiome and autoimmunity: a paradigm from the gut-liver axis. Cell Mol Immunol 2018;15(6):595–609.

68. Zhou YJ, Ying GX, Dong SL, et al. Gut microbial profile of treatment-naive patients with primary biliary cholangitis. Front Immunol 2023;14:1126117.
69. Martinez-Gili L, Pechlivanis A, McDonald JAK, et al. Bacterial and metabolic phenotypes associated with inadequate response to ursodeoxycholic acid treatment in primary biliary cholangitis. Gut Microbes 2023;15(1):2208501.
70. Yurkovetskiy L, Burrows M, Khan AA, et al. Gender bias in autoimmunity is influenced by microbiota. Immunity 2013;39(2):400–12.
71. Markle JGM, Frank DN, Mortin-Toth S, et al. Sex differences in the gut microbiome drive hormone-dependent regulation of autoimmunity. Science 2013;339(6123):1084–8.
72. Schwinge D, Carambia A, Quaas A, et al. Testosterone suppresses hepatic inflammation by the downregulation of IL-17, CXCL-9, and CXCL-10 in a mouse model of experimental acute cholangitis. J Immunol 2015;194(6):2522–30.
73. Bischoff SC, Barbara G, Buurman W, et al. Intestinal permeability–a new target for disease prevention and therapy. BMC Gastroenterol 2014;14:189.
74. Randal Bollinger R, Everett ML, Palestrant D, et al. Human secretory immunoglobulin A may contribute to biofilm formation in the gut. Immunology 2003;109(4):580–7.
75. Floreani A, Baragiotta A, Pizzuti D, et al. Mucosal IgA defect in primary biliary cirrhosis. Am J Gastroenterol 2002;97(2):508–10.
76. Lleo A, Wang G, Gershwin ME, et al. Primary biliary cholangitis. The Lancet 2020;396(10266):1915–26.

Autoimmune Markers in Primary Biliary Cholangitis

Shivani K. Shah, MD, Christopher L. Bowlus, MD*

KEYWORDS

- Anti-mitochondrial antibody • AMA • Antinuclear antibody • ANA • Sp100 • gp210
- Primary biliary cholangitis

KEY POINTS

- The most common biomarker in primary biliary cholangitis (PBC) is the anti-mitochondrial antibody (AMA).
- Other, novel, biomarkers exist that may improve diagnostic accuracy of PBC, especially in patients with a negative AMA.
- Improvements in available laboratory techniques to evaluate for antibodies have led to improvements in sensitivity, specificity, and total time required to complete testing.

INTRODUCTION/BACKGROUND

Primary biliary cholangitis (PBC) is a chronic cholestatic liver disease characterized by inflammation and destruction of the intrahepatic bile ducts, affecting predominately women in their fifth to sixth decade of life. Descriptions of chronic cholestatic or obstructive liver disease akin to PBC date back to the 1850s[1]; however, the term "primary biliary cirrhosis" was not introduced until 1949 as a defined disease characterized by an inflammatory reaction of the intrahepatic ducts.[2] More recently, the nomenclature has shifted from primary biliary cirrhosis to PBC due to the advent of novel autoimmune markers specific to PBC, which allow patients to be diagnosed before the development of cirrhosis. In fact, autoimmune markers of PBC may precede clinical disease manifestations. The purpose of this article will be to discuss current autoimmune markers used in the diagnosis of PBC.

Anti-mitochondrial Antibody

The most common autoimmune marker in PBC is the anti-mitochondrial antibody (AMA), found in approximately 95% of PBC patients (**Table 1**).[3] AMA was first described in 1965, by Dame Sheila Sherlock and colleagues.[4] In this seminal paper,

Division of Gastroenterology and Hepatology, University of California Davis School of Medicine, 4150 V Street, PSSB 3500, Sacramento, CA 95817, USA
* Corresponding author.
E-mail address: clbowlus@ucdavis.edu

Clin Liver Dis 28 (2024) 93–101
https://doi.org/10.1016/j.cld.2023.07.002
1089-3261/24/© 2023 Elsevier Inc. All rights reserved.

Table 1
Comparison of methods for detection of anti-mitochondrial antibodies

	Mechanism	Advantages	Disadvantages
Immunofluorescence (IIF)	• Primary antibody binds to a target molecule. A second antibody carrying a fluorophore binds to the primary antibody resulting in a specific staining pattern. • AMA has a cytoplasmic coarse pattern (now termed reticular pattern) • Reported as a dilution	• Most specific test available	• Time and labor intensive • Observer dependent
Enzyme-linked immunosorbent assay (ELISA)	• Reported as a titer • Requires the presence of an antigen (eg, the M2 antigen) affixed to a microtiter plate. • Antigen is then interfaced with an antibody linked to a reporter enzyme via incubation	• More sensitive than IIF	• Less specific than IIF • Detection is based on a reaction, thus readout must be done within a short period of time • Observer dependent
Immunoblotting	• Nonquantitative • Electrophoresis used to target proteins via an induced antigen-antibody reaction	• Rapid test • More sensitive than IIF	• Less specific than IIF • Risk of antibody interacting with non-intended proteins, or false positives • Costly
Bead-based assay	• Antigen is coated on a bead which can be detected by a cytometer in the bead-based assay	• Eliminates operator variability • Rapid • Automated • May identify more mitochondrial antigens, thus reducing the number of patients with true AMA-negative PBC.	• Relatively novel

the sera of all 32 patients with PBC included in the study demonstrated a coarse granular cytoplasmic fluorescence on unfixed sections of thyroid gland, stomach, kidney, and lymphocytes. The preferential staining for cells rich in mitochondria gave a clue to the target of the autoantibodies and was confirmed by pre-absorption of sera with rat liver mitochondria which abolished the staining. The findings from this study were later expounded on, by a series of papers confirm reactivity of PBC sera to rat liver, pig kidney, and beef heart exclusively to mitochondria[5]; localizing the reactivity to the inner mitochondrial membrane and the mitochondrial fraction containing succinate dehydrogenase[6–8]; and confirmation that the antigen is a protein.[9] Ultimately, reactivity was found to be with a non-organ-specific ATPase-associated antigen within the M2 fraction of mitochondria.[10] The M2 antigen was found to be highly specific to PBC, whereas other disease states which may also demonstrate reactivity to mitochondrial antigens, such as syphilis, pseudo-lupus syndrome, and myocarditis did not react to the M2 fraction.[11] However, the M2 fraction is composed of multiple enzyme-based polypeptides leaving the identity of the PBC-specific antigen unknown.

In 1987, Eric Gershwin and colleagues[12] cloned the mitochondrial antigen recognized by patients with PBC, which at the time could only be demonstrated to be similar to the dihydrolipoamide acetyltransferase of the *Escherichia coli* pyruvate dehydrogenase multienzyme complex (PDC-E2), notably with a conserved the lipoyl-binding site.[13] Work from the Gershwin laboratory later demonstrated that the antigen was the dihydrolipoamide acetyltransferase component of the PDC-E2[14] and that reactivity was could also be demonstrated against additional mitochondrial autoantigens sharing similar structures including branched chain 2-oxo acid dehydrogenase complex (BCOADC-E2) and 2-oxoglutarate dehydrogenase (OGDC-E2).[15] Epitope mapping demonstrated that the immunodominant epitopes of PDC-E2, BCOADC-E2, and OGDC-E2 are all conformational lipoic acid-binding sites[16,17] and require lipoic acid conjugation to the PDC-E2 complex for recognition by PBC antibodies.[18]

The role of AMA as an etiologic agent of PBC or an epiphenomenon has long been debated. AMA has no prognostic value, nor does the presence or titer of AMA correlate with the severity or progression of PBC.[19] In addition, AMA may be present without clinical features of PBC, though in patients with AMA positivity and normal alkaline phosphatase, approximately one in six will develop signs of PBC over the course of 5 years[20] suggesting that the loss of tolerance to PDC-E2 is an early event in the development of PBC. In addition to a genetic predisposition involving variants in the human leukocyte antigen region and interleukin (IL)-12 pathway,[21] environmental exposures including to *E coli*, smoking, and xenobiotics have been implicated in the development of AMA and PBC.[22–26]

A central enigma to the potential role of AMA in PBC has been the specific targeting of the small intrahepatic bile duct cells by an immune response to a ubiquitous antigen found in essentially all cells. The well-described recurrence of PBC after transplantation suggests that the biliary epithelial cell is an innocent bystander and that there is not an innate defect in the biliary epithelial cells of PBC patients. The specificity of the targeting of AMA to PDC-E2 subunits in biliary epithelial cells can be best explained by the "apoptotic bleb theory." Although PDC-E2 is present in all cells with mitochondria, only biliary epithelial cells appear to not degrade PDC-E2 subunit after undergoing apoptosis. Ex vivo studies demonstrated that apoptotic bleb from cultured human intrahepatic biliary epithelial cells (HIBEC) but not blebs from other epithelial cells contained intact PDC-E2.[27] In addition, apoptotic bodies from HIBEC in the presence of AMA and mature monocyte derived macrophages from patients with PBC demonstrated a 10-fold higher level of secreted tumor necrosis factor

(TNF)-α, and a twofold increase in other pro-inflammatory cytokines, such as IL-6, IL-10, macrophage inflammatory protein (MIP)-1b, and IL12p40 compared with control experiments substituting each of the three components (apoptotic bleb, sera, or macrophage).[28]

Clinical methods of identifying and quantifying AMA include the original indirect immunofluorescence (IIF) in clinical laboratories performed on HEp-2 cells and enzyme-linked immunosorbent assays (ELISA) with either the mitochondrial M2 fraction or a triple-expression hybrid clone coined pMIT3 which contains recombinant proteins from PDC-E2, BCOADC-E2, and OGDC-E2 acting as the antigen (**Table 2**).[15] HEp-2 cells are the substrate for both antinuclear antibodies (ANAs) and AMA detection. IIF works by binding of the primary antibody to the target molecule, followed by a secondary antibody, which carries a fluorophore, binding to the primary antibody. For AMA, the resultant staining is a cytoplasmic coarse or now termed reticular pattern.[24] Serial dilutions of sera starting at 1:40 until the fluorophore is no longer visible provide the resultant titer commonly reported. Any titer of AMA is considered a positive result. IIF is highly sensitive, identifying 85% of patients with a clinical diagnosis of PBC, but it is more time and labor intensive and is observer dependent, thus prompting the development of other assays.

In contrast to IIF, ELISA, immunoblot, bead-based assays are based on reactivity of sera to an antigen, such as the M2 antigen, which is immobilized to a substrate and detected by a secondary antibody linked to a reporter enzyme. In the case of ELISA, the antigen is coated on a microtiter plate while immunoblotting, or Western blotting, uses target proteins separated by electrophoresis. As implied by the name, antigen is coated on a bead which can be detected by a cytometer in the bead-based assay. In contrast to a dilution as reported by IIF, these methods report a "unit" based on the signal generated by the reporter enzyme. References are typically set for negative, indeterminate, and positive levels of the resulting enzyme activity.

In comparing ELISA to IIF, IIF was more specific (99% versus 85%–97%) than ELISA,[29] whereas ELISA and immunoblotting were more sensitive than IIF in the detection of AMA.[30] In a study of 164 patients with PBC, AMA was positive by IIF in 147 (89.6%) compared with positive results in 155 (94.5%) by immunodot to purified M2 antigen and 146 (89.0%) by ELISA using MIT3.[31] In contrast, in a study of 103 patients with PBC including 27 patients negative for AMA by IIF, an MIT3-based ELISA significantly increased AMA detection from 63.1% by a conventional anti-M2 ELISA and 73.7% by IIF to 79.6% by the MIT3-based ELISA[32] with similar results validated in a separate cohort.[33] A bead-based assay with the three recombinant antigens identified all 90 previously known AMA-positive patients and 20% of 30 rigorously defined AMA-negative patients.[34] Together, these results demonstrate in that for most patients with PBC, all methods are adequate to detect AMA, but for those that test negative with an M2-based ELISA, additional testing by IIF and MIT3 may be considered.

Primary Biliary Cholangitis-Specific Antinuclear Antibodies

Approximately 50% of patients with PBC have positive ANAs,[3,35] a phenomenon recognized during the same era as the identification of AMA.[36] The most common IIF pattern of ANA produced in patients with PBC is the nuclear-rim and multiple nuclear dots patterns,[37,38] subsequently shown to react specifically to the nuclear pore complex protein gp210 and the nuclear protein Sp100, respectively.[39]

A meta-analysis of 25 studies concluded that both Sp100 and gp210 have high specificity but low sensitivity for PBC. Sensitivity and specificity of gp210 for the diagnosis of PBC were 27.2% and 98.5%, respectively, and 23.1% and 97.7% for Sp100, respectively.[40] The implications of Sp100 and gp210 positivity with respect to prognosis or

Table 2
Comparison of sensitivity and specificity of autoantibody tests for primary biliary cholangitis

Antibody Test	Sensitivity	Specificity	Comments
Anti-mitochondrial antibody by immunofluorescence (IIF)	85%	99%	
Antinuclear antibodies (a). Sp100 (b). gp210	23.1% 27.2	97.7% 98.5%	Sp100 is the only autoantibody associated with PBC which seems to change over time and these changes are associated with disease progression
Anti-kelch-12 antibody	75% (immunoblotting)[a] 68.5% (ELISA)	98%	Anti-kelch-12 and anti-hexokinase-1 antibodies both have higher sensitivities than Sp100 and gp210.
Anti-hexokinase-1 antibody	75% (immunoblotting)[a] 68.5% (ELISA)	93%	Both anti-kelch-12 and anti-hexokinase-1 antibodies have been found in 10%–35% of patients with AMA-negative PBC.

[a] Refers to sensitivities in AMA-negative PBC.

outcomes have not been established, but some studies suggested that Sp100 and gp210 are associated with more advanced disease and poor prognosis.[41,42] Interestingly, Sp100 is the only autoantibody associated with PBC which seems to change over time and these changes are associated with disease progression.[43,44]

Immunoglobulin M

Elevated levels of immunoglobulin M (IgM) levels are commonly found in autoimmune diseases as a response to an underlying antigen response. With respect to hepatobiliary diseases, monoclonal IgM levels are uniquely elevated in cholestatic liver disease, more so in patients with PBC rather than primary sclerosing cholangitis. Elevated IgM is found in approximately 80% of patients with PBC.[45] Although IgM is not part of the diagnostic algorithm for PBC, studies have shown that IgM improves with treatment of PBC with ursodeoxycholic acid[46] and obeticholic acid.[47] Thus, IgM may be of clinical relevance in patient populations with diagnosed PBC but normal alkaline phosphatase and can be used to monitor response to therapy.

Anti-Kelch-Like-12 and Anti-Hexokinase-1 Antibodies

Two relatively recent biomarkers, kelch-like 12 and hexokinase-1 autoantibodies, have been associated with PBC.[48] When evaluated by immunoblot and ELISA, the markers were found to have $\geq$ 95% specificity for PBC and had a higher sensitivity than both anti-gp210 and anti-sp100 antibodies. Furthermore, these autoantibodies were present in 10% to 35% of AMA-negative PBC patients. The addition of these markers improved the sensitivity of AMA-negative PBC to 75% from 55% in immunoblotting assays and 68.5% from 48.3% in ELISA, thus further improving the available diagnostics for patients with suspected PBC who are AMA-negative.[49] Interestingly, the presence of these antibodies may be associated with worse disease severity.[50,51]

SUMMARY

PBC is a chronic cholestatic disease characterized by the destruction of small, intrahepatic bile ducts. Approximately 90% to 95% of patients will have a positive AMA. AMA can be evaluated by different methods of detection (IIF, ELISA, immundot, or bead) which a variety of source of the autoantigen. For the remaining 5% to 10% of patients that have suspected PBC, but are negative for AMA, further supportive testing may include sp100 and gp210 ANA-specific ANAs, IgM, and anti-kelch-like-12 and anti-hexokinase-1 antibodies. Together, these tests allow for the diagnosis of PBC with a high degree of accuracy and sensitivity limiting the need for diagnostic liver biopsy in nearly all cases of PBC. In contrast, the utility of autoantibodies as markers of prognosis remains to be validated, though levels of IgM as an adjunct to alkaline phosphatase may be beneficial when evaluating treatment response.

CLINICS CARE POINTS

- Anti-mitochondrial antibody (AMA) is positive in approximately 90% to 95% of patients.
- If AMA testing is negative, but the suspicion for primary biliary cholangitis (PBC) remains, further testing with ANA-specific antibodies sp100 and gp210 may be considered.
- Anti-kelch-like-12 and anti-hexokinase-1 antibodies are biomarkers that may also assist in the diagnosis of PBC, significantly improving the diagnosis of patients with AMA-negative PBC.

DISCLOSURES

S.K. Shah has nothing to disclose. C.L. Bowlus has received grants from Boston Scientific, United States, Calliditas Therapeutics, ChemoMab, Cour Pharmaceuticals, United States, CymaBay Therapeutics, United States, Gilead Sciences, United States, GSK Pharmaceuticals, Hanmi Pharmaceuticals, Intercept Pharmaceuticals, United States, Ipsen Bioscience, Mirum Pharmaceuticals, Novo Nordisk, United States, Pliant Therapeutics, and Viking Therapeutics and has been an advisor for Cymabay Therapeutics, GSK Pharmaceuticals, Invea Therapeutics, and Ipsen Bioscience.

REFERENCES

1. Addison T, Gull W. On a certain affection of the skin vitiligoidea- α plana, β tuberosa. Guy's Hosp Rep 1851;7:265–76.
2. Dauphinee JA, Sinclair JC. Primary biliary cirrhosis. Can Med Assoc J 1949; 61(1):1–6.
3. Kaplan MM, Gershwin ME. Primary biliary cirrhosis. N Engl J Med 2005;353(12): 1261–73.
4. Walker JG, Doniach D, Roitt IM, et al. Serological tests in diagnosis of primary biliary cirrhosis. Lancet 1965;1(7390):827–31.
5. Baum H, Berg PA. The complex nature of mitochondrial antibodies and their relation to primary biliary cirrhosis. Semin Liver Dis 1981;1(4):309–21.
6. Berg PA, Doniach D, Roitt IM. Mitochondrial antibodies in primary biliary cirrhosis. I. Localization of the antigen to mitochondrial membranes. J Exp Med 1967; 126(2):277–90.
7. Berg PA, Muscatello U, Horne RW, et al. Mitochondrial antibodies in primary biliary cirrhosis. II. The complement fixing antigen as a component of mitochondrial inner membranes. Br J Exp Pathol 1969;50(2):200–8.
8. Bianchi FB, Penfold PL, Roitt IM. Mitochondrial antibodies in primary biliary cirrhosis. V. Ultrastructural localization of the antigen to the inner mitochondrial membrane using a direct peroxidase conjugate. Br J Exp Pathol 1973;54(6): 652–7.
9. Berg PA, Roitt IM, Doniach D, et al. Mitochondrial antibodies in primary biliary cirrhosis. IV. Significance of membrane structure for the complement-fixing antigen. Immunology 1969;17(2):281–93.
10. Lindenborn-Fotinos J, Sayers TJ, Berg PA. Mitochondrial antibodies in primary biliary cirrhosis. VI. Association of the complement fixing antigen with a component of the mitochondrial F1-ATPase complex. Clin Exp Immunol 1982;50(2): 267–74.
11. Berg PA, Klein R, Lindenborn-Fotinos J. Antimitochondrial antibodies in primary biliary cirrhosis. J Hepatol 1986;2(1):123–31.
12. Gershwin ME, Mackay IR, Sturgess A, et al. Identification and specificity of a cDNA encoding the 70 kd mitochondrial antigen recognized in primary biliary cirrhosis. J Immunol 1987;138(10):3525–31.
13. Coppel RL, McNeilage LJ, Surh CD, et al. Primary structure of the human M2 mitochondrial autoantigen of primary biliary cirrhosis: dihydrolipoamide acetyltransferase. Proc Natl Acad Sci U S A 1988;85(19):7317–21.
14. Van de Water J, Turchany J, Leung PS, et al. Molecular mimicry in primary biliary cirrhosis. Evidence for biliary epithelial expression of a molecule cross-reactive with pyruvate dehydrogenase complex-E2. J Clin Invest 1993;91(6):2653–64.
15. Moteki S, Leung PS, Dickson ER, et al. Epitope mapping and reactivity of autoantibodies to the E2 component of 2-oxoglutarate dehydrogenase complex in

primary biliary cirrhosis using recombinant 2-oxoglutarate dehydrogenase complex. Hepatology 1996;23(3):436–44.

16. Leung PS, Chuang DT, Wynn RM, et al. Autoantibodies to BCOADC-E2 in patients with primary biliary cirrhosis recognize a conformational epitope. Hepatology 1995;22(2):505–13.

17. Surh CD, Coppel R, Gershwin ME. Structural requirement for autoreactivity on human pyruvate dehydrogenase-E2, the major autoantigen of primary biliary cirrhosis. Implication for a conformational autoepitope. J Immunol 1990;144(9): 3367–74.

18. Briand JP, Andre C, Tuaillon N, et al. Multiple autoepitope presentation for specific detection of antibodies in primary biliary cirrhosis. Hepatology 1992;16(6): 1395–403.

19. Invernizzi P, Crosignani A, Battezzati PM, et al. Comparison of the clinical features and clinical course of antimitochondrial antibody-positive and -negative primary biliary cirrhosis. Hepatology 1997;25(5):1090–5.

20. Dahlqvist G, Gaouar F, Carrat F, et al. Large-scale characterization study of patients with antimitochondrial antibodies but nonestablished primary biliary cholangitis. Hepatology 2017;65(1):152–63.

21. Hirschfield GM, Liu X, Xu C, et al. Primary biliary cirrhosis associated with HLA, IL12A, and IL12RB2 variants. N Engl J Med 2009;360(24):2544–55.

22. Yang Y, Choi J, Chen Y, et al. E. coli and the etiology of human PBC: antimitochondrial antibodies and spreading determinants. Hepatology 2022;75(2):266–79.

23. Naiyanetr P, Butler JD, Meng L, et al. Electrophile-modified lipoic derivatives of PDC-E2 elicits anti-mitochondrial antibody reactivity. J Autoimmun 2011;37(3): 209–16.

24. Chan EK, Damoiseaux J, Carballo OG, et al. Report of the first international consensus on standardized nomenclature of antinuclear antibody HEp-2 cell patterns 2014-2015. Front Immunol 2015;6:412.

25. Gershwin ME, Selmi C, Worman HJ, et al. Risk factors and comorbidities in primary biliary cirrhosis: a controlled interview-based study of 1032 patients. Hepatology 2005;42(5):1194–202.

26. Chen RC, Naiyanetr P, Shu SA, et al. Antimitochondrial antibody heterogeneity and the xenobiotic etiology of primary biliary cirrhosis. Hepatology 2013;57(4): 1498–508.

27. Lleo A, Selmi C, Invernizzi P, et al. Apotopes and the biliary specificity of primary biliary cirrhosis. Hepatology 2009;49(3):871–9.

28. Lleo A, Bowlus CL, Yang GX, et al. Biliary apotopes and anti-mitochondrial antibodies activate innate immune responses in primary biliary cirrhosis. Hepatology 2010;52(3):987–98.

29. Patel D, Egner W, Gleeson D, et al. Detection of serum M2 anti-mitochondrial antibodies by enzyme-linked immunosorbent assay is potentially less specific than by immunofluorescence. Ann Clin Biochem 2002;39(Pt 3):304–7.

30. Tanaka A, Miyakawa H, Luketic VA, et al. The diagnostic value of anti-mitochondrial antibodies, especially in primary biliary cirrhosis. Cell Mol Biol (Noisy-le-grand) 2002;48(3):295–9.

31. Gaiani F, Minerba R, Picanza A, et al. Optimization of laboratory diagnostics of primary biliary cholangitis: when solid-phase assays and immunofluorescence combine. J Clin Med 2022;11(17). https://doi.org/10.3390/jcm11175238.

32. Gabeta S, Norman GL, Liaskos C, et al. Diagnostic relevance and clinical significance of the new enhanced performance M2 (MIT3) ELISA for the detection of

IgA and IgG antimitochondrial antibodies in primary biliary cirrhosis. J Clin Immunol 2007;27(4):378–87.

33. Han E, Jo SJ, Lee H, et al. Clinical relevance of combined anti-mitochondrial M2 detection assays for primary biliary cirrhosis. Clin Chim Acta 2017;464:113–7.

34. Oertelt S, Rieger R, Selmi C, et al. A sensitive bead assay for antimitochondrial antibodies: chipping away at AMA-negative primary biliary cirrhosis. Hepatology 2007;45(3):659–65.

35. Muratori P, Muratori L, Ferrari R, et al. Characterization and clinical impact of antinuclear antibodies in primary biliary cirrhosis. Am J Gastroenterol 2003;98(2):431–7.

36. Doniach D, Roitt IM, Walker JG, et al. Tissue antibodies in primary biliary cirrhosis, active chronic (lupoid) hepatitis, cryptogenic cirrhosis and other liver diseases and their clinical implications. Clin Exp Immunol 1966;1(3):237–62.

37. Powell F, Schroeter AL, Dickson ER. Antinuclear antibodies in primary biliary cirrhosis. Lancet 1984;1(8371):288–9.

38. Lozano F, Pares A, Borche L, et al. Autoantibodies against nuclear envelope-associated proteins in primary biliary cirrhosis. Hepatology 1988;8(4):930–8.

39. Sternsdorf T, Guldner HH, Szostecki C, et al. Two nuclear dot-associated proteins, PML and Sp100, are often co-autoimmunogenic in patients with primary biliary cirrhosis. Scand J Immunol 1995;42(2):257–68.

40. Hu SL, Zhao FR, Hu Q, et al. Meta-analysis assessment of GP210 and SP100 for the diagnosis of primary biliary cirrhosis. PLoS One 2014;9(7):e101916.

41. Mytilinaiou MG, Meyer W, Scheper T, et al. Diagnostic and clinical utility of antibodies against the nuclear body promyelocytic leukaemia and Sp100 antigens in patients with primary biliary cirrhosis. Clin Chim Acta 2012;413(15–16):1211–6.

42. Haldar D, Janmohamed A, Plant T, et al. Antibodies to gp210 and understanding risk in patients with primary biliary cholangitis. Liver Int 2021;41(3):535–44.

43. Gatselis NK, Zachou K, Norman GL, et al. Clinical significance of the fluctuation of primary biliary cirrhosis-related autoantibodies during the course of the disease. Autoimmunity 2013;46(7):471–9.

44. Tana MM, Shums Z, Milo J, et al. The significance of autoantibody changes over time in primary biliary cirrhosis. Am J Clin Pathol 2015;144(4):601–6.

45. MacSween RN, Horne CH, Moffat AJ, et al. Serum protein levels in primary biliary cirrhosis. J Clin Pathol 1972;25(9):789–92.

46. Poupon RE, Balkau B, Eschwege E, et al. A multicenter, controlled trial of ursodiol for the treatment of primary biliary cirrhosis. UDCA-PBC Study Group. N Engl J Med 1991;324(22):1548–54.

47. Hirschfield GM, Mason A, Luketic V, et al. Efficacy of obeticholic acid in patients with primary biliary cirrhosis and inadequate response to ursodeoxycholic acid. Gastroenterology 2015;148(4):751–761 e8.

48. Hu CJ, Song G, Huang W, et al. Identification of new autoantigens for primary biliary cirrhosis using human proteome microarrays. Mol Cell Proteomics 2012;11(9):669–80.

49. Norman GL, Yang CY, Ostendorff HP, et al. Anti-kelch-like 12 and anti-hexokinase 1: novel autoantibodies in primary biliary cirrhosis. Liver Int 2015;35(2):642–51.

50. Liu ZY, Xu L, Liu B. Detection of anti-kelch-like 12 and anti-hexokinase 1 antibodies in primary biliary cholangitis patients in China. Rev Esp Enferm Dig 2021;113(8):585–90.

51. Reig A, Norman GL, Garcia M, et al. Novel anti-hexokinase 1 antibodies are associated with poor prognosis in patients with primary biliary cholangitis. Am J Gastroenterol 2020;115(10):1634–41.

Treatment of Primary Biliary Cholangitis including Transplantation

Yasameen Muzahim, MD[a], Ali Wakil, MD[a], Mehak Bassi, MD[b],
Nikolaos Pyrsopoulos, MD, PhD, MBA[a],*

KEYWORDS

- PBC treatment • Ursodeoxycholic acid • FXR agonoist • Obeticholic acid

KEY POINTS

- The first-line treatment of primary biliary cholangitis (PBC) is weight-based ursodeoxycholic acid (UDCA) given daily with monitoring response after 6 to 12 months using various prognostic scores.
- The second-line treatment of patients with PBC who either fail to achieve the adequate treatment response to UDCA or are intolerant to obeticholic acid.
- Fibrates can be used in selective patients with PBC as an additive therapy with close monitoring. Multiple ongoing trials are evaluating farsenoid X receptor agonists (such as seladelpar and saroglitazar) and other agents in patients with PBC who are not responsive to first-line therapy. Patients with decompensated PBC cirrhosis or refractory cholestatic pruritus should be considered for liver transplant evaluation.

CURRENT APPROVED PRIMARY BILIARY CHOLANGITIS THERAPY

Once PBC diagnosis is established, treatment should be initiated with the goal of improving liver enzymes and biomarkers, slowing progression of hepatic fibrosis/cirrhosis, and preventing complications of portal hypertension (**Fig. 1**). Currently, only ursodeoxycholic acid (UDCA) and obeticholic acid (OCA) are approved for the treatment of PBC in the United States.

Ursodeoxycholic Acid

The first-line agent for PBC treatment is UDCA, which possesses cytoprotective, immunomodulatory, and anti-inflammatory properties. UDCA is a hydrophilic, viscosity-reducing, bile acid that enhances bile flow and prevents injury to the hepatocytes and the biliary epithelial lining from cholestasis. This in turn reduces

---

[a] Division of Gastroenterology and Hepatlogy, Rutgers New Jersey Medical School, 185 South Orange Avenue, MSB H Rm - 536, Newark, NJ 07101, USA; [b] Division of Gastroenterology and Hepatoloy, Saint Peter's University Hospital, 254 Easton Avenue, New Brunswick, NJ 08901, USA
* Corresponding author. 185 South Orange Avenue, MSB H Room - 536, Newark, NJ 07101-1709.
E-mail address: pyrsopni@njms.rutgers.edu

Clin Liver Dis 28 (2024) 103–114
https://doi.org/10.1016/j.cld.2023.07.003
1089-3261/24/© 2023 Elsevier Inc. All rights reserved.

liver.theclinics.com

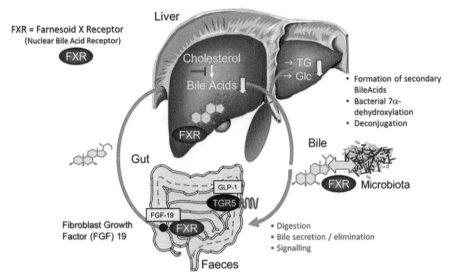

Fig. 1. Mechanism of action of different PBC therapeutic targets. (Trauner, Michael; Fuchs, Claudia Daniela; Halilbasic, Emina; Paumgartner, Gustav. New therapeutic concepts in bile acid transport and signaling for management of cholestasis. Hepatology 65(4):p 1393-1404, April 2017. DOI: 10.1002/hep.28991.)

hepatocellular injury through altering adhesion molecules (Lymphocyte Function Associated Antigen [LFA-I, LFA-II], and Intercellular Adhesion Molecule- I [ICAM-I]), human leukocytes antigen class I and class II expression in the liver and cytokine production.[1]

Before the extensive adoption of UDCA, nearly half of the patients with PBC (49%) would progress to cirrhosis. However, with long-term use of UDCA, the likelihood of progression to cirrhosis has been shown to significantly decrease to approximately 13%. Data has demonstrated UDCA's ability to slow the progression to cirrhosis, reverse fibrosis, and increase transplant-free survival at 5, 10, and 15 years compared with nontreated individuals. Its effect is more profound in younger individuals, patients with earlier histological changes, and higher alkaline phosphatase (ALP) levels. UDCA may be used in patients with advanced disease, where it may help in avoiding or delaying liver transplantation (LT) and has shown a benefit in survival. Several studies have shown consistent evidence in improvement of liver enzymes with the use of UDCA.[2]

The recommended dose is usually 13 to 15 mg/kg/d given in 2 to 3 divided doses; however, UDCA can be given as a once-daily dose to improve compliance. No dose adjustment is needed for renal or liver disease. UDCA absorption can be affected either by bile acid sequestrants such as cholestyramine or by other anion-exchanging resins such as cholestyramine or colestipol. Therefore, UDCA should be given 1 hour before or 4 hours after these agents to enhance absorption.[3] Antacids such as aluminum hydroxide can form complexes with UDCA making it nonabsorbable. There are inconsistent but published data in liver and heart transplant patients that report increased cyclosporin bioavailability with concomitant usage of UDCA administration.[4]

Although evidence is lacking, UDCA is generally used in intrahepatic cholestasis of pregnancy and is considered safe before and during the first trimester of pregnancy.[5] It is unknown whether UDCA is excreted in breast milk; and therefore, it is not approved during lactation.[6] Large-scale, long-period trials have not demonstrated serious adverse effects of UDCA administration. Weight gain in the first 3 months, hair loss, flatulence, and diarrhea are the most frequent side effects reported.[7] The rate of recurrence of PBC after LT is considered to be high, leading perhaps to impaired survival of the patient. A large international study recently demonstrated reduced disease recurrence and graft loss, as well as improved liver-related and all-cause mortality by using preventive UDCA after LT.[8] If tolerated, UDCA is recommended to be used lifelong. Approximately 60% of UDCA-treated patients will have an adequate response after 6 to 12 months of therapy. In patients with an inadequate response to UDCA, a second-line therapy is indicated.[9]

Monitoring response to ursodeoxycholic acid

Biochemical values, especially ALP, are a surrogate marker of treatment efficacy in PBC. A liver biopsy is not indicated to monitor response. Patients who respond to UDCA within 1 year have an excellent prognosis comparable to healthy, unaffected individuals. Improvements on UDCA are seen within a few weeks, even as early as 1 to 2 weeks, and 90% of the response is seen between 6 to 9 months. About 20% of patients will have normal biochemistries after 2 years. Several prognostic scores have been developed to monitor response to UDCA in PBC. These scores help to predict those patients with PBC at an increased risk of death or LT (**Table 1**). The earliest score to predict outcome in late-stage PBC was the Mayo PBC risk score. It showed that after 6 months of UDCA therapy, patients with serum alkaline phosphatase levels less than twice normal ($P < .04$) were more likely to respond favorably to treatment over 2 years. Another prognostic score, the Barcelona criteria, defines the response to treatment by ALP decreased by more than 40% from baseline values or normal levels after 1 year of treatment. A large group of experts from individual centers developed a single score known as the PBC Globe score, which predicts long-term (10-year) survival (**Table 2**). It used the variables of ALP, bilirubin, age, platelet count, and albumin. The transplant-free survival rate during a 10-year period for individuals with a GLOBE score higher than 0.30 is 60%. In contrast, those with a GLOBE score of 0.30 or lower have a notably higher survival rate of 92%.[10]

Obeticholic Acid

OCA is a semisynthetic bile acid analog, 6-ethyl chenodeoxycholic acid, which acts as a farsenoid X receptor (FXR) agonist. OCA is known to be 100 times more effective than endogenous chenodeoxycholic acid. FXR is highly expressed in hepatocytes and enterocytes. FXR signaling directly affects bile acid absorption, secretion, and excretion. OCA stimulation also increases the release of fibroblast growth factor 19 (FGF-19), a cytokine infused into the portal blood, which triggers the inhibitory pathways for cholesterol 7-α-hydroxylase, the rate-limiting enzyme in bile acid synthesis. In addition, OCA has antifibrotic and anti-inflammatory properties.[11]

A phase-2 trial evaluated 3 doses of OCA (10, 25, and 50 mg) compared with placebo in a treatment lasting 3 months. Compared with a 3% reduction in the placebo group, a 21% to 25% reduction in ALP was achieved in the OCA group.[10] The large

Table 1	
Primary biliary cholangitis scoring prediction	
Risk Scoring System	**Included Parameter**
UKC PBC	ALP, bilirubin, and AST (ALT) for 12 months Albumin and platelet count at baseline
Globe Score	ALP, albumin, bilirubin, and platelet count at 12 months Age at diagnosis

Table 2
Ursodeoxycholic acid response monitoring scores

UDCA Response Criteria	Definition of Biochemical Response
Rochester	ALP 2 × ULN
Barcelona	Reduction in ALP 40% from baseline or normalization of ALP after 1 y of treatment
Paris I	ALP < 3 × ULN; AST < 2 × ULN Bilirubin < 1 mg/dL
Rotterdam	Bilirubin <1 × ULN and albumin >1 × lower limit of normal
Toronto	ALP 1.67 × ULN or ALP < 1.76 after 2 y of UDCA
Paris II	ALP 1.5 × ULN; AST 1.5 × ULN after 2 y of UDCA
Rochester	ALP 2 × ULN

phase 3 POISE trial showed significant improvement in alkaline phosphatase at OCA doses of 5 mg or 10 mg compared with placebo (46% vs 47% vs 10%, respectively; $P < .001$). After 1 year of usage, serum ALP less than 1.67 times the upper limit of normal (ULN) was reached in 47% of patients on 10 mg/d and 46% of the patients who were started on 5 mg and increased to 10 mg/d. Additional liver chemistries and inflammatory markers also showed improvement.[12]

OCA is approved as a second-line agent in patients with PBC with either an inadequate response to UDCA or intolerant of UDCA. Inadequate response is defined as by the modified Toronto criteria as ALP greater than 1.67 × ULN and/or elevated bilirubin greater than >2 × ULN after 1-year therapy with UDCA.[11] Approximately 40% of UDCA treated patients will have an inadequate response.

OCA is associated with dose-dependent pruritus, leading to its discontinuation in 1% to 10% of treated patients. Pruritus secondary to can be successively treated with over-the-counter topical treatments, antihistamines, bile acid sequestrants, drug holiday, and other standard treatments of pruritus secondary PBC. With these interventions, discontinuation of therapy is markedly decreased from the published literature. OCA is known to exhibit alterations in serum lipid levels, leading to a mild decrease in HDL in some patients. Its long-term effects on cardiovascular risk factors are unknown.

The recommended dose for initiation in patients without advanced liver disease or compensated Child-Pugh class A is 5 mg/d, with an increase to 10 mg/d if the drug is well tolerated and ALP does not decrease after 3 months of usage. In patients with Child–Pugh class B or C cirrhosis, dosage beyond 5 mg/wk is associated with adverse effects such as liver failure and death. Due to observations of worsening liver disease in these patient groups, the FDA added a black box warning with instructions not to use OCA in patients with advanced cirrhosis with portal hypertension (eg, gastro-esophageal varices, ascites, and persistent thrombocytopenia) or with current or earlier evidence of hepatic dysfunction (coagulopathy and encephalopathy). Therefore, these patients should be referred for LT. Furthermore, it is recommended to carefully monitor any patient with cirrhosis receiving OCA, even if the cirrhosis is not advanced. Long-term efficacy and survival benefits have yet to be proven for OCA.[12]

Investigational Compounds

Many clinical trials are investigating new treatment strategies targeting different stages of the pathogenesis of PBC have been conducted.[13,14]

Peroxisome proliferator-activated receptor agonists

Peroxisome proliferator-activated receptors (PPARs) are nuclear receptors that play a major role in gene transcription and are involved in inflammatory, oncogenic, and metabolic pathways that are considered essential molecular focus in PBC. There are 3 isotypes of PPARs (PPAR-α, PPAR-γ, PPAR-β/δ). PPAR-α in hepatocytes acts as a regulator of bile acid homeostasis, β-oxidation, glucose production, and lipid transport.[15–17]

PPAR-γ, in Kupffer cells, is an immunomodulator for anti-inflammatory activity, which inhibits the production of tumor necrosis factor-α and interleukin-1β. PPAR-β/δ is ubiquitous and mainly found in hepatocytes, cholangiocytes, hepatic Stellate cells, and Kupffer cells. Activation of PPAR-β/δ in Kupffer cells leads to a robust anti-inflammatory response, hepatic carcinogenesis prevention and decreases the rate of liver steatosis. In addition,[18,19] saroglitazar is a dual PPAR α/γ agonist that has potent mechanism in PBC patients. In a proof-of-concept phase II trial, 37 patients with PBC were randomized to saroglitazar 4 mg (n = 13), saroglitazar 2 mg (n = 14), and placebo (n = 10) daily for 16 weeks. Results showed remarkable reduction in mean ALP levels started on week 4 throughout the study duration in both the saroglitazar 4 mg and 2 mg groups ($P < .001$), compared with placebo group (Clinical Trial: NCT03112681).

Bezafibrate is an agonist of all 3 PPAR isoforms. Several studies have shown that bezafibrate was effective in reducing ALP, gamma-glutamyl transferase. (GGT), and immunoglobulin M (IgM), as stand-alone therapy or an add-on to UDCA.[20–22] Clinical trials using fenofibrate suggested that the combination therapy of UDCA and fenofibrate was successful in reducing ALP, GGT, and IgM levels. Other clinical trials have attempted to treat refractory PBC with triple therapy (UDCA, OCA, and fibrates) with higher risks of adverse events despite a remarkable improvement in serological markers.[23,24]

However, *Elafibranor*, a PPARα/δ agonist, has been evaluated in a phase II placebo-controlled trial of 45 patients with PBC who had incomplete response to UDCA. Patients were randomly assigned to elafibranor 80 mg, elafibranor 120 mg, or placebo. The primary endpoint was the relative change of ALP at 12 weeks (NCT03124108). Results showed significant reduction in ALP by 48.3 $\pm$ 14.8% in the elafibranor 80 mg group ($P < .001$ vs placebo) and by 40.6 $\pm$ 17.4% in the elafibranor 120 mg group ($P < .001$) compared with 3.2 $\pm$ 14.8% increase in the placebo group. Levels of Gamma- Glutamyl Transpeptidase (GGTP) decreased by 37.0 $\pm$ 25.5% in the elafibranor 80 mg group ($P < .001$) and 40.0 $\pm$ 24.1% in the elafibranor 120 mg group ($P < .01$) compared with no change in the placebo group.[25]

To the date of this publication, fibrates are not approved for use in PBC in the United States.

Biological and immunosuppressive agents

Multiple immune-suppressive therapies such as corticosteroids, azathioprine, cyclosporine, methotrexate, and mycophenolate mofetil have been used in clinical trials to treat PBC and have not show any therapeutic impact.[26] Similarly, several biologic agents that are known to be standard therapy in other autoimmune conditions such as rituximab,[27–29] ustekinumab,[30] abatacept,[31] and baricitinib have shown no therapeutic effectiveness.

LIVER TRANSPLANT IN PRIMARY BILIARY CHOLANGITIS

Current approved PBC therapies have significantly improved overall disease survival. For those patients who progress to decompensated liver disease, LT is the mainstay of treatment. Interestingly, the number of patients with PBC needing LT has dramatically decreased during the last several decades in developed countries.[13]

The most common indications for LT in patients with PBC are decompensated cirrhosis complicated by portal hypertension with gastroesophageal variceal bleeding, refractory ascites, spontaneous bacterial peritonitis, hepatic encephalopathy, and moderate hepatopulmonary syndrome. Uncontrolled and intolerable pruritus is a special indication for LT in patients with PBC. There is no reported age limit for LT; however, the average age listed for LT in patients with PBC ranges between 53 and 55 years. A retrospective analysis of the United Network for Organ Sharing database for patients undergoing LT between 2002 and 2006 showed that among PBC transplant recipients for living donor LT, the estimated 1-year, 3-year, and 5-year patient survival rates were 93%, 90%, and 86%, respectively, and 90%, 87%, and 85%, respectively.[32–35]

RECURRENT PRIMARY BILIARY CHOLANGITIS

The recurrence rate of PBC in patients who had LT ranges between 21% and 37% at 10 years post-LT. Median time to graft loss secondary to recurrent primary biliary cholangitis (rPBC) showed no difference in survival between those with and without recurrent disease.[36,37]

Many risk factors for rPBC have been studied and results suggest a positive correlation between younger recipient age and a higher rate of recurrence. However, Silveira and colleagues study showed higher risk of recurrence in older patients at the time of LT. The role of HLA mismatch on the recurrence rate remains controversial. Another study showed that patterns alleles such as B48 in donors and recipients were more associated with rPBC.[13,32,36]

Donor age greater than 65 years is associated with a recurrence rate if the recipient is on tacrolimus immunosuppression. Cold ischemic time was found to be a risk factor for recurrence while warm ischemic time was not.[38,39]

The definitive diagnosis of rPBC depends on histopathological findings unlike diagnosing de novo PBC where clinical and serological findings are especially useful. Sylvestre and colleagues[39] showed that one-third to one-half of patients with a definitive histological diagnosis of rPBC had normal ALP levels at the time of biopsy. In rPBC, the histologic hallmarks of the recurrence are damage to the bile ducts, lymphoid aggregate formations, and the presence of mononuclear inflammatory infiltrate or epithelioid granulomas. If 2 or 4 of these characteristics are present in the liver biopsy, a diagnosis of rPBC is highly probable. The diagnosis is definitive if all the 4 characteristics are recognized.[32]

To date, the only available effective treatment of rPBC is UDCA. There are several observational studies that show reinduction of UDCA leads to biochemical improvement. Moreover, recently published studies even suggest a beneficial effect of UDCA use post-LT for the prevention of rPBC progression.[40,41] Further studies in the future are needed to address the preventive effect of UDCA on rPBC extensively and to officialize its use as a prophylactic therapy post-LT.

MANAGEMENT OF SPECIFIC PRIMARY BILIARY CHOLANGITIS SYMPTOMS
Fatigue

The majority of PBC patients experience fatigue at some point during the disease course. The management of fatigue should include an evaluation for causes of fatigue such as hypothyroidism, anemia, and sleep disorders. Modafinil, a neurostimulator approved for the treatment of narcolepsy, showed encouraging results in open-label trials[42]; however, it failed to impact fatigue in larger randomized control trials.[43] Other serotonin receptor agents, such as ondansetron (a 5-HT3 inhibitor) and fluoxetine/fluvoxamine (selective serotonin reuptake inhibitors), have failed to improve fatigue in clinical studies.[44,45] Despite not being extensively tested for fatigue in patients with PBC, a trial of caffeine intake could be recommended because it is readily available, can increase energy levels, and has antifibrotic effects in slowing fibrosis/cirrhosis progression.[46]

Pruritus

The lack of a clear understanding of the exact mechanism of pruritus in PBC makes treatment challenging. A stepwise approach is recommended to achieve clinical response and improve the quality of life for the patient. Cholestyramine—a bile acid resin binder—is the first-line therapy. The recommended dose is 4 grams per dose taken 1 to 4 times a day, 1 hour before or 4 hours after other medications, to avoid absorption inhibition. Cholestyramine has a long track record of clinical efficacy but clinical trials were small.[47,48] Colesevelam is an oral bile acid binder that had no clinical efficacy in a randomized clinical trial.[49]

Rifampicin is a second-line agent for pruritus given in 150 mg to 300 mg once a day. Multiple meta-analyses that showed improvement in cholestatic pruritus in multiple clinical trials.[50,51] Rifampin is cytochrome P450 induced and has multiple drug–drug interactions. Side effects include nephrotoxicity, hemolysis, and potential drug-induced liver injury with jaundice. Rifampicin should be given with caution with close monitoring and is usually not advised in patients with a serum bilirubin level greater than 2.5 mg/dL.[52] Rifampicin can lead to yellow–red urine, which is related to its metabolism and is not of clinical concern. It also may turn other body fluids such as tears orange–red, which may cause contact lenses to become discolored. Naltrexone, an opioid antagonist that can decrease endogenous opioids, is a third-line agent used to treat the pruritus of PBC. A large study compared naltrexone and nalmefene to placebo and revealed significant improvement in pruritus.[53] The high circulating endogenous opioid levels seen in patients with PBC render patients treated with naltrexone to be at risk for opioid withdrawal symptoms. Barbiturates, such as phenobarbital, can also improve pruritus but are rarely used due to their strong sedative effects, effect of worsening fat-soluble vitamin deficiency, and gingival hyperplasia.[54]

Sertraline, a selective serotonin receptor inhibitor is recommended as fourth-line therapy for the pruritus of PBC. The recommended initial dose is 25 mg every day with increases in 25 mg increments every 4 to 5 days until a dose of 75 to 100 mg is achieved. A small, placebo-controlled trial and retrospective case series showed that sertraline was well tolerated and that it was effective in reducing symptoms of pruritus.[54,55]

Patients whose pruritus does not respond to the interventions above are termed refractory pruritus. Refractory pruritus can be treated with interventions such plasmapheresis, molecular adsorbent recirculating system, or light therapy, although no randomized controlled trials exist to validate their efficacy. Newer agents, such as PAR agonists and inhibitors of the ileal bile acid reabsorption transport, are being investigated for cholestatic pruritus.[56] Patients with severe refractory pruritus nonresponsive to all interventions should be referred for LT even if the liver function is normal.

Hyperlipidemia

In spite of the close association between PBC and hyperlipidemia with pathognomonic xanthelasmas, studies demonstrate no relation between hyperlipidemia and cardiovascular events in patients with PBC.[57,58] A recent meta-analysis challenged this data with an increased pooled risk 1.57 (95% CI 1.21–2.06).[58,59] Treatment of hyperlipidemia in these patients is usually not indicated unless there is a strong family history of cardiovascular events, risk factors for coronary disease, painful xanthelasma, or unfavorable lipoprotein results. 3-Hydroxy-3-methylglutaryl-coenzyme A reductase (HMG-CoA) inhibitors, such as statins, are effective and safe in patients with PBC with mildly elevated liver enzymes, and fibrates were also found to be safe in select patients.[60]

Osteoporosis

PBC can decrease bone formation leading to osteoporosis with an incidence as high as 20% to 40%.[61] Baseline bone densitometry and biannual repeat densitometry thereafter is recommended by most guidelines.[12] Randomized clinical trials for osteoporosis treatment in PBC are scarce, and most recommended therapy is based on data from the treatment of osteoporosis in postmenopausal women. Daily vitamin D supplementation and monitoring of vitamin D levels annually is recommended for all patients with PBC. When osteoporosis is diagnosed, biphosphate is recommended. Alendronate and ibandronate were effective in osteoporosis reversal in patients with PBC.[62,63] Etidronate did not reveal clinical efficacy in patients with PBC.[64] Hormonal replacement therapy has shown some improvement in bone density but is rarely used due to toxicity.[65]

Sicca Syndrome

Treatment of Sicca syndrome in PBC is similar to that of Sicca syndrome. Mild keratoconjunctivitis can be managed with hydroxypropyl methylcellulose eye drops. Moderate and severe keratoconjunctivitis should be evaluated by an ophthalmologist and patients considered for immunosuppressive eyedrops such as cyclosporine drops.[66] Refractory symptoms can be managed with cholinergic agents such as pilocarpine and/or ophthalmological procedures such as punctate blocking or light therapy to prevent the draining of tears. Xerostomia can cause dental caries, so patients should receive regular dental care. Treatment includes frequent water sips and sugar-free gum. Anticholinergic drugs can be used, although patients may experience side effects.[67]

SUMMARY

Treatment of PBC follows a stepwise approach with UDCA as first-line therapy and OCA as second-line treatment. Novel therapies such as PPAR agonists are being investigated for their role in PBC treatment. Management of complications of PBC is symptom specific, and LT remains the mainstay of treatment of decompensated disease although recurrent PBC following transplantation is not uncommon.

DISCLOSURE

Pyrsopoulos, NT is a recipient of research grants paid to institution from GILEAD, SALIX, GRIFOLS, CYTOSORBENT, DURECT, OCELOT which are outside the submitted work. Muzahem, Y., Wakil, A, Bassi, M has no conflict of interests related to this publication.

Funding: None used.

REFERENCES

1. Harms MH, van Buuren HR, Corpechot C, et al. Ursodeoxycholic acid therapy and liver transplant-free survival in patients with primary biliary cholangitis. J Hepatol 2019;71(2):357–65.

2. Pares A, Caballeria J, Rodes J. Excellent long-term survival in patient with primary biliary cirrhosis and biochemical response to ursodeoxycholic acid. Gastroenterology 2006;130:715–20.

3. Caroli-Bosc FX, Iliadis A, Salmon L, et al. Ursodeoxycholic acid modulates cyclosporin A oral absorption in liver transplant recipients. Fundam Clin Pharmacol 2000;14(6):601–9.

4. Kondrackiene J, Beuers U, Kupcinskas L. Efficacy and safety of ursodeoxycholic acid versus cholestyramine in intrahepatic cholestasis of pregnancy. Gastroenterology 2005;129(3):894–901.

5. Rudi J, Schönig T, Stremmel W. Therapie mit Ursodeoxycholsäure bei primär biliärer Zirrhose während der Schwangerschaft [-Therapy with ursodeoxycholic acid in primary biliary cirrhosis in pregnancy-]. Z Gastroenterol 1996;34(3): 188–91.

6. Parés A, Caballería L, Rodés J, et al. Long-term effects of ursodeoxycholic acid in primary biliary cirrhosis: results of a double-blind controlled multicentric trial. UDCA-Cooperative Group from the Spanish Association for the Study of the Liver. J Hepatol 2000;32(4):561–6.

7. Corpechot C, Chazouillères O, Belnou P, et al. Long-term impact of preventive UDCA therapy after transplantation for primary biliary cholangitis. J Hepatol 2020;73(3):559–65. PJ Obeticholic acid for the treatment of primary biliary cirrhosis. Expert Rev Clin Pharmacol 2016).

8. Hirschfield GM, Mason A, Luketic V, et al. Efficacy of obeticholic acid in patients with primary biliary cirrhosis and inadequate response to ursodeoxycholic acid. Gastroenterology 2015;148(4):751–61.e8.

9. Nevens F, Andreone P, Mazzella G, et al, POISE Study Group. A placebo-controlled trial of obeticholic acid in primary biliary cholangitis. N Engl J Med 2016;375(7):631–43.

10. Lindor KD. Primary biliary cholangitis: 2018 practice guidance from the american association for the study of liver diseases. Hepatology 2019;69(1):394–419.

11. Trivedi PJ, Hirschfield GM, Gershwin ME. Obeticholic acid for the treatment of primary biliary cirrhosis. Expet Rev Clin Pharmacol 2016;9(1):13–26.

12. Kowdley KV A randomized trial of obeticholic acid monotherapy in patients with primary biliary cholangitis. Hepatology 2018;67:1890–902.

13. Poupon R. Primary biliary cirrhosis: a 2010 update. J Hepatol 2010;52(5):745–58.

14. Kaplan MM, Gershwin ME. Primary biliary cirrhosis. N Engl J Med 2005;353(12): 1261–73.

15. Aguilar MT, Chascsa DM. Update on emerging treatment options for primary biliary cholangitis. Hepatic Med 2020;12:69–77.

16. Colapietro F, Gershwin ME, Lleo A. PPAR agonists for the treatment of primary biliary cholangitis: old and new tales. Journal of translational autoimmunity 2023;6:100188.

17. Wang C, Shi Y, Wang X, et al. Peroxisome proliferator-activated receptors regulate hepatic immunity and assist in the treatment of primary biliary cholangitis. Front Immunol 2022;13:940688.

18. Li C, Zheng K, Chen Y, et al. A randomized, controlled trial on fenofibrate in primary biliary cholangitis patients with incomplete response to ursodeoxycholic acid. Therapeutic advances in chronic disease 2022;13. 20406223221114198.

19. Willson TM, Brown PJ, Sternbach DD, et al. The PPARs: from orphan receptors to drug discovery. J Med Chem 2000;43(4):527–50.

20. Zhang Y, Chen K, Dai W, et al. Combination therapy of bezafibrate and ursodeoxycholic acid for primary biliary cirrhosis: a meta-analysis. Hepatology research 2015;45(1):48–58.

21. Iwasaki S, Ohira H, Nishiguchi S, et al, Study Group of Intractable Liver Diseases for Research on a Specific Disease, Health Science Research Grant, Ministry of Health, Labour and Welfare of Japan. The efficacy of ursodeoxycholic acid and bezafibrate combination therapy for primary biliary cirrhosis: a prospective, multicenter study. Hepatology research 2008;38(6):557–64.

22. Agrawal R, Majeed M, Attar BM, et al. Effectiveness of bezafibrate and ursodeoxycholic acid in patients with primary biliary cholangitis: a meta-analysis of randomized controlled trials. Annals of gastroenterology 2019;32(5):489–97.

23. Liberopoulos EN, Florentin M, Elisaf MS, et al. Fenofibrate in primary biliary cirrhosis: a pilot study. The open cardiovascular medicine journal 2010;4:120–6.

24. Schattenberg JM, Pares A, Kowdley KV, et al. A randomized placebo-controlled trial of elafibranor in patients with primary biliary cholangitis and incomplete response to UDCA. J Hepatol 2021;74(6):1344–54.

25. Gerussi A, Lucà M, Cristoferi L, et al. New therapeutic targets in autoimmune cholangiopathies. Front Med 2020;7:117.

26. Tsuda M, Moritoki Y, Lian ZX, et al. Biochemical and immunologic effects of rituximab in patients with primary biliary cirrhosis and an incomplete response to ursodeoxycholic acid. Hepatology 2012;55(2):512–21.

27. Myers RP, Swain MG, Lee SS, et al. B-cell depletion with rituximab in patients with primary biliary cirrhosis refractory to ursodeoxycholic acid. Am J Gastroenterol 2013;108(6):933–41.

28. Hirschfield GM, Gershwin ME, Strauss R, et al, PURIFI Study Group. Ustekinumab for patients with primary biliary cholangitis who have an inadequate response to ursodeoxycholic acid: a proof-of-concept study. Hepatology 2016; 64(1):189–99.

29. Bowlus CL, Yang GX, Liu CH, et al. Therapeutic trials of biologics in primary biliary cholangitis: an open label study of abatacept and review of the literature. J Autoimmun 2019;101:26–34.

30. Villarino AV, Kanno Y, O'Shea JJ. Mechanisms and consequences of Jak-STAT signaling in the immune system. Nat Immunol 2017;18(4):374–84.

31. Pinzani M, Luong TV. Pathogenesis of biliary fibrosis. Biochimica et biophysica acta. Molecular basis of disease 2018;1864(4 Pt B):1279–83.

32. Mijic M, Saric I, Delija B, et al. Pretransplant evaluation and liver transplantation outcome in PBC patients. Canadian journal of gastroenterology & hepatology 2022;2022:7831165.

33. Akamatsu N, Sugawara Y. Primary biliary cirrhosis and liver transplantation. Intractable & rare diseases research 2012;1(2):66–80.

34. European Association for the Study of the Liver. EASL clinical practice guidelines: liver transplantation. J Hepatol 2016;64(2):433–85.

35. Lee J, Belanger A, Doucette JT, et al. Transplantation trends in primary biliary cirrhosis. Clin Gastroenterol Hepatol 2007;5(11):1313–5.

36. Neuberger J. Recurrent primary biliary cirrhosis. Liver Transplant 2003;9(6):539–46.

37. Aguilar MT, Carey EJ. Current status of liver transplantation for primary biliary cholangitis. Clin Liver Dis 2018;22(3):613–24.

38. Silveira MG, Talwalkar JA, Lindor KD, et al. Recurrent primary biliary cirrhosis after liver transplantation. Am J Transplant 2010;10(4):720–6.

39. Sylvestre PB, Batts KP, Burgart LJ, et al. Recurrence of primary biliary cirrhosis after liver transplantation: histologic estimate of incidence and natural history. Liver Transplant 2003;9(10):1086–93.

40. Sanchez EQ, Levy MF, Goldstein RM, et al. The changing clinical presentation of recurrent primary biliary cirrhosis after liver transplantation. Transplantation 2003; 76(11):1583–8.

41. Bosch A, Dumortier J, Maucort-Boulch D, et al. Preventive administration of UDCA after liver transplantation for primary biliary cirrhosis is associated with a lower risk of disease recurrence. J Hepatol 2015;63(6):1449–58.

42. Jones DE, Newton JL. An open study of modafinil for the treatment of daytime somnolence and fatigue in primary biliary cirrhosis. Aliment Pharmacol Ther 2007;25(4):471–6, 114.

43. Silveira MG, Gossard AA, Stahler AC, et al. A randomized, placebo-controlled clinical trial of efficacy and safety: modafinil in the treatment of fatigue in patients with primary biliary cirrhosis. Am J Therapeut 2017;24(2):e167–76.

44. Theal JJ, Toosi MN, Girlan L, et al. A randomized, controlled crossover trial of on-dansetron in patients with primary biliary cirrhosis and fatigue. Hepatology 2005; 41(6):1305–12, 111.

45. Prince MI, Mitchison HC, Ashley D, et al. Oral antioxidant supplementation for fatigue associated with primary biliary cirrhosis: results of a multicentre, randomized, placebo-controlled, cross-over trial. Aliment Pharmacol Ther 2003;17(1): 137–43, 112.

46. Kennedy OJ, Roderick P, Buchanan R, et al. Systematic review with meta-analysis: coffee consumption and the risk of cirrhosis. Aliment Pharmacol Ther 2016;43(5):562–74.

47. Van Itallie TB, Hashim SA, Crampton RS, et al. The treatment of pruritus and hypercholesteremia of primary biliary cirrhosis with cholestyramine. N Engl J Med 1961;265:469–74.

48. Tandon P, Rowe BH, Vandermeer B, et al. The efficacy and safety of bile Acid binding agents, opioid antagonists, or rifampin in the treatment of cholestasis-associated pruritus. Am J Gastroenterol 2007;102(7):1528–36.

49. Kuiper EM, van Erpecum KJ, Beuers U, et al. The potent bile acid sequestrant colesevelam is not effective in cholestatic pruritus: results of a double-blind, randomized, placebo-controlled trial. Hepatology 2010;52(4):1334–40.

50. Ghent CN, Carruthers SG. Treatment of pruritus in primary biliary cirrhosis with rifampin. Results of a double-blind, crossover, randomized trial. Gastroenterology 1988;94(2):488–93.

51. Khurana S, Singh P. Rifampin is safe for treatment of pruritus due to chronic cholestasis: a meta-analysis of prospective randomized-controlled trials. Liver Int 2006;26(8):943–8.

52. Prince MI, Burt AD, Jones DE. Hepatitis and liver dysfunction with rifampicin therapy for pruritus in primary biliary cirrhosis. Gut 2002;50(3):436–9.

53. Bergasa NV, Alling DW, Talbot TL, et al. Oral nalmefene therapy reduces scratching activity due to the pruritus of cholestasis: a controlled study. J Am Acad Dermatol 1999;41(3 Pt 1):431–4.

54. Bloomer JR, Boyer JL. Phenobarbital effects in cholestatic liver diseases. Ann Intern Med 1975;82(3):310–7.

55. Mayo MJ, Handem I, Saldana S, et al. Sertraline as a first-line treatment for cholestatic pruritus. Hepatology 2007;45(3):666–74.

56. Parés A, Cisneros L, Salmerón JM, et al. Extracorporeal albumin dialysis: a procedure for prolonged relief of intractable pruritus in patients with primary biliary cirrhosis. Am J Gastroenterol 2004;99(6):1105–10.
57. Van Dam GM, Gips CH. Primary biliary cirrhosis in The Netherlands. An analysis of associated diseases, cardiovascular risk, and malignancies on the basis of mortality figures. Scand J Gastroenterol 1997;32(1):77–83.
58. Allocca M, Crosignani A, Gritti A, et al. Hypercholesterolaemia is not associated with early atherosclerotic lesions in primary biliary cirrhosis. Gut 2006;55(12): 1795–800.
59. Ungprasert P, Wijarnpreecha K, Ahuja W, et al. Coronary artery disease in primary biliary cirrhosis: a systematic review and meta-analysis of observational studies. Hepatol Res 2015;45(11):1055–61.
60. Bader T. The myth of statin-induced hepatotoxicity. Am J Gastroenterol 2010; 105(5):978–80.
61. Danford CJ, Trivedi HD, Papamichael K, et al. Osteoporosis in primary biliary cholangitis. World J Gastroenterol 2018;24(31):3513–20.
62. Zein CO, Jorgensen RA, Clarke B, et al. Alendronate improves bone mineral density in primary biliary cirrhosis: a randomized placebo-controlled trial. Hepatology 2005;42(4):762–71.
63. Guañabens N, Monegal A, Cerdá D, et al. Randomized trial comparing monthly ibandronate and weekly alendronate for osteoporosis in patients with primary biliary cirrhosis. Hepatology 2013;58(6):2070–8.
64. Guañabens N, Parés A, Ros I, et al. Alendronate is more effective than etidronate for increasing bone mass in osteopenic patients with primary biliary cirrhosis. Am J Gastroenterol 2003;98(10):2268–74.
65. Boone RH, Cheung AM, Girlan LM, et al. Osteoporosis in primary biliary cirrhosis: a randomized trial of the efficacy and feasibility of estrogen/progestin. Dig Dis Sci 2006;51(6):1103–12.
66. Tatlipinar S, Akpek EK. Topical ciclosporin in the treatment of ocular surface disorders. Br J Ophthalmol 2005;89(10):1363–7.
67. Mavragani CP, Moutsopoulos HM. Conventional therapy of Sjogren's syndrome. Clin Rev Allergy Immunol 2007;32(3):284–91.

Systemic Complications of Primary Biliary Cholangitis

Mariana Zapata, MD, Hendrick Pagan-Torres, MD,
Marlyn J. Mayo, MD*

KEYWORDS

- PBC • PSC • Dry eyes • Bone • Cholangiocarcinoma • Hepatocellular carcinoma
- Lipoprotein x • Renal

KEY POINTS

- Primary Biliary Cholangitis (PBC) is a disorder in which the immune system impairs the excretion of bile from the liver by damaging the small and medium sized bile ducts responsible for carrying bile from the liver to the intestine.
- Retained bile in the liver refluxes into the plasma and can affect multiple organs throughout the body, such as bone (osteoporosis), kidney (bile cast nephropathy), heart (arrythmias), and the nervous system (fatigue, impaired cognition, and itching).
- Cholesterol, the precursor for bile acid synthesis, accumulates and also refluxes into the plasma leading to dyslipidemia.
- The relative paucity of bile reaching the intestine leads to changes in the microbiome and impairs absorption of fat soluble vitamins.
- The immune-mediated destruction of bile ducts is emulated in the salivary and tear ducts, leading to dry eyes and mouth.
- Progression to cirrhosis is associated with increased risk of hepatobiliary cancers.

INTRODUCTION

Primary biliary cholangitis (PBC) is a progressive inflammatory disorder that results in cholestasis. PBC can lead to clinical consequences related to chronic cholestasis that affect numerous organ systems beyond the liver (**Fig. 1**). For instance, patients with PBC often experience pruritus, fatigue, and cognitive dysfunction, which can have a profound negative effect on patients' quality of life. Throughout the course of the disease, patients with PBC are frequently diagnosed with fat-soluble vitamin deficiencies, osteopenia, osteoporosis, and hyperlipidemia. Patients with PBC are more likely to experience Sicca symptoms. Less-recognized complications of chronic cholestasis

University of Texas Southwestern Medical Center, 5323 Harry Hines Boulevard, Dallas, Texas 75390-8887, USA
* Corresponding author. 5323 Harry Hines Boulevard, Dallas, TX 75390.
E-mail address: Marlyn.mayo@utsouthwestern.edu

Clin Liver Dis 28 (2024) 115–128
https://doi.org/10.1016/j.cld.2023.07.004
1089-3261/24/© 2023 Elsevier Inc. All rights reserved.
liver.theclinics.com

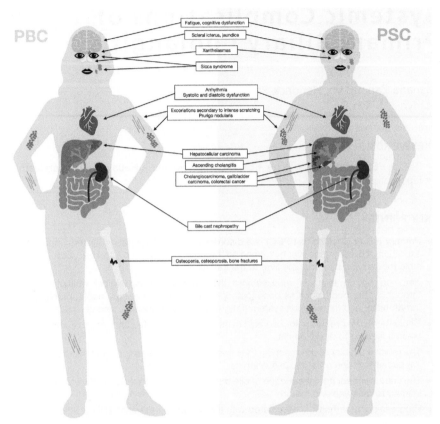

Fig. 1. The systemic consequences of chronic cholestasis in PBC, as compared to those in primary sclerosing cholangitis (PSC).

include cardiac conduction abnormalities, systolic and diastolic cardiac dysfunction as well as bile cast nephropathy and renal tubular acidosis (RTA). In this article, we will discuss the current understanding of the pathophysiology associated with the consequences of chronic cholestasis in PBC as well as therapeutic interventions aimed at improving quality of life and preventing further complications.

Pruritus

Pruritus (itch) associated with PBC can be a disabling symptom that greatly impairs the quality of life. Pruritus occurs in 50% to 80% of patients with PBC. It waxes and wanes and has a poor correlation with disease severity. Pruritus can be present in very early stages of disease and can remain even with normalization of liver enzymes. However, it may also progress with increasing cholestasis and then paradoxically vanish at the very end-stage of disease. It does, however, improve with liver transplantation.[1] Cholestatic pruritus prefers the limbs, palms, and soles, and it follows a circadian rhythm with worsening at night. There is no primary rash but scratching can result in secondary excoriations or prurigo nodularis, a chronic inflammatory skin condition characterized by intensely pruritic, hyperkeratotic nodules.[2] Severe pruritus can result in both physical and mental distress, leading to social isolation, insomnia, and even suicidal ideation.

The pathogenesis of pruritus of cholestasis remains poorly understood. However, it is thought that puritogens bind to receptors on unmyelinated itch C-fibers in the skin and subsequently activate a complex neural cascade leading to the sensation of itch.[3] Puritogen candidates include lysophosphatidic acid, autotaxin, sulfated progesterone metabolites, endogenous opioids, exogenous compounds, bile acids, and others.[3,4] Bile acids have been proposed as the main culprit for cholestatic pruritus for decades. Although there has been no clear correlation between the serum bile acid concentrations and the degree of accumulation in the skin with itch intensity,[3,5] therapies directed at reducing bile acid levels are beneficial. Cholestatic pruritus is not associated with histaminergic activation.

According to the American Association for the Study of Liver Diseases guidelines,[6] treatment options for cholestatic pruritus in PBC include anion exchange resins such as cholestyramine, colestipol, and colesevelam; the pregnane X receptor agonist, rifampicin; the mu-opioid antagonist naltrexone; and serotonin reuptake inhibitor sertraline (**Table 1**). Additionally, patients should be advised to use topical emollients, and to avoid heat, and hot baths. Antihistamines can be helpful, likely due to their sedating effect. However, patients should be counseled on the anticholinergic side effects, which may worsen Sicca syndrome symptoms. For intractable cases, phenobarbital, phototherapy, and plasmapheresis or albumin dialysis have been reported in small cases series as being effective.[6] In rare cases, external biliary drainage or liver transplantation should be considered as a last resort for patients who have failed all other measures. Ursodeoxycholic acid is not a very effective agent to treat cholestatic

Table 1
Evidence-based treatments for cholestatic pruritus associated with primary biliary cholangitis

Medication	Drug Class	Dose (Daily)	Side Effects/ Contraindications	US Guideline-Recommended
Cholestyramine	Anion exchange resin	4–16 g	Impaired drug absorption. Bloating, constipation, diarrhea	Yes
Rifampin	Pregnane X receptor agonist	150–600 mg	Hepatotoxicity, hemolytic anemia, renal failure, thrombotic thrombocytopenia purpura. Avoid if bilirubin >2.5 mg/dL	Yes
Naltrexone	Mu-opioid antagonist	50–100 mg	Patients with high opioidergic tone may experience an opiate withdrawal-like reaction	Yes
Sertraline	Serotonin reuptake inhibitor	75–100 mg	Headache, sleep disturbance	Yes
Phenobarbital	Barbiturate	60–100 mg	Strong sedative. May worsen fatigue. Associated with gingival hyperplasia	Yes
Bezafibrate	Pan-PPAR agonist	400 mg	Renal insufficiency, myopathy	No

pruritus.[7] Notably, clinicians should be aware that obeticholic acid has a dose-dependent increase in pruritus reported in about 40% of patients, which may lead to discontinuation of therapy.[8]

Novel therapeutics being studied for cholestatic pruritus include PPAR agonists, as well as apical sodium-dependent bile acid transporter (ASBT) inhibitors. Bezafibrate, a PPAR agonist, which has been shown to reduce moderate-to-severe pruritus by more than 50% in patients with PBC in a double-blind, randomized, placebo-controlled trial in 2021.[9] The European Association for the Study of the Liver (EASL) clinical practice guidelines for primary sclerosing cholangitis published in 2022 have adapted bezafibrate as a first-line treatment of moderate-to-severe pruritus, although bezafibrate is not yet available in the United States.[10] Linerixibat and volixibat, inhibitors of the ileal bile acid transporter (IBAT, or apical sodium bile acid transporter, ASBT), are under development as a novel treatment of cholestatic pruritus. They interfere with the enterohepatic circulation of bile acids, minimizing the accumulation of bile acids and their associated toxicity. In 2022, a large international, multicenter, phase 2, randomized trial, which included 147 patients with PBC with moderate itching were treated with linerixibat versus placebo. Although linerixibat effect on itch was not significantly different versus placebo in the primary intent-to-treat analysis, it was associated with a significant dose-dependent reduction in itch in the per protocol population. Gastrointestinal distress was the most common side effect.[11] Other ASBT inhibitors have been shown to be beneficial in treating pruritus of pediatric cholestasis disorders, such as Alagille syndrome and progressive familial intrahepatic cholestasis[12,13] and have been approved by regulatory agencies. However, additional investigations are needed in the adult population.

Fatigue and Cognitive Impairment

The feeling of fatigue is characterized by an overwhelming sense of tiredness, lack of energy, and exhaustion.[14] In patients with PBC, fatigue is perhaps the most common symptom affecting more than 50% of the patients, affecting their quality of life. Fatigue does not correlate well with the disease activity and may lead to social isolation, altered mood, loss of appetite sleep disturbances, and it may be associated with decreased overall survival.[6,15,16] Fatigue may be caused by multiple causes other than PBC; hence patients should be evaluated for hypothyroidism, depressive disorders, vitamin D deficiency, anemia, and sleep disorders such as sleep apnea.

The pathophysiological component of fatigue on cholestatic liver disease is unknown, and it is thought to be multifactorial involving liver-CNS inflammatory axis, structural abnormalities in CNS anatomy, autonomic nervous system dysfunction, neurohormonal dysregulation, and microbiome alterations.[17] In PBC, fatigue may present as 2 different entities consisting of peripheral and central fatigue.[14] In peripheral fatigue, neuromuscular manifestations may be seen such as muscle weakness due to a change from aerobic to anaerobic metabolism leading to excessive lactic acid accumulation and therefore accelerated decline in muscle function and prolonged recovery time.[14] Central fatigue is associated with cognitive impairment, poor memory and concentration, sleep–wake disturbances with delayed sleep timing, worse sleep quality, and excessive daytime somnolence, which may be mistaken for hepatic encephalopathy. The underlying mechanisms leading to central fatigue are unknown. A randomized controlled trial of the stimulant, modafinil, in PBC to aid in daytime somnolence showed no benefit.[18] Serotonergic medications have also been studied because one of the theories involves serotonergic and noradrenaline pathways but they have also been unsuccessful.[14–16]

As of right now, there is no recommended therapy for the treatment of fatigue. Although agents such as ursodeoxycholic acid (UDCA), obeticholic acid, fibrates, and budesonide have been explored, none has proven to be effective in treating fatigue.[14–16] Clinicians may emphasize lifestyle changes and coping mechanisms in order to deal with these symptoms. Pruritus, dehydration, and medications such as beta-blockers may also contribute to worsening fatigue. Exercise is encouraged at whatever degree is tolerated by the patient.

Metabolic Bone Disease

Metabolic bone disease can result from cholestasis in a variety of ways, most commonly decreased bone density, with osteopenia, defined as a T score between −1 and –2.5, and osteoporosis, defined as a T score of less than 2.5.[19,20]

Unconjugated bilirubin may contribute to impaired osteoblast proliferative capacity in cultured human osteoblasts, which may play a role in reduced bone formation.[21] Lithocholic acid and unconjugated bilirubin can upregulate osteoblast-induced osteoclastogenesis.[22] UDCA increases osteoblast differentiation and mineralization and neutralizes the detrimental effects of lithocholic acid, bilirubin, and sera from jaundiced patient on human osteoblast cells, thus exerting a possible positive effect on bone in patients with cholestatic liver disease.[23] Clinical trials of UDCA of short duration, however, have not shown improvements in bone density as a secondary endpoint.[23]

Patients with PBC should undergo risk assessment for osteopenia and osteoporosis.[20,24] These risk factors include age, female gender, smoking, excessive alcohol use, low body weight (body mass index <19 kg/m^2) early menopause (before age 45 years), positive family history, and treatment with steroids.[20] If risk factors are identified, intervention is justified, which may include lifestyle changes, adequate nutrition, and weight-bearing exercises.[24] All patients should undergo screening with a bone density scan at the time of diagnosis and repeat bone density scan every 1 to 2 years.[6,15,19,20]

Patients with normal bone density and no history of nephrolithiasis should receive calcium (1000–1200 mg/d) and Vitamin D (1000 U/d). Vitamin D should be measured annually with a goal of greater than 30 ng/mL.[16,19] Treatment of decreased bone density should consider any history of earlier fragility fracture as well as the FRAX score 10-year probability of major osteoporotic fracture.[16,25]

Treatment ideally involves an interdisciplinary approach with an endocrinologist and the patient's primary care provider. Bisphosphonate therapy is the main stay of therapy, which has been shown to increase bone mass in patients with osteoporosis, with major side effects being gastrointestinal complaints, such as pill-induced esophagitis and dyspepsia. Although oral bisphosphonates have not been shown to increase the risk of gastrointestinal bleeding in patients with varices, they do increase endoscopic esophagitis and gastritis,[26] so IV therapy may be preferred in some instances, such as large varices that are untreated or undergoing serial band ligation.[15,16,24] The management of metabolic bone disease is summarized in **Box 1**.[24]

Hyperlipidemia

Serum lipid derangements are common in chronic cholestatic liver diseases, such as PBC. At presentation, 76% of patients diagnosed with PBC have hypercholesterolemia.[27,28] The mechanism for hyperlipidemia in chronic cholestasis stems from poor delivery of bile acids to the ileum and their progressive accumulation in hepatocytes, with subsequent regurgitation into the systemic circulation. Low bile acid concentration in the intestine and high systemic bile acid levels lead to suppression of de novo bile acid synthesis in the liver from its precursor, cholesterol, through a negative feedback loop. Bile is the normal excretory pathway for cholesterol, so both reduced bile

---

Box 1
Management of metabolic bone disease in cholestatic liver disease

Identify risk factors and address:
• Age
• Female Gender
• Tobacco use
• Heavy alcohol consumption
• Underweight
• Family history
• Early menopause
• Treatment with steroids

DEXA scans:
• At diagnosis of PBC and every 2 y
• Calculate FRAX score
• Consider bisphosphonates for t score < −1.5
• Evaluate for varices and determine if IV may be preferred.
• Consider referral to endocrinology for assistance

Start vitamin D and calcium:
• Calcium 1000 to 1200 mg daily
• Vitamin D 1000 IU daily
• Avoid in patients with history of renal stones

Encourage weight-bearing and resistance exercises

Encourage adequate nutrition

---

flow and reduced new bile acid formation leads to the accumulation of cholesterol. In addition, low intestinal bile acids also reduce intestinal absorption of cholesterol. Therefore, there is compensatory endogenous cholesterol synthesis in the liver and decreased uptake of low-density lipoproteins by hepatic receptors. All of these factors lead to high serum cholesterol levels but not fatty liver.[29] In early stages of cholestasis, dyslipidemia is manifested by elevated levels high-density lipoprotein. Later in the disease course, dyslipidemia is characterized by elevated total cholesterol, low-density lipoprotein, high-density lipoprotein, as well as the appearance of the aberrant lipoprotein-X (Lp-X). Lp-X contains a high proportion of nonesterified cholesterol, phospholipids, albumin within its core, and a smaller amount of triglycerides and cholesterol esters (**Fig. 2**).[30] Lp-X is hypothesized to form because of bile regurgitation into the blood.[31,32] However, recent evidence suggests Lp-X is synthesized in the liver and secreted directly into the blood.[30] Both hypercholesterolemia and formation of Lp-X are thought to be a protective mechanism aimed at inactivating the detergent effects of high bile acids concentrations in the systemic circulation.[33] Of note, Lp-X is also present in other causes of intrahepatic and extrahepatic cholestases, lecithin-cholesterol acyltransferase deficiency, and in those receiving intravenous infusions of lipid emulsion.[30] Lp-X is often associated with cutaneous xanthomas. However, fewer than 10% of patients with PBC will have xanthomas on physical examination.[34] Xanthomas regress during a period of months after improvement of hyperlipidemia, as well as with liver transplantation.[30,35]

It remains controversial whether hypercholesterolemia related to chronic cholestasis is associated with increased cardiovascular risk given mixed data in the literature. In one prospective study, the incidence of atherosclerotic death in 312 patients with PBC was not statistically different when compared with the control population.[36] A study by Zhang and colleagues, showed that patients with PBC have the highest

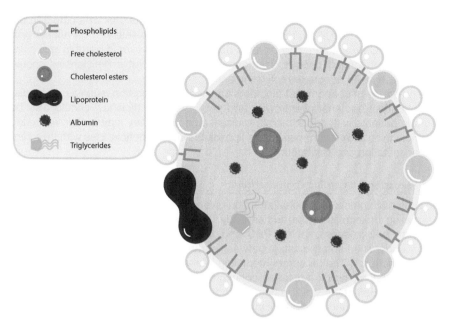

Fig. 2. Lipoprotein-X (Lp-X): Lp-X is an aberrant serum lipoprotein rich in phospholipids and free cholesterol, low in cholesterol esters and triglycerides, and albumin within its core. Lp-X holds apoAI, apoCs, and apoE, and lacks apoB. Lp-X is classified into 3 subfractions based on different biochemical properties. Lp-X1 does not hold apoAI or apoE, unlike Lp-X2-3. Lp-X is present in the plasma of those with extrahepatic and intrahepatic cholestasis, lecithin-cholesterol acyltransferase deficiency, and those receiving intravenous infusion of lipid emulsion.

levels of high-density lipoprotein cholesterol, as well as the lowest degree of hepatic steatosis among those with chronic liver disease, and healthy subjects.[37] The authors hypothesize these findings are protective factors against atherosclerosis and cardiovascular disease in patients with PBC. A systematic review failed to show a significant increase in the risk of cardiovascular disease in patients with PBC, except for those with comorbid metabolic syndrome.[38] However, larger studies suggest there may indeed be a link. Another systematic review and meta-analysis consisting of 3362 patients with PBC showed statistically significant increased risk of cardiovascular disease in this patient population,[39] and an analysis of hospitalizations for immune-mediated disorders in Sweden spanning 1964 to 2008 containing 1852 patients with PBC found that the risk subsequent hospitalization for coronary heart disease within 1 year was increased (standardized incidence ratio 3.32, 95% CI 2.34–4.58).[40]

In the absence of clearly defined risk, a case-by-case approach is recommended in the management of hypercholesterolemia, considering comorbid conditions, as well as family history of cardiovascular disease. It is important to note that ursodeoxycholic acid itself can result in some improvement of dyslipidemia associated with chronic cholestasis[41] but treating with statins and/or fibrates is a more potent and safe approach.

Vitamin Deficiencies

Cholestasis is a major risk factor for the development of fat-soluble vitamin (A, D, E, and K) deficiencies due to reduced intestinal absorption.[41] Malabsorption tends to correlate with degree of elevation in bilirubin levels, with higher risk when the bilirubin levels are greater than 2 mg/dL and with advanced liver disease.[16,24] Patients with controlled PBC do not generally develop deficiencies; however, if bilirubin levels are elevated for prolonged periods, then screening for fat-soluble deficiencies should be done yearly with adequate replenishment.[15,16,24]

The presence of concomitant disorders causing malabsorption, such as celiac disease, intestinal bacterial overgrowth, and pancreatic insufficiency, should also be sought in patients with cholestatic liver disease because they may further worsened the deficiencies. **Box 2** summarizes the liposoluble vitamin deficiencies with their clinical manifestation and treatment.[42]

Nonatherosclerotic Cardiac Complications

Bile acids have gained additional attention given the discoveries of their crucial roles as signaling molecules in the human body. Observational studies of patients with cholestatic liver diseases, such as PBC, and other patients with cirrhotic cardiomyopathy have identified an association between serum bile acid concentrations and cardiac dysfunction.[43] The receptors mediating bile acid signaling are expressed in the cardiovasculature, and[43] increased concentration of bile acids results in electrical conductance defects, such as sinoatrial node dysfunction, decreased cardiac mitochondrial function, and cardiomyocyte apoptosis. Clinically, this presents as PR and QT interval prolongation, leading to arrhythmias, as well as ventricular systolic and diastolic dysfunction. QT prolongation can be found in 64% of Childs Pugh C patients

Box 2
Fat-soluble vitamin deficiencies

Vitamin	Deficiency	Repletion	Comments
A	• Skin changes (hyperkeratosis, poor wound dealing)	• Vitamin A 2,000–200,000 IU/d PO according to severity for 4–8 wk	• If there is no improvement in levels, check for zinc deficiency
	• Ocular changes Poor bone growth		• Due to the risk of toxicity, supplement dosage should be monitored
D	• Bone pain, muscle weakness, osteomalacia, anorexia, hair loss, poor wound healing	• 50,000 IU/wk (D2 or D3) for 8 wk	• Therapeutic target 25-OH vitamin D > 30 ng mL
	• Hypocalcemia, hypophosphatemia	• Followed by maintenance 1500–2000 IU/d	• In individuals with low mineral bone density, calcium should be coadministered
E	• Hemolytic anemia	• α-Tocopherol acetate 400–800IU/d	• Deficiency is much less common than vitamin A or D
	• Neurologic deficits (ataxia, peripheral neuropathy)		• High doses antagonize vitamin A and adversely affect wound healing and platelet function
K	• Bleeding, petechiae, purpura, ecchymosis	• Phytonadione 1–10 mg PO or sub q or IV daily X 3 d	• Deficiencies occur rapidly as it is not stored
	• Prolongation of international normalized ratio (INR)		

with PBC aged older than 63 years,[44] and the left ventricle has impaired ability to respond to orthostasis in PBC.[45] In a 14-year longitudinal study of 580 patients with PBC, cardiac complications were documented in 24 patients (4.1%), including 17 patients (71%) with cardiomyopathy, 21 patients (88%) with arrhythmias, and 14 patients (58%) with both cardiomyopathy and arrhythmias.[46] Studies evaluating cardiac abnormalities in PSC are lacking.

In addition to the increased total serum bile acid concentration, the ratio of cardioprotective hydrophilic bile acids versus cardiotoxic hydrophobic bile acids seems to be crucial in the development of cardiomyopathy. Ursodeoxycholic acid is a relatively hydrophilic bile acid used for the treatment of PBC. Interestingly, ursodeoxycholic acid has been shown to be cardioprotective by preventing cardiomyocyte apoptosis and reversing alterations in cardiac contractility in preclinical and clinical studies.[47]

Malignancy

PBC is associated with a 9-fold increased risk of developing malignancy, both hepatobiliary and potentially extrahepatic.[48,49] PBC patients with cirrhosis are at an increased risk of hepatocellular carcinoma, mainly men with advance age and individuals with portal hypertension.[50] Boonstra and colleagues, in their cohort study also found that patients with PBC have a 5-fold increase in risk for urinary bladder cancer and 1.8-fold breast cancer, although other data has been conflicting regarding breast cancer.[48]

Because of cholestasis, cholangiocytes are overexposed to bile acids, leading to abnormal cell proliferation and cholangiocarcinogenesis. According to experimental models by Werneburg and colleagues, bile acids can phosphorylate epidermal growth receptors in cholangiocarcinoma and immortalized cholangiocyte cell lines, resulting in the proliferation of the cells,[51] which may lead to cholangiocarcinoma.

Renal Complications

Cholestatic liver diseases can cause renal complications in the form of cholemic nephropathy, also known as bile cast nephropathy, which may cause acute kidney injury leading to renal failure. It is sometimes overlooked but typically occurs in patients with severe hyperbilirubinemia in the setting of decompensated end-stage liver disease.[52]

The mechanism by which it occurs is not entirely understood but it is thought that direct toxicity of cholephiles leads to oxidative stress, which damages the tubular cell membranes and impairs regulation of vasoconstriction in the nephrons. Additionally, bile cast formation in nephrons may cause tubular obstruction and epithelial cell damage. Exposure to severe cholestasis (bilirubin of more than 20 mg/dL), in addition to other factors that promote bile cast formation, such as metabolic acidosis and hypoalbuminemia, can enhance bile cast formation and resultant kidney injury.[52] The diagnosis is suggested by an acute decrease in renal function associated with severe cholestasis and the presence of bile casts in the urine. Features of biliary nephropathy may be seen on kidney biopsy, if performed. Treatment focuses on reducing bilirubin levels or bile acid in plasma and urine by treating the underlying cause and limiting bile cast promoting factors.[52]

Another uncommon manifestation of renal involvement in cholestatic liver disease, which can be seen in PBC, is RTA type 1, or distal type RTA.[53,54] Distal RTA is often caused by immune disorders and should be considered in patients with normal anion gap metabolic acidosis with hyperchloremia and hypokalemia, which fails to respond to treatment.[53,54] Another renal complication related to portal hypertension, which is not specific to cholestatic disease, is hepatorenal syndrome.

Sicca Syndrome

Sicca with or without Sjogren syndrome is found in up to 40% of patients with PBC.[55] Keratoconjunctivitis sicca manifests as eye burning, soreness, and even a foreign body sensation,[56] whereas symptoms of xerostomia include halitosis, dysgeusia, dysphagia, odynophagia, difficulty with speech, painful tongue fissures, mucosal ulcers, and excessive cavities.[57] Additionally, vaginal dryness, vulvar pruritus, and dyspareunia are often reported in postmenopausal women with PBC. Early observations associated PBC with lacrimal and salivary gland dysfunction labeled the disease a "dry gland" syndrome.[58] PBC and Sjogren syndrome share similar pathophysiology; both intrahepatic bile ducts and salivary glands undergo immune-mediated destruction from infiltrating lymphocytes, which leads to progressive fibrosis. Notably, antimitochondrial antibody (AMA) has been identified in 22% of patients with Sjogren syndrome, and AMA has been detected in saliva of patients with PBC.[59,60] The salivary gland ducts of patients with PBC manifest PBC-like immunohistochemical staining with a monoclonal AMA specific for the self-antigen PDC-E2.[61] This supports shared pathogenic pathway for the development of autoimmune epitheliitis.

The first-line of therapy for symptomatic management of keratoconjunctivitis sicca is artificial tear drops. Other considerations include topical cyclosporine.[62] In addition, patients should be counseled of avoiding dry or windy environments. Lifitegrast, a lymphocyte function-associated antigen-1 (LFA-1) antagonist eye drop, is FDA approved for the management of dry eyes, but has not been specifically tested in patients with cholestatic liver disease. For xerostomia, salivary substitutes are recommended. The secretagogues, pilocarpine and cevimeline, and muscarinic receptor agonists are effective in reducing symptoms associated with dry mouth and eyes.[63] However, they should not be used in patients with cardiac disease or asthma given risk of bradycardia and bronchospasm. Patients should be counseled on potential side effects, including nausea, flushing, sweating, and urinary frequency. Comanagement with ophthalmology and dentistry is recommended.

DISCUSSION

PBC is a chronic immune-mediated hepatobiliary disease that leads to progressive cholestasis. Repercussions from chronic cholestasis can be recognized systemically, affecting the integumentary, cardiovascular, digestive, nervous, renal, and skeletal systems. The consequences of chronic cholestasis can cause increased morbidity and mortality in patients with PBC; therefore, early identification is paramount. Management of patients with PBC includes not only slowing the progression of disease toward cirrhosis and liver failure but also managing symptoms and preventing extrahepatic complications related to chronic cholestasis. A multidisciplinary approach in treatment of these patients is recommended in order to provide the best quality of care. We aspire that with continued advances in our understanding of the pathophysiology of PBC, additional therapeutics will be aimed at preventing not only progression toward liver transplantation but also the systemic consequences of cholestasis.

CLINICS CARE POINTS

- Fatigue is perhaps the most common complaint in patients with cholestatic liver disease.
- Dyslipidemia associated with chronic cholestasis is characterized by the appearance of the aberrant Lp-X.

- Controversy remains regarding atherogenicity related to cholestatic dyslipidemia.
- Chronic cholestasis is associated with QT prolongation, as well as systolic and diastolic cardiac dysfunction.
- Keratoconjunctivitis sicca, xerostomia, and vaginal dryness are commonly experienced by patients with PBC.
- Osteopenia and osteoporosis are common consequences of chronic cholestasis.
- Renal consequences of severe cholestasis include bile cast nephropathy.
- Chronic cholestasis is a major risk factor for the development of fat-soluble vitamin deficiencies.

DISCLOSURE

Dr M. Zapata and Dr H. Pagan-Torres have nothing to disclose. Dr M.J. Mayo discloses clinical trial agreements with Intercept, CymaBay, Target, Genfit, GSK, Mirum, and advisory agreements with Mallinckrodt, CymaBay, Genfit, GSK, and Intra Sana Laboratories.

REFERENCES

1. Nietsche TR, Dotta G, Barcaui CB, et al. Cholestatic pruritus: a knowledge update. An Bras Dermatol 2022;97(3):332–7.
2. Huang AH, Williams KA, Kwatra SG. Prurigo nodularis: epidemiology and clinical features. J Am Acad Dermatol 2020;83(6):1559–65.
3. Beuers U, Wolters F, Oude Elferink RPJ. Mechanisms of pruritus in cholestasis: understanding and treating the itch. Nat Rev Gastroenterol Hepatol 2023;20(1):26–36.
4. De Vloo C, Nevens F. Cholestatic pruritus : an update. Acta Gastroenterol Belg 2019;82(1):75–82.
5. Kremer AE, Martens JJ, Kulik W, et al. Lysophosphatidic acid is a potential mediator of cholestatic pruritus. Gastroenterology 2010;139(3):1008–18.
6. Bowlus CL, Arrive L, Bergquist A, et al. AASLD practice guidance on primary sclerosing cholangitis and cholangiocarcinoma. Hepatology 2023;77(2):659–702.
7. Rudic JS, Poropat G, Krstic MN, et al. Ursodeoxycholic acid for primary biliary cirrhosis. Cochrane Database Syst Rev 2012;12(12):CD000551.
8. Levy C, Manns M, Hirschfield G. New treatment paradigms in primary biliary cholangitis. Clin Gastroenterol Hepatol 2023. https://doi.org/10.1016/j.cgh.2023.02.005.
9. de Vries E, Bolier R, Goet J, et al. Fibrates for itch (FITCH) in fibrosing cholangiopathies: a double-blind, randomized, placebo-controlled trial. Gastroenterology 2021;160(3):734–743 e6.
10. European Association for the Study of the Liver. Electronic address eee, European association for the study of the L. EASL clinical practice guidelines on sclerosing cholangitis. J Hepatol 2022;77(3):761–806.
11. Levy C, Kendrick S, Bowlus CL, et al. GLIMMER: a randomized phase 2b dose-ranging trial of linerixibat in primary biliary cholangitis patients with pruritus. Clin Gastroenterol Hepatol 2022. https://doi.org/10.1016/j.cgh.2022.10.032.
12. Gonzales E, Hardikar W, Stormon M, et al. Efficacy and safety of maralixibat treatment in patients with Alagille syndrome and cholestatic pruritus (ICONIC): a randomised phase 2 study. Lancet 2021;398(10311):1581–92.

13. Thompson RJ, Arnell H, Artan R, et al. Odevixibat treatment in progressive familial intrahepatic cholestasis: a randomised, placebo-controlled, phase 3 trial. Lancet Gastroenterol Hepatol 2022;7(9):830–42.
14. Lynch EN, Campani C, Innocenti T, et al. Understanding fatigue in primary biliary cholangitis: from pathophysiology to treatment perspectives. World J Hepatol 2022;14(6):1111–9.
15. European Association for the Study of the Liver. Electronic address eee, European Association for the Study of the L. EASL Clinical Practice Guidelines: the diagnosis and management of patients with primary biliary cholangitis. J Hepatol 2017;67(1):145–72.
16. Lindor KD, Bowlus CL, Boyer J, et al. Primary biliary cholangitis: 2018 practice guidance from the American association for the study of liver diseases. Hepatology 2019;69(1):394–419.
17. Kosnik A, Wojcicki M. Fatigue in chronic liver disease patients: prevalence, pathophysiology, and management. Prz Gastroenterol 2022;17(1):21–7.
18. Silveira MG, Gossard AA, Stahler AC, et al. A randomized, placebo-controlled clinical trial of efficacy and safety: modafinil in the treatment of fatigue in patients with primary biliary cirrhosis. Am J Ther 2017;24(2):e167–76.
19. Pedersen MR, Mayo MJ. Managing the symptoms and complications of cholestasis. Clin Liver Dis 2020;15(3):120–4.
20. Raszeja-Wyszomirska J, Miazgowski T. Osteoporosis in primary biliary cirrhosis of the liver. Prz Gastroenterol 2014;9(2):82–7.
21. Janes CH, Dickson ER, Okazaki R, et al. Role of hyperbilirubinemia in the impairment of osteoblast proliferation associated with cholestatic jaundice. J Clin Invest 1995;95(6):2581–6.
22. Ruiz-Gaspa S, Martinez-Ferrer A, Guanabens N, et al. Effects of bilirubin and sera from jaundiced patients on osteoblasts: contribution to the development of osteoporosis in liver diseases. Hepatology 2011;54(6):2104–13.
23. Dubreuil M, Ruiz-Gaspa S, Guanabens N, et al. Ursodeoxycholic acid increases differentiation and mineralization and neutralizes the damaging effects of bilirubin on osteoblastic cells. Liver Int 2013;33(7):1029–38.
24. Assis DN. Chronic complications of cholestasis: evaluation and management. Clin Liver Dis 2018;22(3):533–44.
25. Camacho PM, Petak SM, Binkley N, et al. American association of clinical endocrinologists/American college of endocrinology clinical practice guidelines for the diagnosis and treatment of postmenopausal osteoporosis-2020 update. Endocr Pract 2020;26(Suppl 1):1–46.
26. Santos LAA, Lima TB, de Carvalho Nunes HR, et al. Two-year risedronate treatment for osteoporosis in patients with esophageal varices: a non-randomized clinical trial. Hepatol Int 2022;16(6):1458–67.
27. Longo M, Crosignani A, Battezzati PM, et al. Hyperlipidaemic state and cardiovascular risk in primary biliary cirrhosis. Gut 2002;51(2):265–9.
28. Sinakos E, Abbas G, Jorgensen RA, et al. Serum lipids in primary sclerosing cholangitis. Dig Liver Dis 2012;44(1):44–8.
29. Ahoussougbemey Mele A, Mahmood R, Ogbuagu H, et al. Hyperlipidemia in the setting of primary biliary cholangitis: a case report and review of management strategies. Cureus 2022;14(11):e31411.
30. Miida T, Hirayama S. Controversy over the atherogenicity of lipoprotein-X. Curr Opin Endocrinol Diabetes Obes 2019;26(2):117–23.
31. Fellin R, Manzato E. Lipoprotein-X fifty years after its original discovery. Nutr Metab Cardiovasc Dis 2019;29(1):4–8.

32. Manzato E, Fellin R, Baggio G, et al. Formation of lipoprotein-X. Its relationship to bile compounds. J Clin Invest 1976;57(5):1248–60.
33. Reshetnyak VI, Maev IV. Features of lipid metabolism disorders in primary biliary cholangitis. Biomedicines 2022;10(12). https://doi.org/10.3390/biomedicin es10123046.
34. Carey EJ, Ali AH, Lindor KD. Primary biliary cirrhosis. Lancet 2015;386(10003): 1565–75.
35. Harris J, Cao S, Hile G, et al. Diffuse xanthomas in a patient with primary biliary cholangitis and lipoprotein X. JAAD Case Rep 2021;7:30–2.
36. Crippin JS, Lindor KD, Jorgensen R, et al. Hypercholesterolemia and atherosclerosis in primary biliary cirrhosis: what is the risk? Hepatology 1992;15(5):858–62.
37. Zhang Y, Hu X, Chang J, et al. The liver steatosis severity and lipid characteristics in primary biliary cholangitis. BMC Gastroenterol 2021;21(1):395.
38. Suraweera D, Fanous C, Jimenez M, et al. Risk of cardiovascular events in patients with primary biliary cholangitis - systematic review. J Clin Transl Hepatol 2018;6(2):119–26.
39. Ungprasert P, Wijarnpreecha K, Ahuja W, et al. Coronary artery disease in primary biliary cirrhosis: a systematic review and meta-analysis of observational studies. Hepatol Res 2015;45(11):1055–61.
40. Zoller B, Li X, Sundquist J, et al. Risk of subsequent coronary heart disease in patients hospitalized for immune-mediated diseases: a nationwide follow-up study from Sweden. PLoS One 2012;7(3):e33442.
41. Angelin B, Eusufzai S. Effects of ursodeoxycholic acid on plasma lipids. Scand J Gastroenterol Suppl 1994;204:24–6.
42. Lai JC, Tandon P, Bernal W, et al. Malnutrition, frailty, and sarcopenia in patients with cirrhosis: 2021 practice guidance by the American association for the study of liver diseases. Hepatology 2021;74(3):1611–44.
43. Vasavan T, Ferraro E, Ibrahim E, et al. Heart and bile acids - clinical consequences of altered bile acid metabolism. Biochim Biophys Acta, Mol Basis Dis 2018;1864(4 Pt B):1345–55.
44. Wang Z, Qian R, Wang Y, et al. QTc interval prolongation in the patients with primary biliary cholangitis. Ann Noninvasive Electrocardiol 2022;27(1):e12925.
45. Jones DE, Hollingsworth K, Fattakhova G, et al. Impaired cardiovascular function in primary biliary cirrhosis. Am J Physiol Gastrointest Liver Physiol 2010;298(5): G764–73.
46. Bian S, Chen H, Wang L, et al. Cardiac involvement in patients with primary biliary cholangitis: a 14-year longitudinal survey-based study. PLoS One 2018;13(3): e0194397.
47. Hanafi NI, Mohamed AS, Sheikh Abdul Kadir SH, et al. Overview of bile acids signaling and perspective on the signal of ursodeoxycholic acid, the most hydrophilic bile acid, in the heart. Biomolecules 2018;8(4). https://doi.org/10.3390/biom8040159.
48. Hrad V, Abebe Y, Ali SH, et al. Risk and surveillance of cancers in primary biliary tract disease. Gastroenterol Res Pract 2016;2016:3432640.
49. Boonstra K, Bokelaar R, Stadhouders PH, et al. Increased cancer risk in a large population-based cohort of patients with primary biliary cirrhosis: follow-up for up to 36 years. Hepatol Int 2014;8(2):266–74.
50. Gossard AA. Care of the cholestatic patient. Clin Liver Dis 2013;17(2):331–44.
51. Werneburg NW, Yoon JH, Higuchi H, et al. Bile acids activate EGF receptor via a TGF-alpha-dependent mechanism in human cholangiocyte cell lines. Am J Physiol Gastrointest Liver Physiol 2003;285(1):G31–6.

52. Tinti F, Umbro I, D'Alessandro M, et al. Cholemic nephropathy as cause of acute and chronic kidney disease. Update on an under-diagnosed disease. Life 2021; 11(11). https://doi.org/10.3390/life11111200.
53. Goutaudier V, Szwarc I, Serre JE, et al. Primary sclerosing cholangitis: a new cause of distal renal tubular acidosis. Clin Kidney J 2016;9(6):811–3.
54. Dong KH, Fang YN, Wen XY, et al. Primary biliary cirrhosis with refractory hypokalemia: a case report. Medicine (Baltim) 2018;97(48):e13172.
55. Tsianos EV, Hoofnagle JH, Fox PC, et al. Sjogren's syndrome in patients with primary biliary cirrhosis. Hepatology 1990;11(5):730–4.
56. Foulks GN, Forstot SL, Donshik PC, et al. Clinical guidelines for management of dry eye associated with Sjogren disease. Ocul Surf 2015;13(2):118–32.
57. Baer AN, Walitt B. Sjogren syndrome and other causes of sicca in older adults. Clin Geriatr Med 2017;33(1):87–103.
58. Epstein O, Thomas HC, Sherlock S. Primary biliary cirrhosis is a dry gland syndrome with features of chronic graft-versus-host disease. Lancet 1980;1(8179): 1166–8.
59. Zurgil N, Bakimer R, Moutsopoulos HM, et al. Antimitochondrial (pyruvate dehydrogenase) autoantibodies in autoimmune rheumatic diseases. J Clin Immunol 1992;12(3):201–9.
60. Reynoso-Paz S, Leung PS, Van De Water J, et al. Evidence for a locally driven mucosal response and the presence of mitochondrial antigens in saliva in primary biliary cirrhosis. Hepatology 2000;31(1):24–9.
61. Tsuneyama K, Van de Water J, Nakanuma Y, et al. Human combinatorial autoantibodies and mouse monoclonal antibodies to PDC-E2 produce abnormal apical staining of salivary glands in patients with coexistent primary biliary cirrhosis and Sjogren's syndrome. Hepatology 1994;20(4 Pt 1):893–8.
62. Selmi C, Gershwin ME. Chronic autoimmune epithelitis in sjogren's syndrome and primary biliary cholangitis: a comprehensive review. Rheumatol Ther 2017;4(2): 263–79.
63. Vivino FB, Al-Hashimi I, Khan Z, et al. Pilocarpine tablets for the treatment of dry mouth and dry eye symptoms in patients with Sjogren syndrome: a randomized, placebo-controlled, fixed-dose, multicenter trial. P92-01 Study Group. Arch Intern Med 1999;159(2):174–81.

Primary Sclerosing Cholangitis
Epidemiology, Diagnosis, and Presentation

Aalam Sohal, MD[a], Sanya Kayani, MD[b], Kris V. Kowdley, MD[a,c],*

KEYWORDS

• Primary sclerosing cholangitis • Epidemiology • Diagnosis • Presentation

KEY POINTS

• The incidence of primary sclerosing cholangitis is on the rise because of the use of imaging modalities.
• The incidence and prevalence are highest in North America and Europe, while lowest in Asia and the Mediterranean region.
• Most patients are asymptomatic on presentation, but some can present with signs and symptoms of advanced liver disease or bacterial cholangitis.

BACKGROUND

Primary sclerosing cholangitis (PSC) is a chronic, cholestatic liver disease characterized by idiopathic inflammation and fibrosis of intra- and extrahepatic bile ducts.[1] Many hypotheses have been proposed regarding the etiology of PSC, the most widely recognized of which is that PSC is an immune-mediated disease triggered by an environmental factor leading to hepatocyte injury and inflammation in genetically predisposed individuals.[2–7] PSC is associated with other immune-mediated diseases in the same patient or first-degree relatives.[8–10] Roughly 80% of patients with PSC have concomitant inflammatory bowel disease (IBD).[10,11] Among patients with PSC and IBD, 80% have ulcerative colitis (UC), while the remaining patients have unspecified IBD or Crohn disease (CD).[12]

The natural history of PSC is variable, but in most patients, progressive inflammation, fibrosis, and stricturing of the bile ducts result in cirrhosis and complications of liver disease. The median survival from diagnosis to liver transplantation or death from liver disease has been estimated to be 18 years.[13] Multiple subpopulations within

Conflict of interest: None.
[a] Liver Institute Northwest, , 3216 Northeast 45th Place, Suite 212, Seattle, WA 98105, USA; [b] Avera McKennan Hospital and University Health Center, Sioux Falls, SD, USA; [c] Elson Floyd College of Medicine, Spokane, WA, USA
* Corresponding author. Liver Institute Northwest, 3216 Northeast 45th Place, Suite 212, Seattle, WA 98105.
E-mail address: kkowdley@liverinstitutenw.org

Clin Liver Dis 28 (2024) 129–141
https://doi.org/10.1016/j.cld.2023.07.005
1089-3261/24/© 2023 Elsevier Inc. All rights reserved.

liver.theclinics.com

PSC have been described, namely large-duct PSC, small-duct PSC, and PSC with elevated immunoglobulin G (IgG).[14,15] PSC is a radiological diagnosis characterized by stricturing and beaded appearance of bile ducts.[16] This appearance can be attributed to multifocal stenoses combined with normal or dilated bile duct segments.[16] Patients with small-duct PSC may have normal imaging, and histologic diagnosis is required in the absence of macroscopic bile duct abnormalities.[17]

The only curative treatment for patients with PSC is liver transplantation (LT), which is reserved for patients with advanced and decompensated liver disease.[18] There is an urgent unmet need to find medical therapies to combat PSC, as the incidence of PSC is on the rise as per recent epidemiologic data.[19,20] This article describes the epidemiology, diagnosis, and presentation of PSC.

EPIDEMIOLOGY
Incidence and Prevalence

Population-based epidemiologic studies have investigated the incidence of PSC[19,20] and have reported the incidence of PSC to be increasingly likely because of the regular use of imaging modalities.[21–24] Trivedi and colleagues reported the global mean and median incidence of PSC to be between 0.7 and 0.8 cases per 100,000 population and the mean prevalence to be 10 cases per 100,000 population.[20] The PSC incidence rate (IR) was higher in Northern Europe and North America compared with Asia and the Mediterranean basin.[20]

North America

Mehta and colleagues, in their meta-analysis examining population-based studies of PSC, reported that the IR of PSC in the United States ranges from 0.2 to 0.92 cases per 100,000 persons, while the prevalence ranges from 0 to 13.6 cases per 100,000 persons.[25–28] The lowest IR was reported in Alaska, when Hurlburt and colleagues, in their study of clinical records of 36 years, reported no PSC cases in Alaskan Natives.[26] On the contrary, a study by Bakhshi and colleagues on a population cohort in Olmsted County reported the age- and sex-adjusted IR to be 1.11.[21] Their study reported that the incidence rate nearly doubled during 2001 to 2017 compared to 1976 to 2000, with an increased incidence of patients with milder phenotypes, possibly because of earlier detection of PSC secondary to more frequent laboratory testing and routine use of cross-sectional imaging. Toy and colleagues reported the incidence and prevalence of PSC to be 0.41 cases per 100,000 person-years and 4.03 cases per 100,000 people in northern California, lower than that reported in Minnesota.[21,27] Toy and colleagues attributed these differences to ethnic disparities in these 2 regions.[27] **Table 1** describes the incidence and prevalence of PSC in various regions as per the published literature. **Figs. 1** and **2** describe the incidence and prevalence of the published literature.

Europe

Multiple studies examining the incidence and prevalence of PSC have been conducted in Europe. The crude incidence rate in the United Kingdom has been reported to be between 0.41 to 0.64 cases per 100,000 person-years, while the prevalence rate has been estimated to be between 3.85 and 5.58 cases per 100,000 persons.[25] The IR in Wales was noted to be higher than in the United Kingdom.[30] The lowest IR and prevalence of PSC in Europe was reported in Spain, whereas the highest has been reported in Finland (31.7 cases per 100,000 persons).[31,32]

Asia

There appears to be a lower prevalence of PSC in Asia. A questionnaire-based retrospective study in 2007 estimated the prevalence of PSC to be 0.95 cases per 100,000

Table 1
Incidence and prevalence in different regions of the world

	Study Period	Incidence	Prevalence
North America			
Alaska[26]	1984–2000	0	0
Northern California[27]	2000–2006	0.41	4.15
Minnesota[21]	1976–2018	1.11	23.99
Utah[28]	1986–2011	0.2	1.5
Calgary, Canada[29]	2000–2005	0.91	N/A
Europe			
Norway[33]	1985–1994	0.7	5.6
Oslo, Norway[34]	1985–1995	1.3	8.5
Netherlands[22]	2000–2007	0.5	6
Italy[35]	1985–2014	0.1	N/A
United Kingdom[23]	1991–2001	0.41	3.85
Spain[31]	1984–1988	0.04	0.22
South Wales, United Kingdom[30]	1984–2003	0.91	12.7
United Kingdom[36]	1998–2014	0.68	5.58
Sweden[24]	1992–2005	1.22	16.2
Finland[32]	1990–2015	1.58	31.7
Asia			
Japan[37]	2007–2008	N/A	0.95
Israel[38]	1998–2012	N/A	4
Australia			
Melbourne[39]	2000–2021	0.27	5.9
New Zealand[40]	2008–2016	0.92	13.17
South America		N/A	N/A
Africa		N/A	N/A

persons.[37] By contrast, Israel was noted to have a higher prevalence (4 cases per 100,000 persons) than Japan.[38] Currently, there is a paucity of epidemiologic data on the incidence of PSC in India and China.

Australia
A study by Tan and colleagues reported an annual incidence of 0.27 cases per 100,000 person-years in the greater Melbourne region.[39] Their study also estimated the prevalence to be 5.9 cases per 100,000 inhabitants. A study in New Zealand reported an annual incidence of 0.92 cases per 100,000 population and a prevalence of 13.17 for PSC, higher than that in Australia.[40]

Other continents
There are limited data on the incidence or prevalence of PSC in South America or Africa.

Age of Onset
The median age of diagnosis in patients with PSC is reported to be between 30 and 40 years.[22,41] However, some studies in Japan and North America have reported a second peak in cases after the age of 50 years.[42,43] The phenotype in patients diagnosed above the age of 50 differs from patients diagnosed between 30 and 40 years of

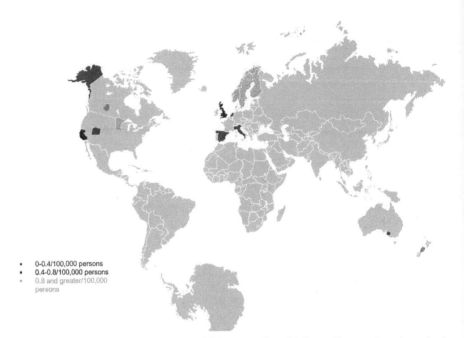

Fig. 1. Incidence of PSC as per reported literature. If multiple studies are done in a single region, the highest reported incidence is described in the figure.

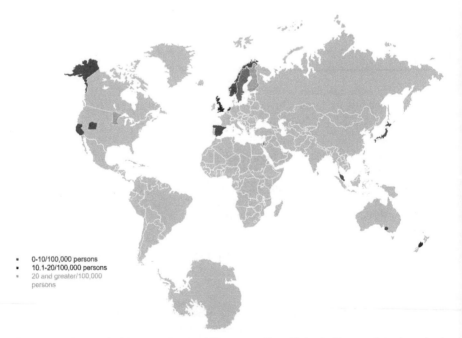

Fig. 2. Prevalence of PSC as per reported literature. If multiple studies are done in a single region, the highest reported prevalence is described in the figure.

age.[43] Patients diagnosed with PSC at over age 50 have a weaker association with ulcerative colitis, lower serum immunoglobulin M (IgM), and higher serum immunoglobulin E (IgE) levels.[42,43] Furthermore, patients with late-onset PSC have been noted to have a higher incidence of cholangiocarcinoma (CCA).[43] In patients with late-onset disease, decreased transplantation-free survival from the time of diagnosis has been noted.[43] Rupp and colleagues suggested that these differences can be attributed to an increased incidence of infectious complications in patients with late-onset PSC.[43] Their study also noted a higher incidence of biliary dilatation therapy and recurrent cholangitis in patients with late-onset PSC.[43]

Sex

Contrary to other autoimmune liver diseases, the prevalence of PSC has been noted to be higher in men than women.[21,24] A study in Sweden on a large regional population noted significant differences in the incidence of PSC among men and women.[24] Men were reported to have a higher incidence and point prevalence than women (1.8 versus 0.7 and 24 versus 9 cases per 100,000 population). Other studies have also noted a higher prevalence in men.[5,21,24] The proportion of cases in men has ranged from 51% to 71%, depending on the region.[21,40] Among patients with late-onset PSC, there is a female predominance.[43,44] The reason for these differences is unclear, and further studies are needed.

Race

Studies have reported that the patient's race seems to play a role in the development of PSC.[44–46] Kelly and colleagues, in their study of 166 patients with ulcerative colitis, reported that women of African or Caribbean descent were more likely to develop PSC.[44] A recent study by Are and colleagues reported that African Americans are diagnosed at a younger age compared with Caucasians.[45] They also reported that African Americans suffer from higher liver-related mortality. Bayable and colleagues evaluated patients with PSC and end-stage liver disease undergoing liver transplants and noted that African Americans had worse outcomes than Caucasians.[46]

Primary Sclerosing Cholangitis in Inflammatory Bowel Disease

A strong link has been suggested between inflammatory bowel disease (IBD) and PSC.[10–12,47,48] It has been estimated that 50% of patients with IBD may develop extraintestinal manifestations, including primary sclerosing cholangitis.[49] A meta-analysis by Barberio and colleagues reported that the pooled prevalence of PSC in patients with IBD is 2.16%. Their study also documented a higher prevalence in patients with ulcerative colitis (UC), 2.47%, compared with 0.96% in Crohn disease.[50] Regional differences have also been noted in the prevalence of PSC in IBD. The prevalence was noted to be lowest in Southeast Asia at 0.60% and the highest in South America, at 3.83%.[50] This study also reported differences in the prevalence of PSC depending on the severity of IBD.[50] In patients with UC, the pooled prevalence was higher in patients with the extensive disease compared with left-sided UC (5.38% versus 0.8%, respectively). In patients with CD, the prevalence of PSC was noted to be higher in patients with colonic (7.02%) and ileocolonic (6.81%) disease, compared to patients with only ileal disease (3.78%).[50]

PRESENTATION

The clinical presentation of PSC can range from asymptomatic cases to advanced stages of liver disease. About 15% to 40% of patients are asymptomatic.[51] In many patients, abnormal laboratory tests are the only finding on presentation.[29] A multi-center retrospective cohort study by Guerra and colleagues in patients with PSC and IBD reported that pruritus was the most common clinical finding (10.8%), followed by abdominal pain (8.3%) and jaundice (8.3%).[52] Other symptoms early during the course of the disease include weight loss and depression.[53,54] Dyson and colleagues, in their study of 40 nontransplanted PSC patients, reported higher fatigue scores than the general population.[55] Kuo and colleagues surveyed 811 patients with PSC and noted that more than half of the patients had significant pruritus, abdominal pain, fatigue, or sleep disturbances.[56] Patients with PSC also report significant fatigue.[56] Another study by Kaplan and colleagues reported abdominal pain, pruritus, jaundice, and fatigue to be common among patients with PSC.[29]

PSC patients are at high risk of fat-soluble deficiencies and can present with steatorrhea and osteopenia.[57] Thus, patients with advanced liver disease should be screened for vitamin A, D, K, and E deficiencies.[17] Typical clinical signs include hepatomegaly (44%) and splenomegaly (39%).[58] Some patients may present with gallstones or acute cholecystitis.[59] Some patients may develop bacterial cholangitis, characterized by fever, chills, and right upper quadrant abdominal pain.[60]

Late presentations of the disease include complications of advanced liver disease, such as variceal bleeding, ascites, and hepatic encephalopathy. PSC patients have an increased risk of cholangiocarcinoma (CCA) and gall bladder carcinoma.[58–60] Patients with cirrhosis are at increased risk of hepatocellular carcinoma (HCC). Thus, vigilant monitoring for HCC and gallbladder cancer is of vital importance.[17] Studies have shown that patients with PSC and IBD have a significantly increased risk of developing colorectal cancer, and regular colonoscopy monitoring is recommended.[17,61]

DIAGNOSIS
Liver Biochemical Tests

A cholestatic pattern of liver injury may be the only sign of PSC in patients presenting during an earlier stage of the disease.[44] The predominantly elevated enzyme is alkaline phosphatase (ALP).[17,62] Modest elevations could be noted in alanine transaminase (ALT) and aspartate aminotransferase (AST), but levels higher than 5 times the upper limit of normal (ULN) lend more significant consideration to autoimmune hepatitis (AIH), which responds well to steroids.[17] Gamma-glutamyl transferase (GGT) is also frequently elevated.[63] Serum bilirubin levels are usually normal on presentation, and elevated bilirubin greater than 2 times ULN on presentation is a poor prognostic marker.[64]

Serum Immunoglobulin G4 Levels and Immunologic Markers

ACG guidelines recommend testing at least once for IgG4 levels for patients with PSC.[17] Roughly 10% of patients with PSC have elevations in serum IgG4 level.[65] These patients have been reported to have higher severity of the disease and shorter time to liver transplantation.[65] Patients with elevated IgG4 and greater than 5 times the upper limit of normal (ULN) of ALT and AST should be screened with antismooth muscle antibodies (ASMAs) to rule out primary sclerosing cholangitis-autoimmune overlap syndrome (PSC-AIH).[17] Included in the differential diagnosis of elevated IgG4 and cholangitis is IgG4-associated sclerosing cholangitis (IAC), which is more commonly seen in elderly patients and is associated with multiorgan involvement.[66]

Patients with PSC also frequently undergo testing for auto-antibodies, although no immunologic or serologic marker has been reported to be sensitive or specific for PSC.[67] The antinuclear antibody (ANA) and ASMA levels may be elevated, with studies reporting wide variability.[68–70] This testing is beneficial in ruling out additional causes of liver disease.

Radiography

In cases of chronic cholestasis, diagnostic imaging usually begins with abdominal ultrasound or computed tomography (CT).[71,72] Ultrasound can be beneficial in the visualization and evaluation of dilated extrahepatic bile ducts. However, intrahepatic disease cannot be excluded in these patients.[72,73] A study by Majoie and colleagues reported a good correlation between mural thickening of the common bile duct on ultrasound and stenosis on endoscopic retrograde cholangiopancreatography (ERCP) in patients with PSC.[72] PSC is also a known risk factor for gallbladder pathology, and some patients may have findings of gallbladder polyps, stones, or sludge on the ultrasound.[59] Patients with PSC have a higher incidence of gallbladder carcinoma, and thus regular screening with the ultrasound is recommended for these patients.[17]

Imaging with a CT scan reveals beading and stricturing without an associated mass lesion.[71] CT is most beneficial in excluding other anatomic causes of cholestasis, such as hepatic or pancreatic lesions.[71] Both CT and ultrasound are beneficial in diagnosing portal hypertension and ascites in patients with advanced-stage liver disease.[71,72] In the past decade, magnetic resonance cholangiopancreatography (MRCP) has been recognized as the preferred diagnostic procedure for patients with PSC.[74] It is noninvasive and less costly compared with ERCP.[74] MRCP displays the typical beaded appearance of PSC owing to short repetitive strictures in the biliary ducts interspersed with areas of either normal or mild wall thickening leading to dilatations.[75,76] The pruned tree appearance on MRCP is seen in the late stages of PSC when the sclerotic nature of the disease has obliterated smaller peripheral ducts, and they are no longer visible.[75] Other common findings of PSC on MRI include intrahepatic bile duct dilatation, stenosis, beading, extrahepatic bile duct stenosis, and thickening.[77] A lesser-known finding on MRCP is outpouchings of the biliary ducts leading to the formation of diverticula that occur between strictures.[78] When multiple such findings are present, the diagnosis of PSC is generally secure.

Direct Cholangiography

ERCP is used in cases where MRCP is not diagnostic or when therapeutic intervention is needed, such as for dominant strictures.[79] Dominant strictures are stenotic areas present in the common bile duct measuring up to 1.5 mm in diameter and up to 1 mm in the common hepatic duct.[80] ERCP can be used for brush cytology or biopsy to investigate such dominant strictures, as these are associated with an increased risk of CCA.[79,81] ERCP can also be used therapeutically for the dilation of strictures and biliary stent placement.[82] However, ERCP carries a 10% risk of hospitalization in PSC patients along with exposure to radiation.[83] Furthermore, ERCP can be difficult to conduct in the late stages of PSC because of numerous biliary strictures.[83]

Percutaneous transhepatic cholangiography (PTC) is an invasive but occasionally useful tool for producing high-quality images of the biliary tree.[84] It may be of therapeutic benefit, as it can aid in the removal of biliary stones and decompression of the biliary tree in cases of bacterial cholangitis when ERCP is not feasible.[84] As PTC accesses the biliary system through the liver, this procedure may be complicated by liver abscesses, biblio-cutaneous fistulas, and cholangitis.[85] PTC is typically used when ERCP has failed because of excessive stricture formation.

Peroral cholangioscopy and SpyGlass are the other 2 techniques that are beneficial in the direct visualization of suspected filling ducts discovered during ERCP.[86,87] SpyGlass, a single-operator peroral cholangioscopic system, has been reported to have greater sensitivity in the assessment of the biliary system compared with that of ERCP alone.[86] SpyGlass-targeted biopsy has been noted to have superior diagnostic yield compared with brush cytology in patients undergoing ERCP because of better visualization of the target lesion.[87]

Liver Stiffness

Transient elastography has emerged in recent years as a noninvasive tool for assessing the degree of liver fibrosis.[88] This procedure can be performed in a few minutes, and the added benefit is no exposure to radiation. Liver stiffness, measured using transient elastography, has been shown to correlate with the degree of liver fibrosis in various chronic liver diseases.[88] Other noninvasive imaging methods include shear-wave elastography and magnetic resonance elastography (MRE).[89,90] MRE is not routinely available, and it is associated with significant cost. However, it is being used more frequently in the staging and diagnosing liver fibrosis, as it is more accurate than transient elastography.[91]

Liver Biopsy

In some cases where imaging does not yield results, but suspicion for PSC remains high, small duct PSC is a consideration.[17] Roughly 12% to 25% of small duct PSC patients will eventually develop large duct PSC.[92] In small duct PSC, the disease process is confined to the intrahepatic biliary ducts too minute to be seen on cholangioscopy, necessitating a biopsy.[17] A liver biopsy is also helpful when IAC or PSC-AIH is suspected.[93] A classic histologic finding on liver biopsy of PSC patients is the onion skin finding caused by concentric periductal fibrosis, yet it is seen in less than 40% of cases.[94] Histology can vary based on the disease stage.[94] As the disease progresses, the duct lumen becomes irregular, and alterations occur in the epithelium and basement membrane.[94] Extensive periductular fibrosis with obliteration of bile ducts results in onion skinning.[94] In patients with advanced fibrosis, the duct is replaced by a nodular scar called tombstone, a pathognomonic sign of PSC.[94]

SUMMARY

Although the incidence and prevalence of PSC continue to increase, there are currently no medical therapies approved for this condition. Multiple drugs are under clinical trials. It is hoped that if these drugs are found to be efficacious in the management of the disease, the natural history of the disease can be altered, and the patients will experience fewer symptoms and longer transplant-free survival.

CLINICS CARE POINTS

- The incidence and prevalence of primary sclerosing cholangitis are rising with the majority of the cases diagnosed when asymptomatic.
- MRCP has replaced liver biopsy as a preferred modality for the diagnosis of the disease.
- Measurement of liver stiffness using transient elastography and magnetic resonance elastography has been beneficial in assessing the degree of liver fibrosis.

REFERENCES

1. Rabiee A, Silveira MG. Primary sclerosing cholangitis. Transl Gastroenterol Hepatol 2021;6:29.

2. Eaton JE, Juran BD, Atkinson EJ, et al. A comprehensive assessment of environmental exposures among 1000 North American patients with primary sclerosing cholangitis, with and without inflammatory bowel disease. Aliment Pharmacol Ther 2015;41(10):980–90.
3. Dyson JK, Blain A, Foster Shirley MD, et al. Geo-epidemiology and environmental co-variate mapping of primary biliary cholangitis and primary sclerosing cholangitis. JHEP Rep 2020;3(1):100202.
4. Tanaka A, Leung PS, Gershwin ME. Environmental basis of primary biliary cholangitis. Exp Biol Med (Maywood) 2018;243(2):184–9.
5. Boberg KM, Lundin KE, Schrumpf E. Etiology and pathogenesis in primary sclerosing cholangitis. Scand J Gastroenterol Suppl 1994;204:47–58.
6. O'Mahony CA, Vierling JM. Etiopathogenesis of primary sclerosing cholangitis. Semin Liver Dis 2006;26:3–21.
7. Aron JH, Bowlus CL. The immunobiology of primary sclerosing cholangitis. Semin Immunopathol 2009;31(3):383–97.
8. Bergquist A, Lindberg G, Saarinen S, et al. Increased prevalence of primary sclerosing cholangitis among first-degree relatives. J Hepatol 2005;42:252–6.
9. Lamberts LE, Janse M, Haagsma EB, et al. Immune-mediated diseases in primary sclerosing cholangitis. Dig Liver Dis 2011;43(10):802–6.
10. de Vries AB, Janse M, Blokzijl H, et al. Distinctive inflammatory bowel disease phenotype in primary sclerosing cholangitis. World J Gastroenterol 2015;21:1956–71.
11. Palmela C, Peerani F, Castaneda D, et al. Inflammatory bowel disease and primary sclerosing cholangitis: a review of the phenotype and associated specific features. Gut Liver 2018;12:17–29.
12. Loftus EV Jr, Harewood GC, Loftus CG, et al. PSC-IBD: a unique form of inflammatory bowel disease associated with primary sclerosing cholangitis. Gut 2005;54:91–6.
13. Ponsioen CY, Vrouenraets SM, Prawirodirdjo W, et al. Natural history of primary sclerosing cholangitis and prognostic value of cholangiography in a Dutch population. Gut 2002;51(4):562–6.
14. Culver EL, Chapman RW. Systematic review: management options for primary sclerosing cholangitis and its variant forms - IgG4-associated cholangitis and overlap with autoimmune hepatitis. Aliment Pharmacol Ther 2011;33:1273–91.
15. Manganis CD, Chapman RW, Culver EL. Review of primary sclerosing cholangitis with increased IgG4 levels. World J Gastroenterol 2020;26(23):3126–44.
16. Pria HD, Torres US, Faria SC, et al. Practical guide for radiological diagnosis of primary and secondary sclerosing cholangitis. Semin Ultrasound CT MR 2022;43(6):490–509.
17. Lindor, Keith D, Kowdley KV, et al. ACG clinical guideline: primary sclerosing cholangitis. Am J Gastroenterol 2015;110(5):646–59.
18. Gow PJ, Chapman RW. Liver transplantation for primary sclerosing cholangitis. Liver 2000;20(2):97–103.
19. Molodecky NA, Kareemi H, Parab R, et al. Incidence of primary sclerosing cholangitis: a systematic review and meta-analysis. Hepatology 2011;53(5):1590–9.
20. Trivedi PJ, Bowlus CL, Yimam KK, et al. Epidemiology, natural history, and outcomes of primary sclerosing cholangitis: a systematic review of population-based studies. Clin Gastroenterol Hepatol 2022;20(8):1687–700.e4.
21. Bakhshi Z, Hilscher MB, Gores GJ, et al. An update on primary sclerosing cholangitis epidemiology, outcomes and quantification of alkaline phosphatase variability in a population-based cohort. J Gastroenterol 2020;55(5):523–32.

22. Boonstra K, Weersma RK, van Erpecum KJ, et al. Population-based epidemiology, malignancy risk, and outcome of primary sclerosing cholangitis. Hepatology 2013;58(6):2045–55.

23. Card TR, Solaymani-Dodaran M, West J. Incidence and mortality of primary sclerosing cholangitis in the UK: a population-based cohort study. J Hepatol 2008; 48(6):939–44.

24. Lindkvist B, Benito de Valle M, Gullberg B, et al. Incidence and prevalence of primary sclerosing cholangitis in a defined adult population in Sweden. Hepatology 2010;52(2):571–7.

25. Mehta TI, Weissman S, Fung BM, et al. Global incidence, prevalence and features of primary sclerosing cholangitis: a systematic review and meta-analysis. Liver Int 2021;41(10):2418–26.

26. Hurlburt KJ, McMahon BJ, Deubner H, et al. Prevalence of autoimmune liver disease in Alaska natives. Am J Gastroenterol 2002;97(9):2402–7.

27. Toy E, Balasubramanian S, Selmi C, et al. The prevalence, incidence and natural history of primary sclerosing cholangitis in an ethnically diverse population. BMC Gastroenterol 2011;11:83.

28. Deneau M, Jensen MK, Holmen J, et al. Primary sclerosing cholangitis, autoimmune hepatitis, and overlap in Utah children: epidemiology and natural history. Hepatology 2013;58(4):1392–400.

29. Kaplan GG, Laupland KB, Butzner D, et al. The burden of large and small duct primary sclerosing cholangitis in adults and children: a population-based analysis. Am J Gastroenterol 2007;102(5):1042–9.

30. Kingham JG, Kochar N, Gravenor MB. Incidence, clinical patterns, and outcomes of primary sclerosing cholangitis in South Wales. United Kingdom. Gastroenterology 2004;126(7):1929–30.

31. Escorsell A, Pares A, Rodes J, et al. Epidemiology of primary sclerosing cholangitis in Spain. Spanish association for the study of the liver. J Hepatol 1994;21(5): 787–91.

32. Barner-Rasmussen N, Pukkala E, Jussila A, et al. Epidemiology, risk of malignancy and patient survival in primary sclerosing cholangitis: a population-based study in Finland. Scand J Gastroenterol 2020;55:74–81.

33. Berdal JE, Ebbesen J, Rydning A. [Incidence and prevalence of autoimmune liver diseases]. Tidsskr Nor Laegeforen 1998;118(29):4517–9.

34. Boberg KM, Aadland E, Jahnsen J, et al. Incidence and prevalence of primary biliary cirrhosis, primary sclerosing cholangitis, and autoimmune hepatitis in a Norwegian population. Scand J Gastroenterol 1998;33(1):99–103.

35. Carbone M, Kodra Y, Rocchetti A, et al. Primary sclerosing cholangitis: burden of disease and mortality using data from the national rare diseases registry in Italy. Int J Environ Res Public Health 2020;17(9):3095.

36. Liang H, Manne S, Shick J, et al. Incidence, prevalence, and natural history of primary sclerosing cholangitis in the United Kingdom. Medicine (Baltim) 2017; 96(24):e7116.

37. Tanaka A, Mori M, Matsumoto K, et al. Increase trend in the prevalence and male-to-female ratio of primary biliary cholangitis, autoimmune hepatitis, and primary sclerosing cholangitis in Japan. Hepatol Res 2019;49(8):881–9.

38. Yanai H, Matalon S, Rosenblatt A, et al. Prognosis of primary sclerosing cholangitis in Israel is independent of coexisting inflammatory bowel disease. J Crohns Colitis 2015;9(2):177–84.

39. Tan N, Ngu N, Worland T, et al. Epidemiology and outcomes of primary sclerosing cholangitis: an Australian multicentre retrospective cohort study. Hepatol Int 2022;16:1094–104.
40. Lamba M, Ngu JH, Stedman CAM. Trends in incidence of autoimmune liver diseases and increasing incidence of autoimmune hepatitis. Clin Gastroenterol Hepatol 2021;19(3):573–9.e1.
41. Broome U, Olsson R, Loof L, et al. Natural history and prognostic factors in 305 Swedish patients with primary sclerosing cholangitis. Gut 1996;38:610–5.
42. Hirano K, Tada M, Isayama H, et al. Clinical features of primary sclerosing cholangitis with onset age above 50 years. J Gastroenterol 2008;43:729–33.
43. Rupp C, Rössler A, Zhou T, et al. Impact of age at diagnosis on disease progression in patients with primary sclerosing cholangitis. United European Gastroenterol J 2018;6(2):255–62.
44. Kelly P, Patchett S, McCloskey D, et al. Sclerosing cholangitis, race and sex. Gut 1997;41(5):688–9.
45. Are VS, Vilar-Gomez E, Gromski MA, et al. Racial differences in primary sclerosing cholangitis mortality is associated with community socioeconomic status. Liver Int 2021;41(11):2703–11.
46. Bayable A, Ohabughiro M, Cheung R, et al. Ethnicity-specific differences in liver transplant outcomes among adults with primary sclerosing cholangitis: 2005-2017 United Network for Organ Sharing/Organ Procurement and transplantation Network. J Clin Exp Hepatol 2021;11(1):30–6.
47. Mertz A, Nguyen NA, Katsanos KH, et al. Primary sclerosing cholangitis and inflammatory bowel disease comorbidity: an update of the evidence. Ann Gastroenterol 2019;32(2):124–33.
48. Xie Y, Chen X, Deng M, et al. Causal linkage between inflammatory bowel disease and primary sclerosing cholangitis: a two-sample Mendelian randomization analysis. Front Genet 2021;12:649376.
49. Vavricka SR, Schoepfer A, Scharl M, et al. Extraintestinal manifestations of inflammatory bowel disease. Inflamm Bowel Dis 2015;21(8):1982–92.
50. Barberio B, Massimi D, Cazzagon N, et al. Prevalence of primary sclerosing cholangitis in patients with inflammatory bowel disease: a systematic review and meta-analysis. Gastroenterology 2021;161(6):1865–77.
51. Talwalkar JA, Lindor KD. Primary sclerosing cholangitis. Inflamm Bowel Dis 2005; 11:62–72.
52. Guerra I, Bujanda L, Castro J, et al. Clinical characteristics, associated malignancies and management of primary sclerosing cholangitis in inflammatory bowel disease patients: a multicentre retrospective cohort study. J Crohns Colitis 2019;13(12):1492–500.
53. Jorge AD, Esley C. Primary sclerosing cholangitis. Endoscopy 1985;17(1):11–4.
54. Ranieri V, Kennedy E, Walmsley M, et al. The Primary Sclerosing Cholangitis (PSC) Wellbeing Study: understanding psychological distress in those living with PSC and those who support them. PLoS One 2020;15(7):e0234624.
55. Dyson JK, Elsharkawy AM, Lamb CA, et al. Fatigue in primary sclerosing cholangitis is associated with sympathetic over-activity and increased cardiac output. Liver Int 2015;35(5):1633–41.
56. Kuo A, Gomel R, Safer R, et al. Characteristics and outcomes reported by patients with primary sclerosing cholangitis through an online registry. Clin Gastroenterol Hepatol 2019;17(7):1372–8.
57. Jorgensen RA, Lindor KD, Sartin JS, et al. Serum lipid and fat-soluble vitamin levels in primary sclerosing cholangitis. J Clin Gastroenterol 1995;20(3):215–9.

58. Tischendorf JJ, Hecker H, Krüger M, et al. Characterization, outcome, and prognosis in 273 patients with primary sclerosing cholangitis: a single center study. Am J Gastroenterol 2007;102:107–14.

59. Said K, Glaumann H, Bergquist A. Gallbladder disease in patients with primary sclerosing cholangitis. J Hepatol 2008;48(4):598–605.

60. Song J, Li Y, Bowlus CL, et al. Cholangiocarcinoma in patients with primary sclerosing cholangitis (PSC): a comprehensive review. Clin Rev Allergy Immunol 2020;58(1):134–49.

61. Kornfeld D, Ekbom A, Ihre T. Is there an excess risk for colorectal cancer in patients with ulcerative colitis and concomitant primary sclerosing cholangitis? A population based study. Gut 1997;41(4):522–5.

62. Poupon R. Liver alkaline phosphatase: a missing link between choleresis and biliary inflammation. Hepatology 2015;61:2080–90.

63. Schrumpf E, Boberg KM. Primary sclerosing cholangitis: challenges of a new millennium. Dig Liver Dis 2000;32:753–5.

64. Haseeb A, Siddiqui A, Taylor LJ, et al. Elevated serum bilirubin level correlates with the development of cholangiocarcinoma, Subsequent liver transplantation, and death in patients with primary sclerosing cholangitis. J Clin Gastroenterol 2016;50(5):431–5.

65. Mendes FD, Jorgensen R, Keach J, et al. Elevated serum IgG4 concentration in patients with primary sclerosing cholangitis. Am J Gastroenterol 2006;101:2070–5.

66. Nakazawa T, Naitoh I, Hayashi K, et al. Diagnosis of IgG4-related sclerosing cholangitis. World J Gastroenterol 2013;19(43):7661–70.

67. Hov JR, Boberg KM, Karlsen TH. Autoantibodies in primary sclerosing cholangitis. World J Gastroenterol 2008;14(24):3781–91.

68. Terjung B, Bogsch F, Klein R, et al. Diagnostic accuracy of atypical p-ANCA in autoimmune hepatitis using ROC- and multivariate regression analysis. Eur J Med Res 2004;9:439–48.

69. Zachou K, Liaskos C, Rigopoulou E, et al. Presence of high avidity anticardiolipin antibodies in patients with autoimmune cholestatic liver diseases. Clin Immunol 2006;119:203–12.

70. Angulo P, Peter JB, Gershwin ME, et al. Serum autoantibodies in patients with primary sclerosing cholangitis. J Hepatol 2000;32:182–7.

71. Khoshpouri P, Habibabadi RR, Hazhirkarzar B, et al. Imaging features of primary sclerosing cholangitis: from diagnosis to liver transplant follow-up. Radiographics 2019;39(7):1938–64.

72. Majoie CB, Smits NJ, Phoa SS, et al. Primary sclerosing cholangitis: sonographic findings. Abdom Imaging 1995;20(2):109–13.

73. Reading C, Jones T, Vangala C, Primary sclerosing cholangitis. SonoWorld 2018. Available at: https://sonoworld.com/Article-Details/Primary_Sclerosing_Cholangitis.aspx?ArticleId=7. Accessed July 2023.

74. Talwalkar JA, Angulo P, Johnson CD, et al. Cost-minimization analysis of MRC versus ERCP for the diagnosis of primary sclerosing cholangitis. Hepatology 2004;40(1):39–45.

75. Vitellas KM, Keogan MT, Freed KS, et al. Radiologic manifestations of sclerosing cholangitis with emphasis on MR cholangiopancreatography. Radiographics 2000;20(4):959–75 [quiz: 1108–1109, 1112].

76. Bader TR, Beavers KL, Semelka RC. MR imaging features of primary sclerosing cholangitis: patterns of cirrhosis in relationship to clinical severity of disease. Radiology 2003;226(3):675–85.

77. Ito K, Mitchell DG, Outwater EK, et al. Primary sclerosing cholangitis: MR imaging features. AJR Am J Roentgenol 1999;172(6):1527–33.
78. Gulliver DJ, Baker ME, Putnam W, et al. Bile duct diverticula and webs: nonspecific cholangiographic features of primary sclerosing cholangitis. AJR Am J Roentgenol 1991;157(2):281–5.
79. European Association for the Study of the Liver. EASL Clinical Practice Guidelines: management of cholestatic liver diseases. J Hepatol 2009;51(2):237–67.
80. Hilscher MB, Tabibian JH, Carey EJ, et al. Dominant strictures in primary sclerosing cholangitis: a multicenter survey of clinical definitions and practices. Hepatol Commun 2018;2(7):836–44.
81. Chapman MH, Webster GJ, Bannoo S, et al. Cholangiocarcinoma and dominant strictures in patients with primary sclerosing cholangitis: a 25-year single-centre experience. Eur J Gastroenterol Hepatol 2012;24(9):1051–8.
82. Dyson JK, Beuers U, Jones DEJ, et al. Primary sclerosing cholangitis. Lancet 2018;391(10139):2547–59.
83. Bangarulingam SY, Gossard AA, Petersen BT, et al. Complications of endoscopic retrograde cholangiopancreatography in primary sclerosing cholangitis. Am J Gastroenterol 2009;104(4):855–60.
84. Yarmohammadi H, Covey AM. Percutaneous biliary interventions and complications in malignant bile duct obstruction. Linchuang Zhongliuxue Zazhi 2016; 5(5):68.
85. Turan AS, Jenniskens S, Martens JM, et al. Complications of percutaneous transhepatic cholangiography and biliary drainage, a multicenter observational study. Abdom Radiol (NY) 2022;47(9):3338–44.
86. Pleskow DK, Parsi MA, Chen YK, et al. Biopsy of Indeterminate biliary strictures: does direct visualization help?—a multicener experience. Gastrointest Endosc 2008;67(5):AB103.
87. Rey JW, Hansen T, Dümcke S, et al. Efficacy of SpyGlass(TM)-directed biopsy compared to brush cytology in obtaining adequate tissue for diagnosis in patients with biliary strictures. World J Gastrointest Endosc 2014;6(4):137–43.
88. Jung KS, Kim SU. Clinical applications of transient elastography. Clin Mol Hepatol 2012;18(2):163–73.
89. Mjelle AB, Fossdal G, Gilja OH, et al. Liver elastography in primary sclerosing cholangitis patients using three different Scanner systems. Ultrasound Med Biol 2020;46(8):1854–64.
90. Hoodeshenas S, Welle CL, Navin PJ, et al. Magnetic resonance elastography in primary sclerosing cholangitis: interobserver agreement for liver stiffness measurement with manual and automated methods. Acad Radiol 2019;26(12):1625–32.
91. Tafur M, Cheung A, Menezes RJ, et al. Risk stratification in primary sclerosing cholangitis: comparison of biliary stricture severity on MRCP versus liver stiffness by MR elastography and vibration-controlled transient elastography. Eur Radiol 2020;30(7):3735–47.
92. Broomé U, Glaumann H, Lindstöm E, et al. Natural history and outcome in 32 Swedish patients with small duct primary sclerosing cholangitis (PSC). J Hepatol 2002;36(5):586–9.
93. Chapman R, Fevery J, Kalloo A, et al. Diagnosis and management of primary sclerosing cholangitis. Hepatology 2010;51(2):660–78.
94. Carrasco-Avino G, Schiano TD, Ward SC, et al. Primary sclerosing cholangitis: detailed histologic assessment and integration using bioinformatics highlights arterial fibrointimal hyperplasia as a novel feature. Am J Clin Pathol 2015; 143(4):505–13.

Phenotypes of Primary Sclerosing Cholangitis and Differential Diagnosis

Brian H. Horwich, MD, MS[a], Douglas T. Dieterich, MD[b],*

KEYWORDS

- Primary sclerosing cholangitis • IgG4-related disease
- Autoimmune overlap syndrome • Secondary sclerosing cholangitis

KEY POINTS

- The diagnosis of PSC can be challenging to make, necessitates extensive evaluation, and sometimes requires histopathologic analysis.
- The anatomic distribution of bile duct involvement (large vs. small duct) provides important prognostic information, with large duct PSC conferring a higher risk of mortality.
- PSC-IBD represents a unique clinical phenotype of both PSC and IBD. For these patients, PSC may be an extraintestinal manifestation of their IBD.
- Some individuals have histologic features of both PSC and AIH, for which a diagnosis of Overlap Syndrome is often assigned.
- PSC is ultimately a diagnosis of exclusion, requiring careful and thorough evaluation of other potential causes of sclerosing cholangitis.

INTRODUCTION, HISTORY, AND BACKGROUND

Primary sclerosing cholangitis (PSC) is a progressive, chronic liver disease driven by a combination of genetic, immunologic, and inflammatory factors. First described in the 1920s, it was characterized as "diffuse contracture" of the extrahepatic biliary tree.[1] Histologic evaluation revealed both loss of bile ducts and periductular fibrosis, termed "obliterative cholangitis".[2] Over the following half-century, the disease would be further defined and ultimately termed a distinct disorder known as primary sclerosing cholangitis.[3–6] While PSC has a more indolent course in some, the diagnosis carries significant long-term health implications. The median transplant-free survival is estimated

---

[a] Division of Gastroenterology, Icahn School of Medicine at Mount Sinai, 1 Gustave L. Levy Place, PO Box 1076, New York, NY 10029, USA; [b] Division of Liver Diseases, Institute for Liver Medicine, Icahn School of Medicine at Mount Sinai, 1468 Madison Avenue, Annenberg 5-04, New York, NY 10029, USA
* Corresponding author.
E-mail address: Douglas.Dieterich@mountsinai.org

Clin Liver Dis 28 (2024) 143–155
https://doi.org/10.1016/j.cld.2023.07.006
1089-3261/24/© 2023 Elsevier Inc. All rights reserved.

to be between 12 and 18 years, with mortality primarily driven by the development of cholangiocarcinoma (CCA).[7,8]

Due to its relatively low prevalence—estimated to be 20.3 and 6.3 in 100,000 for men and women in the United States, respectively—it was not until larger cohort studies that multiple phenotypes were identified.[9,10] Though numerous potential phenotypes have been described, the most widely characterized are defined by the distribution of duct involvement, concomitant presence of IBD, association with IgG4-positive plasma cells, and overlap with other autoimmune liver disease (**Fig. 1**). The identification of secondary causes of biliary structures such as critical illness, trauma, drugs, malignancy, and infections has also allowed for further specificity in defining PSC as a unique entity. Consequently, the presence of biliary strictures on imaging or cholestatic liver injury represents a broad differential diagnosis.

DEFINITIONS AND DIAGNOSIS OF PRIMARY SCLEROSING CHOLANGITIS

Despite recent progress in the understanding of PSC, there remains no universally accepted diagnostic criteria. As there is no single pathognomonic finding of *primary sclerosing cholangitis*, the diagnosis is made based on a combination of clinical and histopathologic features. Current guidance states that the diagnosis of PSC can be made with characteristic cholangiogram or histopathology after eliminating secondary causes.[11,12] In turn, phenotypes of PSC are primarily based on clinical observations and their corresponding outcomes.

Symptoms

Common symptoms of PSC are thought to be driven by obstructive cholestasis. Chronic biliary obstruction results in fatigue and pruritus, adversely impacting quality of life. Patients may also experience intermittent or chronic abdominal pain from cholangitis, which can result in fevers and systemic inflammatory response.[8] Anxiety and

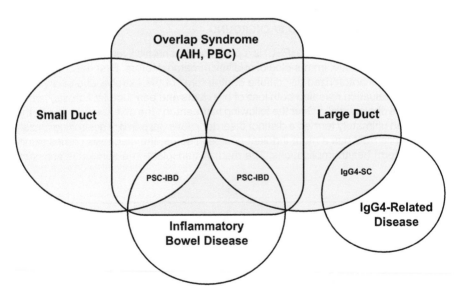

Fig. 1. Overlapping clinical phenotypes of primary sclerosing cholangitis. AIH, autoimmune hepatitis; IgG4-SC, IgG4-associated sclerosing cholangitis; PBC, primary biliary cholangitis; PSC-IBD, primary sclerosing cholangitis-inflammatory bowel disease.

depression are common comorbid diagnoses in patients with PSC, and may be present in the absence of other symptoms.[13] The presence of symptoms suggestive of inflammatory bowel disease (IBD)—such as diarrhea, hematochezia, joint pains, and rashes—may also be present but are not understood to be driven by the hepatobiliary involvement.

Serologic Testing

The most common laboratory abnormalities are cholestatic liver injury, with elevated serum alkaline phosphatase and gamma-glutamyl transferase.[14] Guidelines of the American Association for the Study of Liver Disease (AASLD) recommend a diagnosis of PSC be considered in all patients with evidence of cholestasis.[11] However, elevation in serum aminotransferases are also common, and may suggest overlapping features of autoimmune hepatitis (AIH).[15] Autoantibodies such as antinuclear antibodies and anti-smooth muscle antibodies are often present, but have minimal utility in diagnosis.[16] Serum IgG4 is frequently elevated in patients with PSC, with high titers (>5.6 g/L) aiding in differentiation from IgG4-associated sclerosing cholangitis.[17] No single serologic test definitively rules in or eliminates a diagnosis of PSC.

Biliary Imaging

Due to the ambiguity of serologies, anatomic evaluation of the biliary tree provides the foundation upon which a diagnosis of PSC is made. With the development of endoscopic retrograde cholangiopancreatography (ERCP), it became possible to characterize the ducts without intraoperative or post-mortem evaluation.[3] Ducts were have been described as having a "beaded" appearance, with diffuse foci of narrowing with corresponding proximal dilation.[18] Advances in imaging technology have produced magnetic resonance cholangiopancreatography (MRCP) as a non-invasive strategy with comparable diagnostic accuracy.[19] Characteristic MRCP findings in PSC include concomitant bile duct strictures and dilation in a diffuse distribution. An added advantage to MRCP over ERCP is the characterization of the liver parenchyma, which may demonstrate fibrosis and atrophy.[20] Characteristic MRCP findings, congruent clinical history, and elimination of secondary causes are sufficient to make a diagnosis of PSC.[11]

Histopathology

Though not necessary to make a diagnosis of PSC, biopsy with histologic analysis may be warranted if the diagnosis is unclear or there is concern for a different underlying disorder. Tissue examination is highly useful to make a diagnosis of small-duct PSC (SD-PSC) or when overlap with AIH is suspected. The most common histologic features of PSC include bile duct loss, ductular proliferation, and periductal fibrosis.[21] Presence of lymphoplasmacytic infiltrate with interface hepatitis is suggestive of overlap with AIH.[15]

PHENOTYPING BY ANATOMIC DISTRIBUTION
Large Duct (Classic)

From an anatomic standpoint, PSC can be subdivided based on the involvement (or lack thereof) of the extrahepatic or large intrahepatic biliary tree. Termed "large duct" or "classic" PSC, the findings and management of diffuse structuring of large bile ducts were initially described in the surgical literature.[1,22,23] Large duct PSC (LD-PSC) is more common, with estimated incidence 5 times greater than that of small duct disease.[24] It remains unclear whether this disparity represents true difference in clinical prevalence or challenges in diagnosing small duct disease. As the largest PSC cohort studies did not distinguish between large and small duct PSC (SD-PSC), there is limited data specifically regarding the prognosis of LD-PSC.

Due to historical inconsistencies in stricture definitions, a standardized nomenclature has recently been proposed. Perhaps the most pervasive term is *dominant stricture*, which is defined as common bile duct diameter <1.5 mm or hepatic duct diameter <1 mm on ERCP.[25] Even if benign at time of identification, dominant strictures are associated with recurrent cholangitis and high risk of development of CCA.[25-27] The applicability of this definition in the MRCP era is uncertain as ERCP is performed with high-pressure contrast injection that may increase the measured duct size. Additionally, MRCP typically lacks spatial resolution below 1 mm. Consequently, the term *high-grade* stricture (defined as >75% reduction in lumen) on MRCP has been proposed as an alternative.[11] Similar to dominant strictures, high-grade strictures have been shown to be associated with worse outcomes including increased mortality.[28] Further studies are needed to evaluate whether high-grade strictures have equivalent malignant or cholangitic potential.

Recent guidelines have introduced the term *relevant stricture* as a clinically centered term, referring to any stricture of the common bile or hepatic duct that is associated with obstructive cholestasis or cholangitis.[11] This definition is challenging in clinical practice as it may be difficult to demonstrate that a particular stricture is *not* relevant without procedural intervention such as ERCP. Patients with LD-PSC should be monitored closely, with vigilant observation for signs of cholangitis or CCA.

Small Duct

By definition and in contrast, SD-PSC refers to clinical and histopathologic findings consistent with PSC in the absence of large duct involvement. Though there is evidence that SD-PSC is genetically distinct from the large duct phenotype, the driving mechanisms are poorly understood.[29] Imaging and cholangiographic findings are often normal, but MRCP may demonstrate peribiliary enhancement, heterogenous T2 signal intensity, and periportal lymphadenopathy.[30] For this reason, definitive diagnosis generally requires liver biopsy demonstrating histologic findings typical of PSC. When compared to large duct disease, patients with SD-PSC have a longer transplant-free survival and are significantly less likely to develop CCA.[31,32] Individuals with SD-PSC should be frequently monitored early in disease course, as approximately one-quarter will subsequently develop large duct disease.[31]

INFLAMMATORY BOWEL DISEASE-ASSOCIATED

An alternative means of phenotyping PSC is the presence (or absence) of concomitant idiopathic IBD such as ulcerative colitis (UC) and Crohn's disease (CD). There remains some controversy as to whether IBD-associated PSC represents a distinct clinical entity, an extraintestinal manifestation of IBD, or a sequela of the same underlying immunologic process that results in both hepatobiliary and gastrointestinal mucosal inflammation. Prior cohort studies have shown that 16% of individuals with IBD have elevated liver chemistries with 11% having findings consistent with PSC.[33] It is estimated nearly two-thirds of patients with PSC have or subsequently develop IBD.[34-36]

Individuals with concomitant IBD and PSC also demonstrate a unique IBD phenotype, referred to as PSC-IBD. Cohort studies of patients with PSC-IBD have shown that an IBD diagnosis is generally an antecedent of PSC, with only 5% receiving a PSC diagnosis prior.[37] This may be explained by recent evidence suggesting that a significant proportion of individuals with ulcerative colitis (UC) have biliary tree abnormalities on MRCP (14%) despite normal liver chemistries, sometimes referred to as *subclinical* PSC. On follow-up, more than half of this group eventually progressed to clinical cholestasis by 12 years.[38] Once clinical PSC develops, the overwhelming majority have intrahepatic ductal involvement (98%), with 58% demonstrating both intra- and extrahepatic duct abnormalities.[37] The course of PSC in these individuals may be less aggressive due to the higher proportion with SD-PSC, though one large cohort analysis showed similar PSC-related death rates.[39]

The presence of PSC in the setting of IBD also has significant implications in the prognosis and management of the bowel disease. Though luminal and histologic findings are most often consistent with UC, up to one-third of patients with PSC-IBD have CD. Individuals with colonic involvement of their IBD and PSC are more likely to have backwash ileitis and rectal sparing compared to those without PSC.[40] Those affected also tend to be younger at time of presentation, with more quiescent mucosal disease than those with IBD alone.[41] PSC-IBD is associated with a major increased risk of colonic dysplasia and colorectal cancer, with dysplasia surveillance recommended at time of PSC diagnosis.[41] Interestingly, the activity of PSC and IBD appear to be independent. IBD flares have been commonly reported after liver transplantation for PSC, while remission of mucosal disease does not slow progression of liver disease. Yet, individuals with PSC and UC who have undergone proctocolectomy with ileoanal pouch anastomosis are at an increased risk for pouchitis.[41]

IMMUNOGLOBULIN G SUBCLASS 4-ASSOCIATED SCLEROSING CHOLANGITIS

IgG4-associated sclerosing cholangitis (IgG4-SC) is a mimic of PSC with numerous overlapping clinical features. Though its pathophysiologic mechanisms are thought to be distinct, IgG4-SC is often grouped with classic PSC.[42] First identified in patients with autoimmune pancreatitis (AIP), the biliary stricturing of IgG4-SC is now understood to be a hepatobiliary manifestation of the larger cluster of plasma cell-mediated disorders referred to as IgG4-related disease (IgG4-RD).[43–45]

The concomitant presence of biliary abnormalities in individuals with AIP has been long-described, with initial reports in the 1970s.[46] Over the following several decades, it was observed that patients with sclerosing cholangitis and AIP tended to have a milder clinical course.[45] Similar to classic PSC, these individuals presented with cholestasis with associated biliary structuring on ERCP. IgG4-SC tends to primarily involve large ducts, which may explain why patients with IgG4-SC are more frequently symptomatic at presentation when compared to PSC (94% vs. 25%). The most common presenting symptoms of IgG4-SC are abdominal pain (94%) and jaundice (88%).[47] At diagnosis, individuals with IgG4-SC have higher serum transaminase and total bilirubin levels than PSC, with no significant difference in alkaline phosphatase.[47] IgG4-SC is more frequently found in men and diagnosed at older age when compared to PSC.[43] Given these demographics, patients with IgG4-SC may be initially labeled as having pancreatic cancer or CCA and managed with surgical resection.[43] History of tobacco use and prior pancreatitis are significantly more common in IgG4-SC than in PSC.[47]

Despite these distinct observed clinical features, differentiating between classic PSC and IgG4-SC can be challenging. While elevated serum IgG4 concentration >5.6 g/L is highly suggestive, modest elevations are also observed in PSC.[45,48] The ratio of serum IgG4 to IgG1 can be helpful in delineating a diagnosis in cases of modest IgG4 elevation (1.4–2.8 g/dL). For these individuals, an IgG4:IgG1 ratio of <0.24 essentially excludes IgG4-SC.[17] Histologically, IgG4-SC tends to have more significant plasma cell infiltration, typically with >10 IgG4-positive plasma cells per high powered field.[45] It is important to note that the presence of IgG4-positive plasma cells does not exclude a diagnosis of PSC.[49] Additional histopathologic findings that suggest IgG4-SC include storiform fibrosis and obliterative phlebitis which is seen in other organs of patients with IgG4-RD.[50]

Despite difficulties in diagnostic testing to differentiate IgG4-SC from classic PSC, the hallmark of IgG4-SC is its response to corticosteroid therapy.[45] Over 90% of patients with IgG4-SC are able to achieve remission with steroids, though relapse rates approach 75% at 5 years after treatment is withdrawn. Additional agents that have been used in IgG4-SC management include rituximab, mycophenolate mofetil, and azathioprine.[47] To date, there are no prospective studies comparing immunosuppressive regimens.

Given its responsiveness to medical therapy, it is not surprising that IgG4-SC has a milder clinical course than classic PSC. This includes a significantly lower rate of progression to cirrhosis (7% vs. 37%) and CCA (4% vs. 18%). IgG4-SC does have significant associated mortality, with estimated 5-year overall mortality of 11% and a median of 6.5 years from diagnosis to death.[47] While the most common causes of mortality in this cohort were cirrhosis (20%) and CCA (30%), half of the reported deaths were attributed to non-biliary diagnoses.[47]

AUTOIMMUNE OVERLAP SYNDROMES

Due to the ambiguity in diagnosis of PSC and other autoimmune liver diseases, there remains a sizeable population that presents with overlapping features of PSC, AIH, and primary biliary cholangitis (PBC). Collectively referred to as "overlap syndromes", this cluster of disorders most often refers to individuals that have clinical and/or histologic findings of AIH with either PBC or PSC.[15] While there is no clear consensus the presence of PSC-PBC overlap syndrome, it has been hypothesized that SD-PSC and PBC are on the same spectrum of small duct autoimmune biliary disease.[51]

Current diagnostic criteria for AIH include histology that is "compatible with" or "typical of" AIH with the absence of viral hepatitis. These features include plasma cell-rich interface hepatitis and hepatocellular necrosis.[52] However, there is little guidance regarding assigning a diagnosis of PSC should these features be present in addition to clinical or histologic findings of PSC.

For individuals in which PSC is suspected, an overlap syndrome could be considered if there is: mixed cholestatic and hepatocellular pattern of liver injury, cholestatic injury with absent or equivocal imaging findings, or presence of high-titer autoantibodies that suggest another autoimmune liver disease (eg, anti-smooth muscle antibody or anti-mitochondrial antibodies). It is estimated that 7-14% of patients with a diagnosis of PSC share overlapping features with AIH.[15] In individuals with cholangiographic findings consistent with PSC, 8% have histologic findings of either "probable" or "definite" AIH.[53] As AIH is not strongly associated with IBD, the presence of luminal bowel disease may support a diagnosis of PSC alone if histology is unclear.

Data regarding the treatment of individuals with PSC-AIH overlap syndrome are mixed. Some studies have reported responsiveness to AIH treatment such as steroids or azathioprine, while others have suggested treatment failure rates of 80%.[15] As there is no standard definition for PSC-AIH overlap syndrome, data regarding treatment response cannot be readily extrapolated.

DIFFERENTIAL DIAGNOSIS OF SCLEROSING CHOLANGITIS
Identification of Other Potential Causes

The diagnosis of PSC inherently requires the exclusion of other diseases which result in bile duct stricturing. The clinical finding of bile duct abnormalities with a known contributing etiology is termed *secondary sclerosing cholangitis* (SSC). These alternate underlying causes range from anatomic, malignant, drug-associated, ischemic, non-bacterial infectious or other autoimmune (**Table 1**).[11] The primary driver of biliary stricturing may be clinically apparent (eg, critical illness) or may require extensive investigation to identify a rare malignancy or autoimmune disease. Careful history and evaluation are crucial in identifying or eliminating these etiologies in order to make a diagnosis of PSC.

Anatomic and Obstructive

Chronic biliary obstruction due to anatomic changes in the large bile ducts results in stasis and bacterial overgrowth. In turn, the resulting recurrent cholangitis causes ductal scarring and structuring, referred to as "recurrent suppurative cholangitis."[54] While a wide range of pathologies can cause obstruction, some of the more common etiologies include choledocholithiasis, iatrogenic surgical strictures (eg, cholecystectomy, liver transplantation) or extrinsic compression of the duct (eg, Mirrizi syndrome, adjacent mass or aneurysm). Other less common causes include cystic fibrosis-associated liver disease, portal hypertensive biliopathy, and recurrent pancreatitis.[11]

Malignancy

Through a similar mechanism to anatomic causes, malignancy can result in chronic biliary stasis resulting in sclerosing cholangitis. While primary biliary malignancies such as cholangiocarcinoma (including Klatskin tumors), gallbladder adenocarcinoma,

Table 1	
Differential diagnosis of secondary sclerosing cholangitis	
Anatomic & Obstructive	Choledocholithaisis
	Post-surgical (cholecystectomy, liver transplantation)
	Mirrizi Syndomre
	Extrinsic compression (aneurysm, adjacent mass)
	Cystic fibrosis-associated
	Portal hypertensive biliopathy
	Recurrent pancreatitis
Malignant	Cholangiocarcinoma (Klatskin tumor)
	Gallbladder adenocarcinoma
	Diffuse intrahepatic metastatic disease
	Lymphoma
	Langerhans cell histiocytosis
Drug-Associated	Pembrolizumab
	Nivolumab
Ischemia & Critical Illness	Reperfusion cholangiopathy
	Ischemic cholangiopathy
Non-Bacterial Infections	*Cryptosporidium parvum*
	Ascaris lumbricoides
	Clonorchis sinensis
	Fascioliasis sp.
	Opisthorchis sp.
	Schistosomiasis
	Echinococcus
Autoimmune	Leukocytoclastic vasculitis
	Eosinophilic cholangitis
	Eosinophilic cholangitis
	Celiac disease
	Systemic lupus erythematosus

and pancreatic adenocarcinoma are more commonly associated with the development of SSC, it may also be a result of diffuse hepatic metastases from an extrahepatic primary solid tumor.[55] Hematologic malignancies with hepatic infiltration such as lymphoma or Langerhans cell histiocytosis are also rare causes of SSC.

Drug-Associated

While numerous medications have been associated with cholestatic drug-induced liver injury (DILI), rarely does this result in chronic cholestasis and subsequent sclerosis. Checkpoint-inhibitor therapy has given rise to a newly recognized form of drug-associated sclerosing cholangitis.[56] Though the mechanism is not entirely understood, individuals develop an autoimmune-like sclerosing cholangitis after exposure to anti-programmed cell death-1 (PD-1) therapy. The most commonly implicated agents are nivolumab and pembrolizumab.[56]

Ischemia and Critical Illness

As the bile ducts derive their primary blood supply from the hepatic artery, they are more sensitive to ischemic injury than the remainder of the liver parenchyma.[57] Given the extensive collateral blood supply to the liver from the portal venous system, ischemia of the bile ducts due to systemic hypotension is rare. In liver transplantation, the intentional blockade of the hepatic arteries and extracorporeal time can result in severe ischemic injury. After reperfusion, the ducts can become sclerotic, resulting in chronic cholestasis and potential graft loss. In the era of modern intensive care, a similar phenomenon has been observed in critically ill patients—particularly those on long-term mechanical ventilation. Histopathologic analysis of these individuals demonstrates similar pattern of injury with multifocal bile duct stricturing, thought to be related to repeated systemic hypoxia resulting in ischemia.[58]

Non-bacterial Infections

While recurrent bacterial infections of the ducts are considered to be the primary driving mechanism in most forms of sclerosing cholangitis, numerous other non-bacterial sources have been implicated. In patients with uncontrolled human immunodeficiency virus (HIV) resulting in acquired immune deficiency syndrome (AIDS), the bile ducts can become infected with opportunistic organisms such as *Crytposporidium parvum* and microsporidia. It is hypothesized that these microbes synergistically interact with HIV to cause recurrent cholangiocyte apoptosis and eventual scarring.[59] Other parasitic infections in immunocompetent hosts are also a frequently reported cause of SSC. While *Ascaris lumbricoides* and *Clonorchis sinensis* are common, *Fascioliasis* and *Opisthorchis sp.* have also been implicated.[60] In the Middle East, East Asia and South America, schistosomiasis or "liver fluke" infection of the bile duct is a well-documented cause of SSC, resulting in a high burden of cirrhosis and cholangiocarcinoma.[61] Echinococcus, a tapeworm found in dogs and sheep, and associated hydatid cyst formation is yet another parasitic etiology of SSC.[11] SARS-CoV-2 has been identified as a cause of SSC in as many as 15% of infected patients.[62,63] SSC secondary to SARS-CoV-2 is associated with a rapid progression to cirrhosis.[64]

Other Autoimmune Disease

Numerous other autoimmune diseases can present with sclerosing cholangitis by either direct or indirect mechanisms. Systemic vasculitides such as leukocytoclastic vasculitis can result in bile duct injury by a similar means to ischemic cholangitis. Analogous to PSC, eosinophilic cholangitis is an exceedingly rare chronic inflammatory disorder of the biliary tree that is differentiated by marked eosinophil proliferation.[65]

Other autoimmune conditions implicated in SSC include Sjogren's syndrome, celiac disease, systemic lupus erythematosus.[66]

DISCUSSION AND SUMMARY

As the understanding of primary sclerosing cholangitis expands, so will the knowledge of if its various phenotypes. Current phenotypic classification relies solely on clinically observable features such as size of duct involvement, association with IBD, infiltration of IgG4-producing plasma cells, or overlapping features of other autoimmune liver disease. Even when suspected, making a definitive diagnosis of PSC can be challenging. And finally, careful elimination of potential other underlying etiologies—for which a diagnosis of SSC is more appropriate—is critical to management. Further exploration of the pathophysiologic mechanisms of PSC will likely provide more understanding regarding these observed phenotypes and may allow for better directed therapeutic strategies.

CLINICS CARE POINTS

- PSC can be phenotypically categorized by duct size, association with IBD, or evidence of IgG4-related disease.
- The presence of large-duct involvement of PSC is generally a poor prognostic sign, and is associated with increased risk of cholangiocarcinoma.
- Individuals with both PSC and IBD have a high risk of colorectal dysplasia and cancer, independent of PSC disease activity.
- IgG4-associated sclerosing cholangitis is a classic PSC disease mimic but is often responsive to corticosteroid therapy.
- Differentiating between PSC and other autoimmune liver diseases can be challenging, and some people may exhibit features of multiple.
- The differential diagnosis for sclerosing cholangitis is very broad. Careful evaluation and elimination of potential underlying causes including anatomic derangements, ischemia, malignancy, offending medications, non-bacterial infections, or autoimmune disease is crucial.

DISCLOSURE

Dr B.H. Horwich: Nothing to disclose. Dr D.T. Dieterich: Nothing to disclose.

REFERENCES

1. Ransom HK, Malcolm KD. Obstructive jaundice: due to diffuse contracture of the extrahepatic bile ducts. Arch Surg 1934;28(4):713–26.
2. Klemperer P. Chronic intrahepatic obliterating cholangitis. J Mt Sinai Hosp 1937; 4:279.
3. Chapman RW, Arborgh BA, Rhodes JM, et al. Primary sclerosing cholangitis: a review of its clinical features, cholangiography, and hepatic histology. Gut 1980; 21(10):870–7.
4. Ludwig J. Surgical pathology of the syndrome of primary sclerosing cholangitis. Am J Surg Pathol 1989;13:43–9.
5. Chapman RW, Jewell DP. Primary sclerosing cholangitis–an immunologically mediated disease? West J Med 1985;143(2):193–5.

6. Wiesner RH, LaRusso NF. Clinicopathologic features of the syndrome of primary sclerosing cholangitis. Gastroenterology 1980;79(2):200–6.

7. Ponsioen CY. Natural history of primary sclerosing cholangitis and prognostic value of cholangiography in a Dutch population. Gut 2002;51(4):562–6.

8. Broome U, Olsson R, Lööf L, et al. Natural history and prognostic factors in 305 Swedish patients with primary sclerosing cholangitis. Gut 1996;38(4):610–5.

9. Bambha K, Kim WR, Talwalkar J, et al. Incidence, clinical spectrum, and outcomes of primary sclerosing cholangitis in a United States community. Gastroenterology 2003;125(5):1364–9.

10. Lindkvist B, Benito de Valle M, Gullberg B, et al. Incidence and prevalence of primary sclerosing cholangitis in a defined adult population in Sweden. Hepatology 2010;52(2):571–7.

11. Bowlus CL, Arrivé L, Bergquist A, et al. AASLD practice guidance on primary sclerosing cholangitis and cholangiocarcinoma. Hepatology 2023;77(2):659–702.

12. EASL clinical practice guidelines on sclerosing cholangitis. J Hepatol 2022;77(3): 761–806.

13. Kuo A, Gomel R, Safer R, et al. Characteristics and outcomes reported by patients with primary sclerosing cholangitis through an online registry. Clin Gastroenterol Hepatol 2019;17(7):1372–8.

14. Lunder AK, Hov JR, Borthne A, et al. Prevalence of sclerosing cholangitis detected by magnetic resonance cholangiography in patients with long-term inflammatory bowel disease. Gastroenterology 2016;151(4):660–9, e4.

15. Boberg KM, Chapman RW, Hirschfield GM, et al. Overlap syndromes: the international autoimmune hepatitis group (IAIHG) position statement on a controversial issue. J Hepatol 2011;54(2):374–85.

16. Sebode M, Weiler-Normann C, Liwinski T, et al. Autoantibodies in autoimmune liver disease—clinical and diagnostic relevance. Front Immunol 2018;9:609.

17. Boonstra K, Culver EL, de Buy Wenniger LM, et al. Serum immunoglobulin G4 and immunoglobulin G1 for distinguishing immunoglobulin G4-associated cholangitis from primary sclerosing cholangitis. Hepatology 2014;59(5):1954–63.

18. Aabakken L, Karlsen TH, Albert J, et al. Role of endoscopy in primary sclerosing cholangitis: European society of gastrointestinal endoscopy (ESGE) and European association for the study of the liver (EASL) clinical guideline. Endoscopy 2017;49(06):588–608.

19. Dave M, Elmunzer BJ, Dwamena BA, et al. Primary sclerosing cholangitis: meta-analysis of diagnostic performance of MR cholangiopancreatography. Radiology 2010;256(2):387–96.

20. Ruiz A, Lemoinne S, Carrat F, et al. Radiologic course of primary sclerosing cholangitis: assessment by three-dimensional magnetic resonance cholangiography and predictive features of progression. Hepatology 2014;59(1):242–50.

21. Ponsioen CY, Assis DN, Boberg KM, et al. Defining primary sclerosing cholangitis: results from an international primary sclerosing cholangitis study group consensus process. Gastroenterology 2021;161(6):1764–75, e5.

22. Schwartz SI, Dale WA. Primary sclerosing cholangitis; review and report of six cases. AMA Arch Surg 1958;77(3):439–51.

23. Lemmer ER, Bornman PC, Krige JE, et al. Primary sclerosing cholangitis. Requiem for biliary drainage operations? Arch Surg 1994;129(7):723–8.

24. Kaplan GG, Laupland KB, Butzner D, et al. The burden of large and small duct primary sclerosing cholangitis in adults and children: a population-based analysis, *Am J Gastroenterol*, 102 (5), 2007, 1042-1049.

25. Björnsson E, Lindqvist-Ottosson J, Asztely M, et al. Dominant strictures in patients with primary sclerosing cholangitis. Am J Gastroenterol 2004;99(3):502–8.
26. Chapman MH, Webster GJ, Bannoo S, et al. Cholangiocarcinoma and dominant strictures in patients with primary sclerosing cholangitis; a 25 year single centre experience. Eur J Gastroenterol Hepatol 2012;24(9):1051.
27. Rudolph G, Gotthardt D, Klöters-Plachky P, et al. Influence of dominant bile duct stenoses and biliary infections on outcome in primary sclerosing cholangitis. J Hepatol 2009;51(1):149–55.
28. Lemoinne S, Cazzagon N, El Mouhadi S, et al. Simple magnetic resonance scores associate with outcomes of patients with primary sclerosing cholangitis. Clin Gastroenterol Hepatol 2019;17(13):2785–92, e3.
29. Næss S, Björnsson E, Anmarkrud JA, et al. Small duct primary sclerosing cholangitis without inflammatory bowel disease is genetically different from large duct disease. Liver Int 2014;34(10):1488–95.
30. Kozaka K, Sheedy SP, Eaton JE, et al. Magnetic resonance imaging features of small-duct primary sclerosing cholangitis. Abdominal Radiology 2020;45:2388–99.
31. Björnsson E, Olsson R, Bergquist A, et al. The natural history of small-duct primary sclerosing cholangitis. Gastroenterology 2008;134(4):975–80.
32. Bjornsson E, Boberg K, Schrumpf E, et al. Patients with small duct primary sclerosing cholangitis have favorable long term prognosis. Hepatology 2001;34(4):617.
33. Heikius B, Niemelä S, Lehtola J, et al. Hepatobiliary and coexisting pancreatic duct abnormalities in patients with inflammatory bowel disease. Scand J Gastroenterol 1997;32(2):153–61.
34. Garioud A, Seksik P, Chrétien Y, et al. Characteristics and clinical course of primary sclerosing cholangitis in France: a prospective cohort study. Eur J Gastroenterol Hepatol 2010;22(7):842–7.
35. Escorsell A, Parés A, Rodés J, et al. Epidemiology of primary sclerosing cholangitis in Spain. J Hepatol 1994;21(5):787–91.
36. Ataseven H, Parlak E, Yuksel I, et al. Primary sclerosing cholangitis in Turkish patients: characteristic features and prognosis. Hepatobiliary Pancreat Dis Int 2009; 8(3):312–5.
37. Sørensen JØ, Nielsen OH, Andersson M, et al. Inflammatory bowel disease with primary sclerosing cholangitis: a Danish population-based cohort study 1977-2011. Liver Int 2018;38(3):532–41.
38. Culver EL, Bungay HK, Betts M, et al. Prevalence and long-term outcome of subclinical primary sclerosing cholangitis in patients with ulcerative colitis. Liver Int 2020;40(11):2744–57.
39. Boonstra K, Weersma RK, van Erpecum KJ, et al. Population-based epidemiology, malignancy risk, and outcome of primary sclerosing cholangitis. Hepatology 2013;58(6):2045–55.
40. Loftus E, Harewood G, Loftus C, et al. PSC-IBD: a unique form of inflammatory bowel disease associated with primary sclerosing cholangitis. Gut 2005; 54(1):91–6.
41. de Vries AB, Janse M, Blokzijl H, et al. Distinctive inflammatory bowel disease phenotype in primary sclerosing cholangitis. World J Gastroenterol 2015;21(6):1956.
42. Liu Q, Li B, Li Y, et al. Altered faecal microbiome and metabolome in IgG4-related sclerosing cholangitis and primary sclerosing cholangitis. Gut 2022;71(5):899–909.

43. Nakazawa T, Ohara H, Sano H, et al. Clinical differences between primary sclerosing cholangitis and sclerosing cholangitis with autoimmune pancreatitis. Pancreas 2005;30(1):20–5.

44. Ghazale A, Chari ST, Zhang L, et al. Immunoglobulin G4–associated cholangitis: clinical profile and response to therapy. Gastroenterology 2008;134(3):706–15.

45. Kamisawa T, Nakazawa T, Tazuma S, et al. Clinical practice guidelines for IgG4-related sclerosing cholangitis. J Hepato-Biliary-Pancreatic Sci 2019;26(1):9–42.

46. Waldram R, Tsantoulas D, Kopelman H, et al. Chronic pancreatitis, sclerosing cholangitis, and sicca complex in two siblings. Lancet 1975;305(7906):550–2.

47. Ali AH, Bi Y, Machicado JD, et al. The long-term outcomes of patients with immunoglobulin G4-related sclerosing cholangitis: the Mayo Clinic experience. J Gastroenterol 2020;55(11):1087–97.

48. Mendes FD, Jorgensen R, Keach J, et al. Elevated serum IgG4 concentration in patients with primary sclerosing cholangitis. Am J Gastroenterol 2006;101(9): 2070–5.

49. Zhang L, Lewis JT, Abraham SC, et al. IgG4+ plasma cell infiltrates in liver explants with primary sclerosing cholangitis. Am J Surg Pathol 2010;34(1):88–94.

50. Stone JH, Zen Y, Deshpande V. IgG4-Related disease. N Engl J Med 2012; 366(6):539–51.

51. Oliveira EM. Overlapping of primary biliary cirrhosis and small duct primary sclerosing cholangitis: first case report. J Clin Med Res 2012;4(6):429–33.

52. Hennes EM, Zeniya M, Czaja AJ, et al. Simplified criteria for the diagnosis of autoimmune hepatitis. Hepatology 2008;48(1):169–76.

53. Kaya M, Angulo P, Lindor KD. Overlap of autoimmune hepatitis and primary sclerosing cholangitis: an evaluation of a modified scoring system. J Hepatol 2000; 33(4):537–42.

54. Ruemmele P, Hofstaedter F, Gelbmann CM. Secondary sclerosing cholangitis. Nat Rev Gastroenterol Hepatol 2009;6(5):287–95.

55. Estrella JS, Othman ML, Taggart MW, et al. Intrabiliary growth of liver metastases. Am J Surg Pathol 2013;37(10):1571–9.

56. Onoyama T, Takeda Y, Yamashita T, et al. Programmed cell death-1 inhibitor-related sclerosing cholangitis: a systematic review. World J Gastroenterol 2020; 26(3):353–65.

57. Deltenre P, Valla D-C. Ischemic cholangiopathy. J Hepatol 2006;44(4):806–17.

58. Gelbmann CM, Rümmele P, Wimmer M, et al. Ischemic-like cholangiopathy with secondary sclerosing cholangitis in critically ill patients. Am J Gastroenterol 2007; 102(6):1221–9.

59. Naseer M, Dailey FE, Juboori AA, et al. Epidemiology, determinants, and management of AIDS cholangiopathy: a review. World J Gastroenterol 2018;24(7): 767–74.

60. Singh Rana S, Bhasin DK, Nanda M, et al. Parasitic infestations of the biliary tract. Curr Gastroenterol Rep 2007;9(2):156–64.

61. Manzella A, Ohtomo K, Monzawa S, et al. Schistosomiasis of the liver. Abdom Imaging 2008;33(2):144–50.

62. Hartl L, Haslinger K, Angerer M, et al. Progressive cholestasis and associated sclerosing cholangitis are frequent complications of COVID-19 in patients with chronic liver disease. Hepatology 2022;76(6):1563–75.

63. Roth NC, Kim A, Vitkovski T, et al. Post–COVID-19 cholangiopathy: a novel entity, *Am J Gastroenterol*, 116 (5), 2021, 1077-1082.

64. Seifert M, Kneiseler G, Dechene A. Secondary sclerosing cholangitis due to severe COVID-19: an emerging disease entity? Digestion 2023;1–7. https://doi.org/10.1159/000528689.

65. Fragulidis GP, Vezakis AI, Kontis EA, et al. Eosinophilic cholangitis–a challenging diagnosis of benign biliary stricture: a case report. Medicine (Baltim) 2016;95(1): e2394.

66. Abdalian R, Heathcote EJ. Sclerosing cholangitis: a focus on secondary causes. Hepatology 2006;44(5):1063–74.

Diagnostic Tests in Primary Sclerosing Cholangitis

Serology, Elastography, Imaging, and Histology

Clara Y. Tow, MD[a,b], Erica Chung, MD[c], Bindu Kaul, MD[b,d],
Amarpreet Bhalla, MD[b,e], Brett E. Fortune, MD, MSc[a,b],*

KEYWORDS

- Primary sclerosing cholangitis • Cholangiopathy • Cholestasis • Diagnosis
- Elastography • Cholangiogram • Pathology

KEY POINTS

- Primary sclerosing cholangitis (PSC) is a chronic liver disease characterized by inflammation and fibrosis of the bile ducts.
- A diagnosis of PSC is best made based when classic radiographic findings of multifocal strictures with the segmental dilatation of the bile ducts, interspersed with ducts of normal or near-normal caliber are visualized on either MR cholangiography (MRCP) or endoscopic retrograde cholangiopancreatography (ERCP).
- Laboratory studies are often used to help rule out other diseases rather than confirm the diagnosis of PSC.
- Liver biopsy is not recommended in patients with PSC who have characteristic cholangiogram findings and should be reserved for cases of potential small-duct PSC or overlap syndrome.
- Elastography, particularly MR elastography, is a well-accepted modality to non-invasively stage fibrosis in patients with PSC.

INTRODUCTION

Primary sclerosing cholangitis (PSC) remains a diagnostic conundrum and is often discovered years later after first report of symptoms or at later stages of disease. However, recent innovation in imaging technology has led to shifting away from invasive diagnostic tools, such as endoscopic retrograde cholangiopancreatography (ERCP) and liver biopsy, towards less invasive imaging modalities using magnetic resonance

[a] Division of Hepatology, Montefiore Medical Center, 111 East 210th Street, Bronx, NY 10467, USA; [b] Albert Einstein College of Medicine, 1300 Morris Park Avenue, Bronx, NY 10461, USA; [c] Division of Gastroenterology, Montefiore Medical Center, 111 East 210th Street, Bronx, NY 10467, USA; [d] Department of Radiology, Montefiore Medical Center, 111 East 210th Street, Bronx, NY 10467, USA; [e] Department of Pathology, Montefiore Medical Center, 111 East 210th Street, Bronx, NY 10467, USA
* Corresponding author. 111 East 210th Street, Bronx, NY 10467.
E-mail address: bfortune@montefiore.org

Clin Liver Dis 28 (2024) 157–169
https://doi.org/10.1016/j.cld.2023.07.007
1089-3261/24/© 2023 Elsevier Inc. All rights reserved.

liver.theclinics.com

to allow safe and accurate detection of PSC. Future development of PSC-specific bio-markers will further refine the diagnostic algorithm. This review addresses current evidence on the various diagnostic testing used to identify PSC.

SEROLOGY

Patients with PSC classically demonstrate a cholestatic pattern of liver tests with a predominant elevation in alkaline phosphatase and gamma glutamyl transferase relative to AST and ALT. Among patients with longstanding inflammatory bowel disease, one study found that approximately 70% of patients have cholestatic liver tests at the time of radiographic diagnosis of PSC.[1] Early in the disease, subtle elevations in alkaline phosphatase can be appreciated even if the value is within normal range. Bilirubin becomes elevated when biliary obstruction becomes more pronounced and/or hepatic function is poor. Bile acid levels increase though do not necessarily correlate with the severity of pruritus.[2] As the disease advances, the degree of cholestasis can fluctuate in a progressive relapse-remitting pattern caused by periods of intermittent inflammation, obstruction, and/or cholangitis. Due to impaired bile flow, patients develop deficiencies in fat soluble vitamins (A, D, E, and K). Similar to other cholestatic liver diseases, patients with PSC often demonstrate increased hepatic and urinary copper concentrations with low ceruloplasmin, though this is secondary to cholestasis and not related to Wilson disease.[3]

There are no biochemical studies that can confirm a diagnosis of PSC; however, there are several immune markers identified that have been associated with the PSC.[4–8] These markers most commonly include immunoglobulin G (IgG), immunoglobulin M, anti-nuclear antibody, p-ANCA, anti-smooth muscle antibody, anti-cardiolipin, thyroperoxidase, and rheumatoid factor. Anti-mitochondrial antibody (AMA), anti-liver/kidney microsomal antibodies (ALKM), anti-soluble liver antigen (ASLA), anti-saccharomyces cerevisiae (ASCA), anti-biliary epithelial cells (anti-BEC), anti-endothelial cell (AECA), anti-glomerular basement membrane (AGBM) have also been reported. In one study of 73 men with PSC, 97% were found to have at least 1 autoantibody and more than 80% had 3 or more autoantibodies present regardless of whether patients had concomitant IBD.[4] Various HLA haplotypes have been identified, including HLA-DRB1, DQA1, and DQB1.[9–11]

Except immunoglobulin G and anticardiolipin, autoantibodies and titer levels do not correlate with disease severity or prognosis. Anti-cardiolpin positivity has been described in various cholestatic liver diseases. In a cohort of 41 patients with PSC, anti-cardiolipin IgM and/or IgG was detected in 26.8% of patients, which was significantly higher than control subjects (10.8%), though lower than patients with primary biliary cholangitis (46%).[12] Patients expressing anti-cardiolipin notably had longer disease activity and higher alkaline phosphatase. In another study, anti-cardiolipin was associated with increased Mayo Risk Score and fibrosis stage.[4]

Reported prevalence of elevated total immunoglobulin G (IgG) levels is widely reported in the literature, ranging from as low as 4% to as high as 45%.[13–15] The significance of hypergammaglobulinemia in PSC remains unclear. A single-center study published in 2019 retrospectively evaluated 148 patients with PSC over a 30-year period.[14] Patients with elevated IgG ($\geq$14 g/L) were younger but otherwise had similar clinical characteristics (including presence of overlap features and IBD) to those without elevated levels. Researchers found hypergammaglobulinemia to be an independent risk factor for reduced transplant-free survival.

Elevated IgG4 subclass, which is characteristic in IgG4-related disease and can manifest its own form of immune-mediated cholangitis, has also been observed in upwards of one-third of patients with PSC.[16–19] Given the diagnostic dilemma in being able to distinguish between these two entities, small studies suggest evaluating both the absolute value of IgG4 and the IgG4:IgG1 ratio. One study from China found that patients with an absolute high-titer of IgG4 ≥ 1.25 times the upper limit of normal had high 86% sensitivity and 97.9% specificity for IgG4-related disease.[20] A Dutch study, however, suggests that for patients with IgG4 levels between 1 and 2 times the upper limit of normal should also have the IgG4:IgG1 ratio assessed.[13] A low ratio < 0.24 excludes IgG4-related disease and thus suggests PSC as the diagnosis.

In addition to the diagnostic utility of IgG4, several studies have associated elevated IgG4 with worse outcomes among patients with PSC, including higher total bilirubin, alkaline phosphatase, PSC Mayo Risk score and prevalence of cirrhosis.[16,18,19] Patients were also less likely to have IBD and had a shorter time to liver transplantation.[16] Zhang and colleagues[19] performed IgG4 staining on 98 consecutive PSC explants; 23% had positive IgG4 plasma cells, and none had histologic features diagnostic of IgG4-related cholangitis. Positive IgG4 staining correlated with moderate-to-severe periductal lymphoplasmacytic inflammation, shorter time to transplantation, and higher risk of recurrent disease post-transplant.

Atypical perinuclear antineutrophil cytoplasmic antibodies (p-ANCA) may be present in upwards of 94% of patients with PSC.[21] For this reason, there has been much speculation as to the relationship between p-ANCA and the pathogenesis of PSC and possibly IBD. While p-ANCA may be highly sensitive (AUC 0.690 ± 0.04, OR 3.4), its poor specificity precludes it from having significant diagnostic utility in PSC.[22] There is no consensus regarding the prognostic use of p-ANCA in patients with PSC. Multiple small studies with heterogenous patient samples have shown higher rates of biliary complications, including biliary calculi or cholangiocarcinoma, as well as more extensive biliary involvement.[23,24] Other studies have seen higher rates of cirrhosis and need for liver transplantation in patients with p-ANCA.[23,25,26] Another small study of 14 patients with PSC found fluctuating expression of p-ANCA over a 2-year follow-up period. Furthermore, p-ANCA was not associated with clinical activity, liver test elevations, or fibrosis staging on liver biopsy. While there remains a lack of consensus on serologies to assist with PSC detection, future investigation will hopefully elucidate novel PSC-specific biomarkers to help accurately and noninvasively diagnose PSC.

ELASTOGRAPHY

PSC is an insidious and slowly progressive disease that can lead to extensive liver fibrosis and cirrhosis. Higher stages of fibrosis are associated with worse prognosis and have implications for treatment and management. Thus, determining the extent of fibrosis is an important part of the clinical workup. Although liver biopsy has traditionally been considered the reference standard for the assessment of liver fibrosis for many chronic liver diseases, PSC is characterized by high-grade strictures and cholestasis that often lead to patchy distributions of fibrosis throughout the liver, resulting in sampling error on liver biopsies.[27] Liver biopsies are also invasive, associated with procedural risks such as bleeding, have higher costs, and have considerable intra- and inter-observer variability in the interpretation of histology, and is therefore not recommended for fibrosis staging in PSC.[28]

Liver elastography has emerged as a powerful non-invasive method to evaluate liver fibrosis in chronic liver diseases as it allows for the quantification of liver stiffness as an indirect method of assessing fibrosis with high diagnostic accuracy compared with liver biopsy. Several types of elastography have been studied, though somewhat limited in PSC-specific cohorts.

Transient Elastography

The diagnostic performance of vibration-controlled transient elastography (TE) was evaluated in a prospective study of 73 consecutive patients with PSC who underwent both liver biopsy and TE.[29] Liver stiffness measurements (LSM) based on TE were found to correlate strongly with liver fibrosis, especially for the diagnosis of severe fibrosis and cirrhosis, and had higher diagnostic accuracy for the diagnosis of advanced fibrosis and cirrhosis compared to that of other serum markers of liver fibrosis including the APRI score, FIB-4 score, and Mayo risk score. Similar findings were reported in a retrospective analysis that concluded that TE measurements had an overall very good test accuracy for fibrosis stages F2 and F3.[30] TE is a non-invasive, painless, and rapid examination with studies showing reproducible results between operators.[29] However, the performance of TE can be influenced by BMI, presence of significant ascites, or narrow intercostal spaces. Additionally, LSM may be affected by the presence of extrahepatic cholestasis, with one study showing a significant decrease in LSM measured by TE in 13 of 15 patients after successful drainage of biliary obstruction, suggesting that extrahepatic cholestasis be excluded by labs or imaging before interpreting LSM based on TE.[31]

Shear Wave Elastography

A parallel assessment of point shear wave elastography (pSWE) and 2D-shear wave elastography (2D-SWE) was performed to determine their ability to identify and stage liver fibrosis in patients with PSC using TE as the gold standard and showed that both pSWE and 2D-SWE performed well in the identification of advanced fibrosis (F3-F4).[32] Another study showed that shear wave velocity measurements were found to be significantly higher in patients with B-mode ultrasound findings of cirrhosis, suggesting an increased sensitivity in identifying fibrosis in patients with PSC.[33] Ultrasound-based point shear wave elastography also has the added benefit of obtaining simultaneous ultrasound images of the liver and surrounding structures and can also assess for sequela of portal hypertension including splenomegaly and ascites.

Magnetic resonance elastography

Magnetic resonance elastography (MRE) is considered the most accurate non-invasive method for liver fibrosis staging, with studies showing that liver stiffness measured by MRE was able to accurately identify cirrhosis with high sensitivity and specificity in patients with PSC.[34–37] Though more costly and less available than other staging modalities, MRE has several advantages including the ability to perform the test in conjunction with an MRI with MRCP. Additionally, as fibrosis in PSC can be patchy, it is important to encompass large areas of liver parenchyma to get an accurate assessment of liver fibrosis, which is better assessed with MRE than with other staging modalities. Further, MRE is not as affected by BMI as other staging modalities.

IMAGING

Several biliary and liver parenchymal changes can be seen in PSC across various imaging modalities. Transabdominal ultrasound is often the first imaging test performed in the evaluation of abnormal liver tests as it is noninvasive, widely accessible, and inexpensive. In PSC, findings such as bile duct thickening with or without dilatation or brightly echogenic portal triads may be seen (**Fig. 1**A).[38] Similarly, cross-sectional imaging with computed tomography (CT) in PSC may demonstrate thickening or enhancement of the bile ducts, or segments of biliary ductal dilatation (**Fig. 2**A). However, these findings are nonspecific, and both ultrasound and CT are

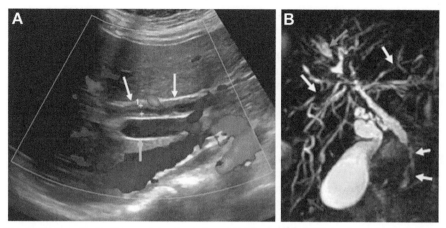

Fig. 1. (*A*) Longitudinal transabdominal ultrasound image of the liver shows a thick-walled nondilated common bile duct (*white arrows*) with patent portal vein seen posteriorly (*green arrow*). (*B*) Coronal MRCP image shows extensive extrahepatic common duct stricturing (*yellow arrows*), and multifocal intrahepatic strictures with areas of signal cut off (*white arrows*) and ductal ectasia (*orange arrow*). Note peripheral intrahepatic ductal pruning (*red arrow*).

limited in their ability to visualize the intrahepatic and small peripheral bile ducts which may be affected in early stages of the disease.[39] Thus, ultrasound and CT are rarely useful in the diagnosis of PSC, though may be helpful in excluding other causes of biliary obstruction such as choledocholithiasis, evaluating for radiographic evidence of cirrhosis or sequelae of portal hypertension, and detecting liver masses, cysts, or gallbladder polyps.[38,40]

A radiographic diagnosis of PSC is established by the presence of typical biliary ductal changes seen on cholangiography. These changes include diffuse, multifocal strictures with the segmental dilatation of the bile ducts, interspersed with ducts of normal or near-normal caliber, creating the typical "beaded" appearance (**Fig. 1**B).

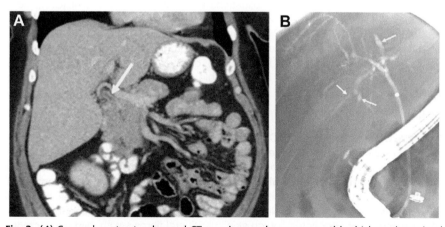

Fig. 2. (*A*) Coronal contrast-enhanced CT scan image shows a smoothly thickened proximal common duct wall with prominent enhancement (*yellow arrow*). (*B*) ERCP image shows multifocal intrahepatic strictures (*white arrow*) and areas of saccular ductal ectasia (*yellow arrows*).

Biliary ductal wall enhancement and thickening are also commonly seen. Both the intrahepatic and extrahepatic bile ducts are affected in most cases. Isolated involvement of the extrahepatic bile ducts is rare (<5%), whereas isolated involvement of the intrahepatic ducts has been reported in 25% of patients.[41] Strictured segments are usually short, though longer strictures may be seen in more advanced disease. Other findings, including hypertrophy of the left lateral lobe, particularly in advanced cirrhosis, periportal and portocaval reactive lymphadenopathy, and perfusion abnormalities associated with inflammation and/or cholangitis can also be seen (**Fig. 3A–C**).

Historically, ERCP was considered the gold standard for the diagnosis of PSC (**Fig. 2B**). However, this is an invasive procedure that carries risks of radiation exposure, bleeding, perforation, pancreatitis, and cholangitis, and hospitalization for the management of severe complications have been reported in over 10% of patients with PSC undergoing ERCP. Post-procedural cholangitis, in particular, has been reported in 0.6-8% of patients with PSC undergoing ERCP, and several studies have noted that the risk of post-ERCP cholangitis is significantly increased in patients with PSC compared to patients with non-PSC.[42–47] While prophylactic periprocedural antibiotics are generally recommended, some studies have still noted a negligible difference in incidence of post-ERCP cholangitis in patients with PSC compared to patients with non-PSC despite the use of prophylactic antibiotics.[43,48]

Magnetic resonance cholangiopancreatography (MRCP) has now largely replaced ERCP for diagnostic cholangiography due to advances in magnetic resonance techniques and the noninvasive nature of the procedure. Several studies have shown that MRCP has high sensitivity (85–88%) and specificity (92–97%) for the diagnosis of PSC, which is comparable to that of ERCP, though may be less sensitive than ERCP in detecting early changes of PSC and less specific in patients with cirrhosis.[49–53] MRCP also has high sensitivity and specificity for the localization of intrahepatic vs extrahepatic disease involvement.[52] Additionally, cost-minimization analyses have shown that use of MRCP as the initial diagnostic test in patients with suspected PSC is associated with a reduced average cost per correct diagnosis compared to ERCP.[54,55] Therefore, as a cost-effective, non-invasive test with high diagnostic accuracy for PSC that avoids the potential adverse effects of radiation exposure and post-procedural complications associated with ERCP, MRCP is now recommended as the initial diagnostic imaging modality of choice in the workup of patients with suspected PSC.[21,28,56] ERCP remains a valuable tool when therapeutic interventions are indicated to relieve biliary obstruction, when tissue samples are required (biopsy when imaging is inconclusive, or to exclude sequelae such as cholangiocarcinoma), or when MRCP is not feasible.

LIVER HISTOLOGY

Due to the wide availability of MRCP or ERCP, liver biopsy is not commonly performed and often reserved to confirm cases of possible small-duct PSC or overlap syndrome. In patients with classic cholangiogram findings of PSC, liver biopsy does not offer additional clinical information that alters the diagnosis or clinical management and is therefore not routinely recommended.[21,28,57]

The classic finding of PSC on liver histology is the fibro-obliterative lesion, which initially presents as concentric "onion skin" periductal fibrosis with mild lymphocytic infiltrate and progresses to complete obliteration of ducts (**Fig. 4A–F**). These findings have a patchy distribution and can be missed despite adequate tissue sampling. The most common findings in PSC are bile ductular reaction and proliferation (see **Fig. 4A**).

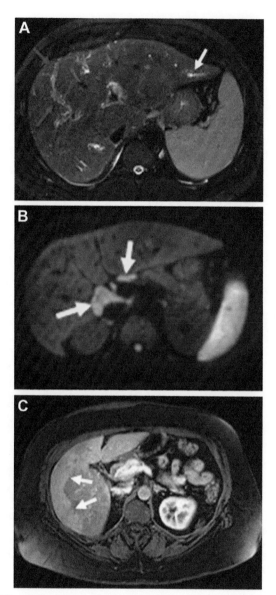

Fig. 3. (*A*) Axial T2-weighted fat-suppressed MR image shows hypertrophy of the lateral segment left lobe (*green asterisk*). Peripheral periportal high signal consistent with periductal fibrosis is seen (*red arrows*) with asymmetric focus of peripheral left lobe ductal ectasia (*yellow arrow*). (*B*) Axial diffusion weighted MR image shows periportal and portocaval reactive lymphadenopathy is present (*yellow arrows*). Hypertrophy of the lateral left lobe segement also seen (*green asterisk*). (*C*) Axial contrast-enhanced T1-weighted MR image shows geographic heterogeneous arterial phase enhancement (*white arrows*) consistent with associated inflammatory perfusion abnormality.

Other findings of chronic cholestasis, including copper deposition, can be observed (see **Fig. 4**E). Copper dry weight of the liver correlates with increasing stage of fibrosis (>150mcg/g dry weight of copper correlates with cirrhosis) and with serum total bilirubin and alkaline phosphatase.[3]

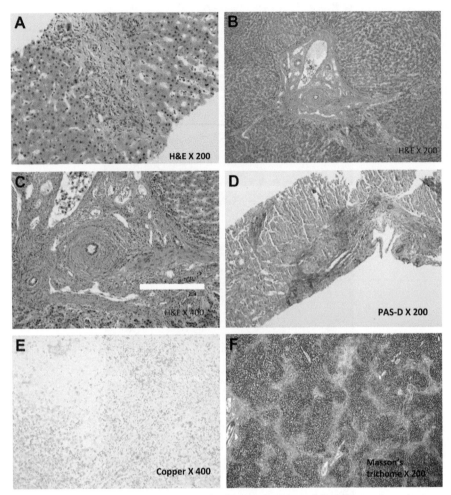

Fig. 4. (*A*) Bile ductular reaction and proliferation with neutrophilic infiltrate in early stages of PSC. (*B, C*) Examples of fibroinflammatory lesions with "onion-skin" periductal fibrosis and duct epithelial damage. (*D*) Thickened basement membranes of bile ducts highlighted with PAS-D stain. (*E*) Copper deposits in periportal hepatocytes in chronic biliary obstruction. (*F*) Portal-portal bridging fibrosis and cirrhosis.

Histologic findings are similar in patients with PSC whether they have extra-hepatic disease alone or intra- and extra-hepatic disease manifestation.[58] Over time, chronic inflammation of the bile ducts leads to fibrosis development. Approximately one-third of patients already have cirrhosis by the time of biopsy (see **Fig. 4**F).

Few histological scoring systems have been adapted for patients with PSC for prognostic purposes. In 2017, a multi-center European study performed liver biopsies in 119 patients with PSC and followed them on average for over 10 years to assess the clinical utility of Ishak, Nakanuma, and Ludwig scoring systems (**Table 1**).[59] During the follow-up period, 29% of patients had a liver-related complication, 9% were diagnosed with cholangiocarcinoma, 26% of patients underwent liver transplantation and 26% of patients died. The Nakanuma scoring system was the best independent predictor of liver-related complications and transplantation and was the only scoring

Table 1		
Histological scoring systems in primary sclerosing cholangitis		
Scoring System	**Score**	**Criteria**
Ishak	0	No fibrosis
	1	Fibrous expansion of some portal areas with or without short fibrous septae
	2	Fibrous expansion of most portal areas, with or without short fibrous septa
	3	Fibrous expansion of most portal areas with occasional portal to portal bridging
	4	Fibrous expansion of portal areas with marked bridging (portal to portal as well as portal to central)
	5	Marked bridging (portal-portal and/or portal-central) with occasional nodules (incomplete cirrhosis)
	6	Cirrhosis, probable or definite
Ludwig	0	No fibrosis
	1	Cholangitis or portal hepatitis
	2	Periportal fibrosis or hepatitis
	3	Septal fibrosis, bridging necrosis or both
	4	Biliary cirrhosis
Nakanuma	*Fibrosis*	
	0	No portal fibrosis or fibrosis limited to portal tracts
	1	Portal fibrosis with periportal fibrosis or incomplete septal fibrosis
	2	Bridging fibrosis with variable lobular disarray
	3	Liver cirrhosis with regenerative nodules and extensive fibrosis
	Bile duct loss	
	0	No bile duct loss
	1	Bile duct loss in less than one-third of portal tracts
	2	Bile duct loss in one-third to two-thirds of portal tracts
	3	Bile duct loss in more than two-thirds of portal tracts
	Deposition of orcein-positive granules	
	0	No deposition of granules
	1	Deposition of granules in a couple of zone 1 hepatocytes at less than one-third of portal tracts
	2	Deposition of granules in a variable number of zone 1 hepatocytes at one-third to two-thirds of portal tracts
	3	Deposition of granules in most zone 1 hepatocytes at more than two-thirds of portal tracts

system associated with the combined outcome of liver transplantation and death. In a smaller Dutch cohort of 64 patients, all three scoring systems had strong associations with transplant-free survival and time to transplant.[60] Sjöblom and colleagues[61] subsequently published research suggesting a modified Nakanuma scoring system, called the PSC histoscore. With the addition of 3 additional parameters, portal inflammation (0–3), portal edema (0–2), and ductular reaction (0–2), the PSC histoscore was more predictive of a combined endpoint of liver transplantation, cholangiocarcinoma and/or liver-related death compared to the Nakanuma scoring system. Further studies are needed to validate these findings.

DIAGNOSTIC APPROACH

The first line diagnostic tool for patients suspected to have PSC is MRI/MRCP.[28] If radiographic findings of biliary strictures with beading are seen, then a diagnosis of PSC can be made in the absence of other secondary causes. If no findings are seen with MRCP, then providers can proceed with liver biopsy to assess for small duct PSC or an alternative etiology. There are no current recommendations on the use of serologies to detect PSC. However, serologies may be useful in the detection of other cholestatic or autoimmune diseases. Elastography may be performed longitudinally to detect for advanced fibrosis as well as disease progression over time.

DISCUSSION

PSC remains a diagnostic challenge and requires clinical acumen to suspect its presence. However, advancements in liver imaging with MRCP has led to an accurate noninvasive modality to detect PSC, reducing the need for invasive tools such as ERCP and liver biopsy. Liver biopsy still carries a role among cases where the diagnosis remains unclear. In addition, elastography technology now allows providers to assess patients' level of hepatic fibrosis and can serially follow for disease progression. Finally, while serologies remain investigative for PSC diagnosis, future research is ongoing to determine novel biomarkers that can accurately capture PSC diagnosis at earlier stages and advance the field.

CLINICS CARE POINTS

- The diagnosis of primary sclerosing cholangitis (PSC) is often delayed and requires providers' clinical consideration in the setting of a patient presenting with abnormal liver tests or liver imaging.
- Laboratory studies are not specific for PSC and MR cholangiopgraphy (MRCP) is the gold standard for diagnosis of PSC. If patients are not able to obtain MR imaging, consideration for alternative imaging or endoscopic cholangiography may need to be considered.
- Noninvasive testing using elastography have been validated to correctly assess hepatic fibrosis in patients with PSC and can be used as an alternative to liver biopsy.

DISCLOSURE

There are no disclosures to report for all authors.

REFERENCES

1. Lunder AK, Hov JR, Borthne A, et al. Prevalence of sclerosing cholangitis detected by magnetic resonance cholangiography in patients with long-term inflammatory bowel disease. Gastroenterology 2016;151:660–9.
2. Freedman MR, Holzbach RT, Ferhuson DR. Pruritis in cholestasis: no direct causative role for bile acid retention. Am J Med 1981;70:1011–6.
3. Kodley K, Knox TA, Kaplan MM. Hepatic copper content is normal in early primary biliary cirrhosis and primary sclerosing cholangitis. Dig Dis Sci 1994;39:2416–20.
4. Angulo P, Peter JB, Gershwin ME, et al. Serum autoantibodies in patients with primary sclerosing cholangitis. J Hepatol 2000;32:182–7.
5. Xu B, Broome U, Ericzon B-G, et al. High frequency of autoantibodies in patients with primary sclerosing cholangitis that bind biliary epithelial cells and induce expression of CD44 and production of interleukin 6. Gut 2002;51:120–7.
6. Zauli D, Schrumpf E, Crespi C, et al. An autoantibody profile in primary sclerosing cholangitis. J Hepatol 1987;5:14–8.

7. Granito A, Muratori P, Muratori L, et al. Antibodies to SS-A/Ro-52kD and centromere in autoimmune liver disease: a clue to diagnosis and prognosis in primary biliary cirrhosis. Aliment Pharmacol Ther 2007;26:831–8.

8. Zauli D, Grassi A, Cassani F, et al. Autoimmune serology of primary sclerosing cholangitis. Dig Liver Dis 2001;33:391–2.

9. Henriksen EKK, Viken MK, Wittig M, et al. HLA haplotypes in primary sclerosing cholangitis patients of admixed and non-European ancestry. HLA 2017;90:228–33.

10. Donaldson PT, Norris S. Evaluation of the role of MHC class II alleles, haplotypes and selected amino acid sequences in primary sclerosing cholangitis. Autoimmunity 2002;35:555–64.

11. Spukland A, Saarinen S, Boberg KM, et al. HLA class II haplotypes in primary sclerosing cholangitis patients from five European populations. Tissue Antigens 1999;53:459–69.

12. Zachou K, Liaskos C, Rigopoulou E, et al. Presence of high avidity anticardiolipin antibodies in patients with autoimmune cholestatic liver diseases. Clin Imunol 2006;119:203–12.

13. Boonstra K, Culver EL, Maillette L, et al. Serum immunoglobulin G4 and immunoglobulin G1 for distinguishing immunoglobulin G4-associated cholangitis from primary sclerosing cholangitis. Hepatology 2014;59:1954–63.

14. Hippchen T, Sauer P, Göppert B, et al. Association between serum IgG level and clinical course in primary sclerosing cholangitis. BMC Gastroenterol 2019;19:153.

15. Lee YM, Kaplan MM. Primary sclerosing cholangitis. N Engl J Med 1995;332:924–33.

16. Mendes FD, Jorgensen R, Keach J, et al. Elevated serum IgG4 concentration in patients with primary sclerosing cholangitis. Am J Gastroenterol 2006;101:2070–5.

17. Hirano K, Kawabe T, Yamamoto N, et al. Serum igG4 concentrations in pancreatic and biliary diseases. Clin Chim Acta 2006;367:181–4.

18. Björnsson E, Chari S, Silveria M, et al. Primary sclerosing cholangitis associated with elevated immunoglobulin G4: clinical characteristics and response to therapy. Am J Therapeut 2001;18:198–205.

19. Zhang L, Lewis JT, Abraham SC, et al. IgG4+ plasma cell infiltrates in liver explants with primary sclerosing cholangitis. Am J Surg Pathol 2010;34:88–94.

20. Lian M, Li B, Xiao X, et al. Comparative clinical characteristics and natural history of three variants of sclerosing cholangitis: IgG4-related SC, PSC/AIH and PSC alone. Autoimmun Rev 2017;16:875–82.

21. European Association for the Study of Liver. EASL clinical practice guidelines on sclerosing cholangitis. J Hepatol 2022;77:761–806.

22. Terjung B, Bogsch F, Klein R, et al. Diagnostic accuracy of atypical p-ANCA in autoimmune hepatitis using ROC-and multivariate regression analysis. Eur J Med Res 2004;9:439–48.

23. Pokorny CS, Norton ID, McCaughan GW, et al. Anti-neutrophil cytoplasmic antibody: a prognostic indicator in primary sclerosing cholangitis. J Gastroenterol Hepatol 1994;9:40–4.

24. Bansi DS, Fleming KA, Chapman RW. Importance of antineutrophil cytoplasmic antibodies in primary sclerosing cholangitis and ulcerative colitis: prevalence, titre, and IgG subclass. Gut 1996;38:384–9.

25. Mulder AH, Horst G, Haagsma EB, et al. Prevalence and characterization of neutrophil cytoplasmic antibodies in autoimmune liver diseases. Hepatology 1993;17:411–7.

26. Roozendaal C, Van Milligen de Wit AW, Haagsma EB, et al. Antineutrophil cytoplasmic antibodies in primary sclerosing cholangitis: defined specificities may be associated with distinct clinical features. Am J Med 1998;105:393–9.

27. Olsson R, Hagerstrand I, Broome U, et al. Sampling variability of percutaneous liver biopsy in primary sclerosing cholangitis. J Clin Pathol 1995;48:933–5.

28. Bowlus CL, Arivé L, Bergquist A, et al. AASLD practice guidance on primary sclerosing cholangitis and cholangiocarcinoma. Hepatology 2023;77(2):659–702.

29. Corpechot C, Gaouar F, El Naggar A, et al. Baseline values and changes in liver stiffness measured by transient elastography are associated with severity of fibrosis and outcomes of patients with primary sclerosing cholangitis. Gastroenterology 2014;146:970–9.

30. Ehlken H, Wroblewski R, Corpechot C, et al. Validation of transient elastography and comparison with spleen length measurement for staging of fibrosis and clinical prognosis in primary sclerosing cholangitis. PLoS One 2016;11:e0164224.

31. Millonig G, Reimann FM, Friedrich S, et al. Extrahepatic cholestasis increases liver stiffness (FibroScan) irrespective of fibrosis. Hepatology 2008;48:1718–23.

32. Mjelle AB, Fossdal G, Gilja OH, et al. Liver elastography in primary sclerosing cholangitis patients using three different scanner systems. Ultrasound 2020;46:1854–64.

33. Mjelle AB, Mulabecirovic A, Hausken T, et al. Ultrasound and point shear wave elastography in livers of patients with primary sclerosing cholangitis. Ultrasound Med Biol 2016;42:2146–55.

34. Singh S, Venkatesh SK, Wang Z, et al. Diagnostic performance of magnetic resonance elastography in staging liver fibrosis: a systemic review and meta-analysis of individual participant data. Clin Gastroenterol Hepatol 2015;13:440–51.e6.

35. Welle CL, Navin PJ, Olson MC, et al. MR elastography in primary sclerosing cholangitis: a pictorial review. Abdom Radiol 2023;48:63–78.

36. Eaton JE, Dzyubak B, Venkatesh SK, et al. Performance of magnetic resonance elastography in primary sclerosing cholangitis. J Gastroenterol Hepatol 2016;31:1184–90.

37. Jhaveri KS, Hosseini-Nik H, Sadoughi N, et al. The development and validation of magnetic resonance elastography for fibrosis staging in primary sclerosing cholangitis. Eur Radiol 2018;29:1039–47.

38. Khoshpouri P, Habibabadi RR, Hazhirkarzar B, et al. Imaging features of primary sclerosing cholangitis: from diagnosis to liver transplant follow-up. Radiographics 2019;39:1938–64.

39. Majoie CB, Smits NJ, Phoa SS, et al. Primary sclerosing cholangitis: sonographic findings. Abdom Imaging 1995;20:109–12.

40. Kim N, Kim SY, Lee SS, et al. Sclerosing cholangitis: clinicopathologic features, imaging spectrum, and systemic approach to differential diagnosis. Korean J Radiol 2016;17(1):25–38.

41. Chapman R, Fevery J, Kalloo A, et al. Diagnosis and management of primary sclerosing cholangitis. Hepatology 2010;51(2):660–78.

42. Natt N, Michael F, Michael H, et al. ERCP-related adverse events in primary sclerosing cholangitis: a systemic review and meta-analysis. Can J Gastroenterol Hepatol 2002;2022:2372257.

43. Bangarulingam SY, Gossard AA, Petersen BT, et al. Complications of endoscopic retrograde cholangiopancreatography in primary sclerosing cholangitis. AJG 2009;104:855–60.

44. Navaneethan U, Jegadeesan R, Nayak S, et al. ERCP-related adverse events in patients with primary sclerosing cholangitis. Gastrointest Endosc 2015;81:410–9.

45. Fung BM, Tabibian JH. Biliary endoscopy in the management of primary sclerosing cholangitis and its complications. Liver Res 2019;3:106–17.
46. Gluck M, Cantone NR, Brandabur JJ, et al. A twenty-year experience with endoscopic therapy for symptomatic primary sclerosing cholangitis. J Clin Gastroenterol 2008;42:1032–9.
47. Etzel JP, Eng SC, Ko CW, et al. Complications after ERCP in patients with primary sclerosing cholangitis. Gastrointest Endosc 2008;67:643–8.
48. Gustafsson A, Enochsson L, Tingstedt B, et al. Antibiotic prophylaxis and its effect on postprocedural adverse events in endoscopic retrograde cholangiopancreatography for primary sclerosing cholangitis. JGH Open 2022;5:24–9.
49. Moff SL, Kamel IR, Eustace J, et al. Diagnosis of primary sclerosing cholangitis: a blinded comparative study using magnetic resonance cholangiography and endoscopic retrograde cholangiography. Gastrointest Endosc 2006;64:219–23.
50. Dave M, Elmunzer BJ, Dwamena BA, et al. Primary sclerosing cholangitis: meta-analysis of diagnostic performance of MR cholangiopancreatography. Radiology 2010;256:387–96.
51. Weber C, Kuhlencordt R, Grotelueschen R, et al. Magnetic resonance cholangiopancreatography in the diagnosis of primary sclerosing cholangitis. Endoscopy 2008;40:739–45.
52. Fulcher AS, Turner MA, Franklin KJ, et al. Primary sclerosing cholangitis: evaluation with MR cholangiography – a case-control study. Radiology 2000;215:71–80.
53. Angulo P, Pearce DH, Johnson CD, et al. Magnetic resonance cholangiography in patients with biliary disease: its role in primary sclerosing cholangitis. J Hepatol 2000;33:520–7.
54. Talwalkar JA, Angulo P, Johnson CD, et al. Cost-minimization analysis of MRC versus ERCP for the diagnosis of primary sclerosing cholangitis. Hepatology 2004;40:39–45.
55. Meagher S, Yusoff I, Kennedy W, et al. The roles of magnetic resonance and endoscopic retrograde cholangiopancreatography (MRCP and ERCP) in the diagnosis of patients with suspected sclerosing cholangitis: a cost-effectiveness analysis. Endoscopy 2007;39:222–8.
56. Chapman MH, Thorburn D, Hirschfield GM, et al. British Society of Gastroenterology and UK-PSC guidelines for the diagnosis and management of primary sclerosing cholangitis. Gut 2019;68:1356–78.
57. Burak KW, Angulo P, Lindo KD. Is there a role for liver biopsy in primary sclerosing cholangitis? Am J Gastroenterol 2003;98:1155–8.
58. Ludwig J, Barham SS, LaRusso NF, et al. Morphologic features of chronic hepatitis associated with primary sclerosing cholangitis and chronic ulcerative colitis. Hepatology 1981;1:632–40.
59. de Vries EMG, de Krijger M, Färkkliä M, et al. Validation of the prognostic value of histologic scoring systems in primary sclerosing cholangitis: an international cohort study. Hepatology 2017;65:907–19.
60. de Vries EMG, Verheij J, Hubscher SG, et al. Applicability and prognostic value of histologic scoring systems in primary sclerosing cholangitis. J Hepatol 2015;63: 1212–9.
61. Sjöblom N, Boyd S, Kautiainen H, et al. Novel histologic scoring for predicting disease outcome in primary sclerosing cholangitis. Histopathology 2002;81: 192–204.

Treatment of Primary Sclerosing Cholangitis Including Transplantation

William H. Wheless, MD, Mark W. Russo, MD, MPH*

KEYWORDS

- Liver • Cholestatic • Therapy • Ursodeoxycholic acid • Investigational

KEY POINTS

- A 12-month course of ursodeoxycholic acid (17–23 mg/kg/day) can be considered for patients with PSC to determine if they will have a treatment response. Higher doses of 28-30 kg/mg/day are not recommended and associated with adverse outcomes.
- A number of drugs are under investigation for PSC, some of which are approved for other indications. Thus far, none have a demonstrated a definitive clinical benefit.
- Endoscopic stenting of strictures is not routinely recommended. Balloon angioplasty should be attempted first for biliary strictures associated with obstruction or cholangitis.
- Liver transplantation is associated with excellent patient and graft survival in patients with end stage liver disease from PSC and acceptable outcomes for patients with unresectable perihilar cholangiocarcinoma.

INTRODUCTION
Epidemiology

Primary sclerosing cholangitis (PSC) is a progressive cholestatic liver disease with no effective medical therapy (**Fig. 1**). The estimated incidence of PSC is 0.1-1.58 individuals per 100,000 and the estimated point prevalence ranges from 0.0 to 31.7 per 100,000.[1,2] Among patient with PSC, 70% have inflammatory bowel disease and among patients with inflammatory bowel disease 5% have PSC.[2] In the United States end stage liver disease from cholestatic liver diseases accounts for approximately 8% of adult liver transplants.[3] Effective medical therapy for PSC has been elusive. The discussion later in discussion focuses on medical therapy for PSC as well as endoscopic therapy followed by a discussion on liver transplantation for PSC.

The authors have no disclosures.
Division of Hepatology, Atrium Health Wake Forest, Charlotte, NC, USA
* Corresponding author. Atrium Health- Morehead Medical Plaza, 1025 Morehead Medical Drive, 6th Floor MMP, Charlotte, NC 28204.
E-mail address: Mark.Russo@atriumhealth.org

Clin Liver Dis 28 (2024) 171–182
https://doi.org/10.1016/j.cld.2023.07.008
liver.theclinics.com

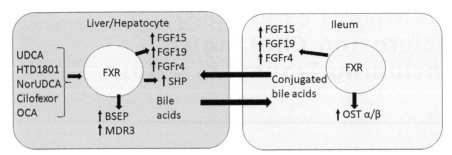

Fig. 1. The nuclear gene farsenoid X receptor encodes genes that regulate bile acid transport. FXR is expressed in the liver and ileum and induces expression of bile acid metabolism and transport. FXR is also expressed in the ileum where conjugated bile acids enter the enterohepatic circulation. BSEP, bile salt export pump; FGR, fibroblast growth factor; FXR, farsenoid X receptor; HTD1801, beberine ursodeoxycholate; MDR3, multidrug resistant 3; norUDCA, norursodeoxycholic acid; OCA, obeticholic acid; OST, organic solute transporter alpha/beta; SHP, small heterodimer partner; UDCA, ursodeoxycholic acid.

DISCUSSION

There are currently no FDA approved medications for PSC. All medications discussed in the article are unapproved and considered "off-label."

Ursodeoxycholic Acid

Ursodeoxycholic acid (UDCA) is a naturally occurring hydrophilic bile acid that accounts for 4% of the bile acid pool. It is formed by colonic bacteria from the epimerization of the primary bile acid chenodeoxycholic acid. UDCA has been described to prevent the production of reactive oxygen species by Kupffer cells and resident macrophages in the liver, thus attenuating oxidative stress in the liver. UDCA can also change the hydrophobicity of the bile acid pool, competitively displacing the more hydrophobic or toxic bile acids.[4]

In a landmark double-blinded, randomized clinical trial,105 patients with PSC were randomized to UDCA (13–15 mg/kg/day) in divided doses or placebo with a median follow-up of 2.2 years.[5] The primary outcome was a composite outcome: death, liver transplantation, histologic progression on liver biopsy or progression to cirrhosis, development of varices, ascites, or encephalopathy, sustained quadrupling of the serum bilirubin concentration, worsening of fatigue or pruritus, inability to tolerate drug or voluntary withdrawal from the study. The mean age of the UDCA group was 41.7 years-old, 13% had cirrhosis, and 77% had inflammatory bowel disease. The mean serum alkaline phosphatase (ALP) and total bilirubin were 1103 U/L and 1.6 mg/dL, respectively. There were no significant differences between the UDCA and placebo groups in treatment failure or transplant free survival. UDCA was associated with a greater reduction in ALP compared to placebo at year 2, -447 U/L and −104 U/L, respectively, p < 0.001. UDCA was well tolerated.

In another clinical trial in patients with PSC, 218 subjects were randomized to 17-23 mg per day or placebo.[6] No statistically significant differences were demonstrated between the two groups in occurrence of liver transplantation. Serum alanine aminotransferase and ALP levels decreased in the UDCA group compared to the placebo group during the first 6 months of treatment, although the differences were not statistically significant. UDCA doses of 17-23 mg/kg were not significantly better than placebo in improving clinical outcomes.

High dose UDCA (28–30 mg./kg/day) was evaluated in 150 adult patients with PSC in a randomized-double blinded controlled trial.[7] The primary outcome was the development of cirrhosis, varices, cholangiocarcinoma, liver transplantation or death. Although biochemical improvement in ALP and AST were seen in the UDCA group compared to the placebo group, clinical outcomes were not better in the UDCA group. In fact, after adjusting for baseline characteristics, UDCA was associated with 2.1-fold increased risk for death, transplantation or minimal listing criteria compared to placebo, $p = 0.038$ and serious adverse events were more common in the UDCA group, 63% and 37%, $p < 0.01$. High dose UDCA has also been associated with a 4.4-fold increased risk of colorectal neoplasia in patients with PSC and ulcerative colitis (UC).[8]

Because several studies have reported that a reduction in ALP less than 1.5 times the upper limit of normal or a 40% reduction or normalization of ALP are associated with better clinical outcomes, the American Association for the Study of Liver Diseases (AASLD) guidance document states that patients with PSC can be considered for a 12 month trial of UDCA.[9–12] UDCA doses of 13-23 mg/kg/d in divided doses are recommended and doses of 28 mg/kg/day and higher should be avoided (**Table 1**). The AASLD recommends monitoring ALP for 6 months prior to initiating UDCA because levels can spontaneously normalize.

Antimicrobials

Antibiotics are an attractive class of medications to study in PSC because alterations in the gut microbiome may have beneficial effects on disease progression. In a randomized trial of 35 adult patients with PSC, vancomycin 125 mg or 250 mg four times a day was compared to metronidazole 250 mg or 500 mg three times a day for 12 weeks.[13] The vancomycin groups had significant declines in ALP compared to baseline while metronidazole was not associated with significant reductions in ALP. A large clinical trial of vancomycin in adult with PSC is ongoing with anticipated study completion in 2024.[14] Other antibiotics that have been associated with reductions in ALP include minocycline and rifaximin.[15,16]

Fibrates

The fibrates are associated with a biochemical improvement in ALP and reduced toxicity of the bile acid pool in patients with cholestatic liver disease. Fenofibrate is a peroxisome proliferator-activated receptor alpha (PPARα) agonist that regulates bile acid metabolism. A study of 19 patients who had PSC of which eight were on UDCA reported the addition of fenofibrate was associated with a reduction or normalization of ALP in 86% of subjects.[17] Fenofibrate was associated with a reduction in total serum bile acids.[17] Fenofibrate was not associated with elevations in serum creatinine or rhabdomyolysis. A study that randomized patients with PSC to fenofibrate 200 mg daily or placebo for 6 months reported 10 (66.7%) subjects in the treatment group compared to 52.8% in the placebo group achieved a 50% reduction or normalization in ALP.[18]

Obeticholic Acid

Obeticholic acid (OCA), an FXR nuclear receptor agonist, is approved for primary biliary cholangitis and has been studied in PSC. In a clinical trial, 76 patients with PSC were randomized to OCA 1.5-3.0 mg daily, 5-10 mg daily or placebo for 24 weeks.[19] In the high dose OCA group, the least square mean reduction in ALP was −83.4 U/L compared to placebo, $p = 0.043$. A significant difference in ALP reduction was not observed between the low dose OCA group and placebo group. Pruritus was more common with high dose OCA compared to placebo 67% and 46%,

Table 1
Off label drugs for PSC

Drug	Outcome	Adverse Events and Limitations
Ursodeoxycholic acid (UDCA)	Doses of 17–23 mg/kg/day associated with improved clinical outcomes if reduction or normalization in ALP achieved	Doses of 28–30 mg/kg/day associated with increased risk of death, transplant, colorectal cancer
Vancomycin	Reduction in ALP with 250 mg qid	Risk of colonization with VRE
Fibrates	Reduction in ALP	Rhabdomyolysis, elevation creatinine, cholestatic liver injury
Obeticholic acid	Reduction in ALP	Pruritus
Statins	Reduction in all cause mortality, and liver transplant	Observational data
Biologics	No effect, except adalimumab may reduce ALP	

respectively. Overall, more patients in the OCA groups experienced a severe adverse event compared to the placebo group, 52% and 17%, respectively.

Other drugs that may hold promise in repurposing for PSC include statins. In an observational population-based study among patients with PSC statins were associated with a 32% reduction in all-cause mortality and 50% reduction in death or transplantation.[20]

Biologics Used for Inflammatory Bowel Disease

A double-blind, randomized clinical trial of infliximab in patients with PSC was terminated early because a significant treatment effect on ALP was not demonstrated.[21] Infliximab, vedolizumab, and adalimumab do not appear to exacerbate liver tests in patients with PSC, however, adalimumab has been associated with reductions in ALP.[22,23]

Investigational drugs
Berberine ursodeoxycholate. Berberine ursodeoxycholate (HTD1801) is an ionic salt of berberine and UDCA, that in addition to the choleretic properties of UDCA, it also has antimicrobial effects. In a clinical trial of 55 patients with PSC, 16, 15, and 24 patients were randomized to placebo, HTD1801 500 mg bid or HTD1801 1000 mg bid, respectively[24] (**Table 2**). After 6 weeks of treatment a significant decrease in ALP was seen with the low and high dose of HTD1801, least mean square −53 U/L and −37 U/L, compared with placebo, 98 U/L, p = 0.019. When subjects in the HTD1801 groups were crossed over to placebo ALP increased. Discontinuation rates were similar among the 3 groups.

Cilofexor. Cilofexor is a nonsteroidal FXR receptor agonist which regulates bile acid synthesis, conjugation, and excretion. In addition, FXR activation results in the release of fibroblast growth factor 19 which decreases bile acid synthesis by downregulating cholesterol 7α-hydroxylase. Fifty-two subjects with PSC without cirrhosis were randomized to cilofexor 100 mg daily, cilofexor 30 mg daily or placebo for 12 weeks.[25] Sixty percent had inflammatory bowel disease and 46% were taking UDCA. The

Table 2
Investigational drugs for PSC

Drug	Mechanism	Outcome
Berberine ursodeoxycholate	Ionic salt of beberine and UDCA, increases choleretic properties and antimicrobial	Decline in serum ALP
Cenicriviroc	Chemokine receptor 2 and 5 receptor antagonist	No significant reduction in serum ALP
Cilofexor	Nonsteroidal FXR receptor agonist	25% reduction from baseline serum ALP more common in 100 mg group. Further study terminated
Simtuzumab	Monoclonal antibody directed against lysl oxidase like-2 (LOXL2)	No significant improvement in hepatic collagen content or clinical outcomes
norUrsodeoxycholic acid	Homologue of UDCA that has superior anti-inflammatory and antifibrotic compared to UDCA	26% reduction from baseline serum ALP over 12 weeks

primary outcome was incidence of treatment emergent adverse events. Exploratory analyses were reported for changes in liver tests, including ALP. Three patients discontinued therapy in the cilofexor 100 mg group due to adverse events compared to one patient each in the 30 mg group and placebo group. A 25% reduction in ALP from baseline was more frequent in the 100 mg group compared to the lower dose cilofexor group and placebo group, 35%, 5.3% and 10%, respectively, p = 0.21. Reductions in ALT and GGT were significantly greater in the cilofexor 100 mg group compared to the placebo, p = 0.009 for ALT and p = 0.003 for GGT.

Results from an open-label extension study of the cilofexor trial were reported on 47 subjects that continued cilofexor 100 mg oral daily.[26] At week 96, an 8.3% reduction in ALP (p = 0.066), 29.8% reduction in GGT (p < 0.001), 29.8% reduction in ALT (p = 0.002) and 16.7% reduction in AST (p = 0.010) were reported with cilofexor. Fifteen (32%) patients discontinued cilofexor prematurely due to pruritus or other adverse events. Despite promising results from the phase 2 trials, the phase 3 study of cilofexor for PSC was discontinued due to a planned review of interim data demonstrating futility.

norUrsodeoxycholic acid (norUDCA). norUDCA is homologue of UDCA that has superior anti-inflammatory and antifibrotic effects compared to UDCA in animal models. In a randomized clinical trial, norUDCA was compared to placebo in 161 patients with PSC who were not on UDCA.[27] Twelve weeks of 500 mg, 1,000 mg, or 1500 mg/d of norUDCA was associated with ALP reductions of −12.3%, −17.3%, and −26.0%, respectively compared to a +1.2% increase in the placebo group, p < 0.0001. Serious adverse events occurred in seven, five, two, and three subjects in the norUDCA 500 mg/d, 1000 mg/d, 1500 mg/d, and placebo groups, respectively.

Other investigational agents being evaluated in PSC include cenicriviroc, simtizumab and curcumin.[28–30] In a single arm open label study cenicriviroc, a chemokine receptor 2 and 5 receptor antagonist, none of the subjects achieved ALP normalization, a 50% decrease in ALP, or ALP <1.5 x ULN.[28] Simtizumab is a monoclonal antibody directed against lysl oxidase like-2 (LOXL2) which regulates fibrogenesis and involved in cross linkage of collagen and elastin. LOXL2 levels are elevated in patients with PSC. Simtizumab was not associated with a significant improvement in hepatic collagen content, Ishak fibrosis score, or liver-related clinical events.[29] Curcumin a principal component of turmeric with anti-inflammatory properties. In a pilot study of 15 patients with PSC, 12 weeks of curcumin 750 mg daily was not associated with a significant reduction in ALP.[30]

PSC may be associated with adverse changes in gut microflora. Fecal microbiota transplantation (FMT) may restore favorable gut microbiome and improve biochemical parameters. Among ten patients with PSC in a pilot study of FMT, three experienced a 50% or greater decrease in ALP.[31]

ENDOSCOPIC THERAPY

For benign dominant strictures that are associated with clinical deterioration, such as worsening jaundice, pruritus, or cholangitis, the American Society of Gastrointestinal Endoscopy and the American College of Gastroenterology recommend ERCP with balloon dilatation and reserving stenting for strictures refractory to balloon dilatation.[32,33] Short term stenting can be considered for severe dominant strictures. The American Association for the Study of Liver Diseases guidance document states the choice between balloon dilatation with or without a stent(s) is left up to the discretion of the endoscopist, but if a stent is placed it should be removed within 4 weeks of placement. Preoperative antibiotic prophylaxis followed by a 3–5 day course post-ERCP should be prescribed to prevent cholangitis.

LIVER TRANSPLANTATION FOR PRIMARY SCLEROSING CHOLANGITIS

Liver transplantation (LT) is the only current definitive treatment for PSC. Indications for LT in patients with PSC are similar to other etiologies of liver disease and include decompensated cirrhosis with complications from portal hypertension. Organs are allocated within each blood type to the candidate with the highest model for end stage liver disease sodium (MELD-Na/MELD 3.0) score. Outcomes after liver transplant for PSC are excellent with 1-year patient and graft survival exceeding 95% and 93%, respectively (**Fig. 2**).

Conditions for MELD exception scores specific to PSC include recurrent bacterial cholangitis, intractable pruritus, and early-stage hilar cholangiocarcinoma[34] (**Table 3**). In select patients with PSC and unresectable perihilar cholangiocarcinoma liver transplantation offers 5-year survival rates from 65% to 75%.[35]

Livers used for transplantation are most frequently recovered from donors with documented brain death (DBD). As more patients are waiting for liver transplant than available deceased donor organs, alternative strategies have been pursued. One such strategy is recovering livers from donors after circulatory death (DCD). Because ischemic biliary complications are higher after DCD transplant, utilization of DCD is lower in PSC compared to other etiologies[36] Despite this, recent data has suggested a mortality benefit with DCD LT compared to DBD LT when adjusted for recipient characteristics.[37] The UK DCD risk score (UKSS) incorporates donor and recipient variables to risk stratify patients into low-risk, high-risk and "futile" categories and has shown promise in identifying candidates at lowest risk for complications after liver transplant from a DCD liver.[38,39] Normothermic machine perfusion may further decrease post-transplant biliary ischemic complications after DCD transplant. A recent multicenter randomized controlled trial found that the use of normothermic

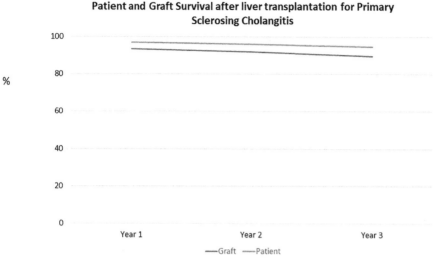

Fig. 2. Patient and graft survival in adults with end stage liver disease from PSC undergoing first liver transplant. (*Data from* the Scientific Registry of Transplant Recipients).

perfusion reduces early allograft dysfunction and ischemic biliary complications which may potentially increase DCD utilization.[40]

Living donor liver transplant (LDLT) may confer reduced wait list morbidity and mortality for the candidate but must be balanced against the risks to the donor. Patients with PSC are four times as likely to receive a LDLT compared to patients with other indications.[41,42] Although a benefit of LDLT is a reduction in wait list mortality, data from a retrospective analysis that included more than 150 centers from Europe demonstrated statistically significant higher recipient mortality more than 90 days after LDLT compared to recipients of DBDs.[43] LDLT recipients had higher primary recurrence rate and biliary complications post-transplant compared to DBD recipients.[43]

Biliary Reconstruction in Liver Transplantation: Hepaticojejunostomy vs. Duct to Duct Anastamosis

Biliary reconstruction by hepaticojejunostomy in LT for PSC has been the standard approach for biliary anastomosis while duct-to-duct (DTD) anastomosis is commonly used for other indications for LT. DTD anastomosis has not been routinely performed in LT for PSC because of the potential for developing cholangiocarcinoma in the recipient duct as well as an increased risk for stricture formation from underlying PSC.[44] However, studies suggest that DTD anastomosis in LT for PSC has comparable patient and graft survival, PSC recurrence rates, a minimal risk of cholangiocarcinoma, a comparable risk of biliary strictures and cholangitis compared to hepaticojejunostomy.[44,45] The type of biliary reconstruction utilized remains at the discretion of the surgical transplant team.

Recurrent Primary Sclerosing Cholangitis After Liver Transplantation

Recurrent PSC (rPSC) after LT occurs in up to 25% of recipients.[46] An increased risk of recurrence has been seen in LDLT compared to deceased donor grafts, which is thought to be in part due to increased shared antigens and susceptibility of alloimmune disease in recipients of related liver donors.[43] rPSC is commonly diagnosed

Table 3
MELD exception points in patients with primary sclerosing cholangitis

Recurrent Cholangitis
  Must meet BOTH of the following criteria:
  1. Candidate admitted to intensive care unit two or more times in a three-month period with hemodynamic instability requiring vasopressors
  2. Candidate has cirrhosis
  Plus ONE of the following criteria:
  • Biliary tract stricture not responsive to treatment by ERCP or percutaneous transhepatic cholangiography (PTC)
  • Diagnosed with highly resistant infectious organism (eg VRE, ESBL producing gram negative, CRE, multi-drug resistant Acinetobacter)
	Median MELD at transplant around donor hospital minus 3

Early stage peri-hilar cholangiocarcinoma (pCCA)
  • Submission of a written protocol
  • Unresectable
  • Documentation excluding metastatic disease
  • Biopsy or cytology demonstrating malignancy
  • Carbohydrate antigen 19–9 greater than 100 U/mL in the absence of cholangitis
  • Aneuploidy
  • Hilar mass less than 3 cm in radial diameter
  • Transperitoneal aspiration of biopsy of the primary tumor by endoscopic ultrasound, operative or percutaneous approach must be avoided due to seeding
	Median MELD at transplant around donor hospital minus 3

by imaging (eg, MRCP) with evidence of non-anastomotic strictures, after the exclusion of other etiologies (eg, hepatic artery thrombosis) and it is associated with decreased survival.[47] Risk factors for rPSC include the presence of inflammatory bowel disease (IBD), cholangiocarcinoma prior to LT, donor age, multiple episodes of acute cellular rejection, and late cellular rejection.[48]

There is currently no effective prophylaxis to prevent rPSC. Although there are reports that colectomy before or after LT is associated with a decreased risk of rPSC, data are insufficient to recommend colectomy to prevent recurrence.[49]

Risk of Colorectal Cancer in Primary Sclerosing Cholangitis Liver Transplant Recipients and Recommendations for Screening

A systematic review of 18 studies reported the pooled incidence rate of colorectal cancer in recipients with PSC after LT was 5.8 per 1000 person-years while in patients with PSC with IBD the pooled incidence rate was 13.5 per 1000 person-years.[50] In a prospective cohort involving 112 patients followed for a median of 7 years with moderate to severe IBD post-LT had a higher rate of colorectal cancer than recipients with mild or no IBD, 21% and 3% respectively.[51] After LT, recipients with PSC and IBD should undergo annual colonoscopy for colorectal cancer surveillance.[12]

Inflammatory Bowel Disease in Recipients with Primary Sclerosing Cholangitis After Liver Transplantation

Transplant recipients with a history of PSC have up to a 30% risk of developing *de novo* IBD.[52] The clinical course of *de novo* IBD post-LT is generally milder than those with pre-existing IBD, with not as many patients requiring colectomies.[53] Risk factors that have been associated with IBD activity post-transplant include advanced age, smoking and IBD activity at time of transplant.[54]

Mouchli and colleagues[52] found that up to 40% of patients with pre-existing IBD and PSC after LT required the escalation of IBD-related therapy despite immunosuppression. Azathioprine was protective against IBD progression and prevented the development of *de novo* IBD. Tacrolimus-based regimens were found to have a higher risk of IBD-flare post-transplant. Almost 40% of patients required colectomy for intractable disease or for evidence of malignancy.

SUMMARY

Developing effective medical therapy for PSC has been challenging. A course of UDCA is recommended at doses of 13-23 mg/kg/day for up to a year and if a decline or normalization in ALP is achieved then treatment with UDCA should be continued. Higher doses of UDCA, 28-30 mg/kg/day have been associated with adverse events and are not recommended. Drugs that are available for other indications that have been associated with biochemical improvement or improved clinical outcomes include vancomycin, fibrates and statins and warrant further study. Investigational drugs that are analogues of UDCA, including norUDCA and beberine ursodeoxycholate show promise and are under investigation. Liver transplantation is the definitive therapy for end stage liver disease secondary to PSC and is associated with excellent patient and graft survival. Recurrence rates are as high as 25% within 5 years after transplantation. Liver transplant recipients with a history of PSC and IBD should undergo annual colonoscopy due to the increased risk of colorectal cancer.

CLINICS CARE POINTS

- A 6-12 month course of UDCA 13-23 mg/kg/day in divided doses can be prescribed to patients with PSC and continued if there is a reduction or normalization if ALP. Higher doses of UDCA 28-30 mg/kg/day should be avoided.

- Drugs with indications other than PSC that have been associated with improvement in ALP or clinical outcomes include fenofibrate, statins and obeticholic acid and warrant further investigation.

- Investigational agents with similar mechanisms of action as UDCA that show promise are beberine ursodeoxycholate and norursodeoxycholic acid.

- Endoscopic stenting of a stricture(s) from PSC is not routinely recommended and balloon dilatation is preferred if the stricture is short and amenable to dilatation. If stenting is necessary, the stent should be exchanged within 4 weeks.

- Liver transplantation is definitive therapy for end stage liver disease from PSC, but recurrence occurs in up to 25% of recipients within 5 years.

- Patients with PSC and perihilar cholangiocarcinoma who are potential liver transplant candidates should not undergo transperitoneal biopsy of the mass via endoscopic ultrasound or percutaneous biopsy due to the risk of tumor seeding.

- Liver transplant recipients with a history of PSC and IBD should undergo annual colonoscopy due to the increased risk of colorectal cancer.

REFERENCES

1. Boonstra K, Beuers U, Ponsioen CY. Epidemiology of primary sclerosing cholangitis and primary biliary cirrhosis: a systematic review. J Hepatol 2012;56(5):1181–8.
2. Trivedi PJ, Bowlus CL, Yimam KK, et al. Epidemiology, natural history, and outcomes of primary sclerosing cholangitis: a systematic review of population-based studies. Clin Gastroenterol Hepatol 2022;20:1687–700.
3. Kwong AJ, Ebel NH, Kim WR, et al. OPTN/SRTR 2020 annual data report: liver. Am J Transplant 2022;22(Suppl 2):204–309.
4. Achufusi TG, Safadi A, Mahabadi N. Ursodeoxyxholic acid. In: StatPearls. Treasure Island (FL): StatPearls Publishing; 2023. Jan 2012 PMID: 31424887.
5. Lindor KD. Ursodiol for primary sclerosing cholangitis. N Engl J Med 1997;336:691–5.
6. Olsson R, Boberg KM, de Muckadell OS, et al. High-dose ursodeoxycholic acid in primary sclerosing cholangitis: a 5-year multicenter, andomized, controlled study. Gastroenterology 2005;129:1464–72.
7. Lindor KD, Kowdley KV, Luketic VAC, et al. High-dose urdodeoxycholic acid for the treatment of primary sclerosing cholangitis. Hepatology 2009;50:808–14.
8. Eaton JE, Silveira MG, Pardi DS, et al. High-dose ursodeoxycholic acid is associated with the development of colorectal neoplasia in patients with ulcerative colitis and primary sclerosing cholangitis. Am J Gastroenterol 2011;106:1638–45.
9. Hilscher M, Enders FB, Carey EJ, et al. Alkaline phosphatase normalization is a biomarker of improved survival in primary sclerosing cholangitis. Ann Hepatol 2016;15(2):246–53.
10. Al Mamari S, Djordjevic J, Halliday JS, et al. Improvement of serum alkaline phosphatase to <1.5 upper limit of normal predicts better outcome and reduced risk of cholangiocarcinoma in primary sclerosing cholangitis. J Hepatol 2013;58:329–34.
11. Lindstrom L, Friis-Liby I, Bergquist A. Association between reduced levels of alkaline phosphatase and survival times of patients sith primary sclerosing cholangitis. Clin Gastroenterol Hepatol 2013;11:841–6.
12. Bowlus CL, Arrive L, Bergquist A, et al. AASLD practice guidance on primary sclerosing cholangitis and cholangiocarcinoma. Hepatology 2023;77:659–702.
13. Tabiban JH, Weeding E, Jorgensen RA, et al. Randomised clinical trial: vancomycin or metronidazole in patients with primary sclerosing cholangitis- a pilot study. Aliment Pharmacol Ther 2013;37:604–12.
14. Available at: www.clinical trials.gov (NCT03710122). (Accessed March 2nd, 2023).
15. Silveira MG, Torok NJ, Gossard AA, et al. Minocycline in the treatment of patients with primary sclerosing cholangitis: results of a pilot study. Am J Gastroenterol 2009;104:83–8.
16. Tabibian JH, Gossard A, El-Youssef M, et al. Prospective clinical trial of rifaximin therapy for patients with primary sclerosing cholangitis. Am J Therapeut 2017;24:e56–63.
17. Hemme CL, Auclair AM, Ghonem NS, et al. Fenofibrate improves liver function and reduces the toxicity of the bile acid pool in patients with primary biliary cholangitis and primary sclerosing cholangitis who are partial responders to ursodiol. Clin Pharmacol Ther 2020;108:1213–23.

18. Hatami B, Mosala M, Hassani AH, et al. Fenofibrate in primary sclerosing cholangitis; a randomized, double-blind, placebo-controlled trial. Pharmacol Res Perspect 2002;10:e00984.
19. Kowdley KV, Vuppalanchi R, Levy C, et al. A randomized, placebo-controlled, phase II study of obeticholic acid for primary sclerosing cholangitis. JHepatol 2020;73:94–101.
20. Stokkeland K, Hoijer J, Bottai M, et al. Statin use is associated with primary sclerosing cholangitis. Clin Gastroenterol Hepatol 2019;17:1860–6.
21. Hommes DW, Erkelens W, Ponsioen C, et al. A double-blind placebo-controlled, randomized study of infliximab in primary sclerosing cholangitis. J Clin Gastroenterol 2008;42:522–6.
22. Hedin CRH, Sado G, Ndegwa N, et al. Effects of tumor necrosis factor antagonists in patients with primary sclerosing cholangitis. Clin Gastroenterol Hepatol 2020;18:2295–304.
23. Lynch KD, Chapman RW, Keshav S, et al. Effects of vedolizumab in patients with primary sclerosing cholangtitis and inflammatory bowel disease. Clin Gastroenterol Hepatol 2020;18:179–87.
24. Kowdley KV, Forman L, Eksteen B, et al. A randomized, dose-finding, proof-of-concept study of berberine ursodeoxycholate in patients with primary sclerosing cholangitis. Am J Gastroenterol 2022;117:1805–15.
25. Trauner M, Gulamhusein A, Hameed B, et al. The nonsteroidal farsenoid X receptor agonist cilofexor (GS-9674) improves markers of cholestasis and liver injury in patients with primary sclerosing cholangitis. Hepatology 2019;70:788–801.
26. Trauner M, Bowlus CL, Gulamhusein A, et al. Safety and sustained efficacy of the farsenoid X receptor (FXR) agonist cilofexor over a 96-week open-label extension in patients with PSC. Clin Gastroenterol Hepatol 2022;70(3):S1542–3565.
27. Fickert P, Hirschfield GM, Denk G, et al. norUrsodeoxycholic acid improves cholestasis in primary sclerosing cholangitis. J Hepatol 2017;67:549–58.
28. Eksteen B, Bowlus CL, Montana-Loza AJ, et al. Efficacy and safety of cenicriviroc in patients with primary sclerosing cholangitis: PERSEUS study. Hepatol Commun 2020;5:478–90.
29. Muir AJ, Levy C, Janssen HLA, et al. Simtizumab for primary sclerosing cholangitis :Phase 2 study results with insights on the natural history of the disease. Hepatolgoy 2019;69:684–98.
30. Eaton JE, Nelson KM, Gossman AA, et al. Efficacy and safety of curcumin in primary sclerosing cholangitis: an open label pilot study. Scand J Gastroenterol 2019;54:633–9.
31. Allegretti J, Kassam Z, Carrellas M, et al. Fecal microbiota transplantation in patients with primary sclerosing cholangitis: a pilot clinical trial. Am J Gastroenterol 2019;114:1071–9.
32. ASGE Standards of Practice Committee. The role of ERCP in benign diseases of the biliary tract. Gastrointest Endosc 2015;81:795–803.
33. Lindor K, Kowdley K, Harrision E. ACG clinical guideline: primary sclerosing cholangitis. Am J Gastroenterol 2015;110:646–59.
34. Guidance to liver transplant programs and the national liver review board for: Adult Meld Exception review. Available at: https://optn.transplant.hrsa.gov/media/2847/liver_guidance_adult_meld_201706.pdf. (Accessed March 4, 2023).
35. Zamora-Valdes D, Heimbach JK. Liver transplant for cholangiocarcinoma. Gastroenterol Clin North Am 2018;47:267–80.
36. Croome KP, Taner CB. The changing landscapes in DCD liver transplantation. Curr Transplant Rep 2020;7:194–204.

37. Taylor R, Allen E, Richards JA, et al. Survival advantage for patients accepting the offer of a circulatory death liver transplant. J Hepatol 2019;70(5):855–65.
38. Schlegel A, Kalisvaart M, Scalera I, et al. The UK DCD Risk Score: a new proposal to define futility in donation-after-circulatory- death liver transplantation. J Hepatol 2018;68(3):456–64.
39. Wu WK, Ziogas IA, Matsuoka LK, et al. Applicability of the UK DCD risk score in the modern era of liver transplantation: a U.S. update. Clin Transplant 2022;36(4):e14579.
40. Markmann JF, Abouljoud MS, Ghobrial RM, et al. Impact of portable normothermic blood-based machine perfusion on outcomes of liver transplant: the OCS Liver PROTECT randomized clinical trial. JAMA Surg 2022;157(3):189–98.
41. Goldberg DS, French B, Thomasson A, et al. Current trends in living donor liver transplantation for primary sclerosing cholangitis. Transplantation 2011;91(10): 1148–52.
42. Fisher RA. Living donor liver transplantation: eliminating the wait for death in end-stage liver disease? Nat Rev Gastroenterol Hepatol 2017;14:373–82.
43. Heinemann M, Liwinski T, Adam R, et al. And the European liver and intestine transplant association (ELITA). Long-term outcome after living donor liver transplantation compared to donation after brain death in autoimmune liver diseases: experience from the European Liver Transplant Registry. Am J Transplant 2022; 22(2):626–33.
44. Sutton ME, Bense RD, Lisman T, et al. Duct-to-duct reconstruction in liver transplantation for primary sclerosing cholangitis is associated with fewer biliary complications in comparison with hepaticojejunostomy. Liver Transpl 2014;20(4):457–63.
45. Pandanaboyana S, Bell R, Bartlett AJ, et al. Meta-analysis of Duct-to-duct versus Roux-en-Y biliary reconstruction following liver transplantation for primary sclerosing cholangitis. Transpl Int 2015;28(4):485–91.
46. Dyson JK, Beuers U, Jones DEJ, et al. Primary sclerosing cholangitis. Lancet 2018;391:2547–59.
47. Visseren T, Erler NS, Polak WG, et al. Recurrence of primary sclerosing cholangitis after liver transplantation – analysing the European Liver Transplant Registry and beyond. Transpl Int 2021;34:1455–67.
48. Steenstraten IC, Sebib Korkmaz K, Trivedi PJ, et al. Systematic review with meta-analysis: risk factors for recurrent primary sclerosing cholangitis after liver transplantation, *Aliment Pharmacol Ther*, 49, 2019, 636–643.
49. Buchholz BM, Lykoudis PM, Ravikumar R, et al. Role of colectomy in preventing recurrent primary sclerosing cholangitis in liver transplant recipients. World J Gastroenterol 2018;24(28):3171–80.
50. Singh S, Edakkanambeth Varayil J, Loftus EV Jr, et al. Incidence of colorectal cancer after liver transplantation for primary sclerosing cholangitis: a systematic review and meta-analysis. Liver Transpl 2013;19(12):1361–9.
51. Peverelle M, Paleri S, Hughes J, et al. Activity of inflammatory bowel disease after liver transplantation for primary sclerosing cholangitis predicts poorer clinical outcomes. Inflamm Bowel Dis 2020;26(12):1901–8.
52. Mouchli MA, Singh S, Boardman L, et al. Natural History of established and de novo inflammatory bowel disease after liver transplantation for primary sclerosing cholangitis. Inflamm Bowel Dis 2018;24(5):1074–81.
53. Indriolo A, Ravelli P. Clinical management of inflammatory bowel disease in the organ recipient. World J Gastroenterol 2014;20:3523–33.
54. Joshi D, Bjarnason I, Belgaumkar A, et al. The impact of inflammatory bowel disease post-liver transplantation for primary sclerosing cholangitis. Liver Int 2013; 33:53–61.

Cholangiocarcinoma Surveillance Recommendations in Patients with Primary Sclerosing Cholangitis

Daniel Saca, MD, Steven L. Flamm, MD*

KEYWORDS

- Primary sclerosing cholangitis • Cholangiocarcinoma • Screening • Surveillance
- CA 19-9 • MRCP

KEY POINTS

- Patients with primary sclerosing cholangitis (PSC) commonly progress to end-stage liver disease, have recurrent bacterial cholangitis and have a higher risk of malignancies such as cholangiocarcinoma (CCA), gallbladder cancer, colorectal adenocarcinoma, and hepatocellular carcinoma.
- CCA in the setting of PSC is not uncommon, is usually diagnosed at an advanced stage, and has extremely high mortality.
- Common diagnostic strategies for CCA include serum tumor markers such as carbohydrate antigen 19–9 (CA 19–9), imaging studies such as MRI/Magnetic resonance cholangiopancreatography (MRCP), and endoscopic-assisted studies such as endoscopic retrograde cholangiopancreatography with brush cytology, biopsy, and fluorescence in situ hybridization testing.
- Surveillance strategies to identify CCA in the setting of PSC are sought because early identification improves patient outcomes.
- Although there are no widely agreed upon surveillance approaches for CCA, periodic measurement of serum CA 19-9 in combination with MRCP is recommended for patients with PSC.

INTRODUCTION

Primary sclerosing cholangitis (PSC) is an autoimmune cholangiopathy in which fibroinflammatory damage of the biliary tree results in multifocal fibrotic biliary strictures. The pathophysiology is not yet clearly elucidated, although interactions between

Rush University Medical School, 1725 West Harrison Street Suite 110, Chicago, IL 60612, USA
* Corresponding author.
E-mail address: Steven_Flamm@Rush.edu

Clin Liver Dis 28 (2024) 183–192
https://doi.org/10.1016/j.cld.2023.07.010

environmental factors and a dysregulated immune system are the prevailing theory. Impaired protective mechanisms to bile acid injury, an exaggerated inflammatory response to microbial antigenic triggers, and/or abnormal gut microbiota have been proposed as pathophysiologic mechanisms associated with chronic bile duct injury.[1] The resulting cholestatic liver damage related to these strictures frequently progresses to end-stage liver disease.

The highest incidence of PSC occurs between the second and fourth decades of life, with men accounting for most of the cases.[2,3] For reasons that are unclear, 60% to 80% of patients who have PSC have concomitant inflammatory bowel disease (IBD).[2,4–6]

PSC usually affects the large extrahepatic biliary ducts.[7] Many patients with PSC are asymptomatic at presentation and are first identified when a cholestatic liver profile is observed on routine blood testing. Others may have symptoms of cholestatic liver disease such as fatigue and pruritus. Some patients may present with complications of end-stage liver disease, symptoms consistent with bacterial cholangitis such as fevers and chills, metabolic bone disease, or with hepatic or extrahepatic malignancy.[8,9] There is an increased risk of malignancy in patients with PSC, with higher rates than expected of cholangiocarcinoma (CCA), colorectal adenocarcinoma, hepatocellular carcinoma, and gallbladder cancer observed.[10–12] Extrahepatic CCA, in particular, is common and is responsible for significant mortality in patients with PSC.[7,11,13,14] Early diagnosis of CCA is challenging. This discussion will focus on surveillance strategies to identify CCA before the development of symptoms and improve patient outcomes.

CHOLANGIOCARCINOMA IN THE SETTING OF PRIMARY SCLEROSING CHOLANGITIS

The incidence of CCA in patients with PSC is up to 1500 times the general population.[3,15] About 30% to 50% of CCA are identified within the first year of diagnosis of PSC and may be the reason that PSC is diagnosed. There should be particular vigilance for CCA after the initial diagnosis.[7,16,17] The 5 year incidence of CCA in the setting of PSC is 7%, and the lifetime risk ranges from 9% to 20%.[17–19]

The pathophysiology of CCA is poorly understood. The development of CCA is thought to result from a progression from inflammation to dysplasia to CCA. In the setting of the inflammatory process and fibrotic biliary strictures of PSC, dysplasia of cholangiocytes may be induced by a combination of chronic biliary infection and accumulation of toxic bile acids, superimposed on predisposing genetic and epigenetic abnormalities.[20–26]

Extrahepatic CCA usually develops from a dominant stricture, defined as a stricture with less than 1.5 mm diameter in the common bile duct or less than 1 mm in the hepatic duct. Dominant strictures are common in PSC and are observed in approximately 50% of patients. However, only a minority are malignant.[2,18,22,27,28] CCA in the setting of PSC is most commonly diagnosed in the fifth decade, although it can occur in younger and older patients.[22,29,30]

Clinical symptoms of CCA include fatigue, pruritus, abdominal pain, and fever due to bacterial cholangitis, jaundice, weight loss, or abnormal imaging suggestive of biliary malignancy.[2,29,31] However, similar symptoms are observed in PSC, making the diagnosis challenging. If there is an abrupt change in a patient's symptoms or the cholestatic liver biochemical profile worsens, there should be concern for the development of CCA.[28,32]

Unfortunately, symptomatic CCA is usually diagnosed at a later stage when surgical resection or liver transplantation is no longer possible.[22,33] When CCA is not amenable to surgical therapy, the median survival time is 5 to 12 months, with or without chemo-therapy.[29,34,35] If CCA is discovered at an early stage, the prognosis is improved, providing the impetus for screening.[36–39]

DIAGNOSIS OF CHOLANGIOCARCINOMA IN THE SETTING OF PRIMARY SCLEROSING CHOLANGITIS

Serum biomarkers, imaging studies, and endoscopic studies are used to diagnose CCA. Biomarkers that have been used include carbohydrate antigen 19-9 (CA 19-9), carcinoembryonic antigen (CEA), and anti-glycoprotein 2 IgA.[40–43]

CA 19-9 is the most commonly used; however, mild elevations are nonspecific as such elevations can be observed with active cholangitis. Further, 7% to 10% of patients do not express Lewis antigen and thus do not have elevated CA 19-9.[28,43–45] Neverthe-less, if there is at least a 3 fold elevation of CA 19-9 (129 U/mL), the sensitivity for the diagnosis of CCA is 79%, and the specificity is 99%.[46] It should be noted that patients with PSC can have elevated CA 19-9 above those levels for prolonged periods of time and not have CCA.[44]

CEA has a high specificity but lower sensitivity for the diagnosis of CCA.[47,48] CEA is not used frequently in clinical practice for the diagnosis of CCA. Other biomarkers including antiglycoprotein 2 IgA are under investigation but do not yet have a defined role for the diagnosis of CCA in this population.

Many imaging modalities have been implemented to diagnose CCA. These include ultrasound, contrast-enhanced ultrasound, computed tomography scan, MRI/MRCP, and PET scan. MRI/MRCP has high specificity (100%) and the highest sensitivity (32%); thus, this is the most useful noninvasive diagnostic modality. Unfortunately, when CCA is visible by imaging modalities, most of the tumors are in an advanced stage.[29,42,49,50]

When there is a concern for a diagnosis of CCA, endoscopic-assisted procedures are used to obtain tissue and confirm the diagnosis. The most commonly implemented procedures include endoscopic retrograde cholangiopancreatography (ERCP), chol-angioscopy, and endoscopic ultrasound (EUS). Cholangiography can reveal suspi-cious extrahepatic strictures. Brush cytology is considered the gold standard, with a specificity of greater than 95%. However, the sensitivity is only 43% to 67%.[51–53] Endobiliary biopsy improves the sensitivity (up to 100%) and also has excellent spec-ificity (>97%).[52,54] Currently, endoscopic brush cytology and biopsy together are the diagnostic test of choice to confirm a diagnosis of CCA.[28,37] Fluorescence in situ hy-bridization (FISH) in combination with brush cytology further increases the sensitivity for detecting CCA. FISH positivity has an approximately 60% sensitivity in the setting of negative brush cytology.[55–59] EUS with FNA is an effective technique for the diag-nosis of distal CCA in the setting of PSC; however, there is concern for needle tracking of tumor so it may not be ideal if curative surgical resection or liver transplantation is under consideration.[60–62]

SURVEILLANCE FOR CHOLANGIOCARCINOMA IN THE SETTING OF PRIMARY SCLEROSING CHOLANGITIS

As patients with PSC are at increased risk for CCA, and symptomatic CCA is typically diagnosed in the advanced stage with an extremely poor prognosis, surveillance stra-tegies to identify CCA at an early stage to improve outcomes have been advocated. When devising a surveillance strategy, patients should be selected who are truly at increased risk of the disease. For PSC, children rarely develop CCA, and thus surveil-lance is not recommended.[18,63] Furthermore, patients with small duct PSC, as well as those with IgG4-associated sclerosing cholangitis, are not at increased risk for CCA, and surveillance is not recommended in these settings.[64–66]

For adult patients with PSC, societies generally recommend surveillance for CCA, although surveillance recommendations differ (**Table 1**). Surveillance should include an approach that uses diagnostic testing that is safe, reproducible, cost-effective, and has a high sensitivity and high specificity. For CCA, no currently available strategies have optimal sensitivity. For instance, imaging alone is challenging when the tumor is small or multiple strictures are present.[42]

In clinical practice, usage of CA 19-9 and MRCP in combination every 6 to 12 months offers the safest approach, with the best sensitivity and specificity.[37,70] ERCP is not performed for surveillance purposes as it is expensive and is fraught with complications such as pancreatitis and bacterial cholangitis.

Clinical practice guidelines regarding the surveillance for CCA have no uniformity, but the long-term impact on the morbidity and mortality of successful surveillance has grown in recognition. A recent retrospective study highlights the importance of

Table 1	
Society screening recommendations for cholangiocarcinoma in patients with primary sclerosing cholangitis	
Society	**CCA**
AASLD[67]	CCA and gallbladder carcinoma surveillance should be performed annually and include abdominal imaging, preferably by MRI/MRCP with or without serum CA 19-9. Surveillance is not recommended for patients with PSC under 18 y of age or with small-duct PSC. Intraductal tissue sampling for cytology and FISH should be performed routinely during ERCP for relevant strictures.
EASL[68]	Surveillance with ultrasound and/or MRI/MRCP for CCA and gallbladder malignancy is suggested at least yearly in patients with large duct disease regardless of disease stage. CA 19-9 is not suggested for surveillance purposes due to its insufficient accuracy (LoE 3, weak recommendation, 96% consensus). Surveillance for hepatobiliary malignancy is suggested every 6 mo in the presence of cirrhosis (LoE 3, weak recommendation, 93% consensus).
ACG[18]	Screening for CCA with cross-sectional imaging with ultrasound or MR every 6–12 mo and serial CA 19-9.
BSG[69]	We suggest that an elevated CA 19.9 may support a diagnosis of suspected CCA but has a low diagnostic accuracy. Routine measurement of serum CA 19.9 is not recommended for surveillance for CCA in PSC (strength of recommendation: WEAK; quality of evidence: MODERATE). We recommend that when a diagnosis of CCA is clinically suspected, referral for specialist MDM review is essential (strength of recommendation: STRONG; quality of evidence: MODERATE). We recommend that where CCA is suspected, contrast-enhanced, cross-sectional imaging remains the initial preferred investigation for diagnosis and staging (strength of recommendation: STRONG; quality of evidence: HIGH). Confirmatory diagnosis relies on histology with the approach to tissue sampling guided by MDM review. Options include ERCP-guided biliary brush cytology/FISH/endobiliary biopsy/cholangioscopy/EUS-guided biopsy and/or percutaneous biopsy (strength of recommendation: STRONG; quality of evidence: HIGH).

Abbreviations: AASLD, American Association for the Study of Liver Diseases; ACG, American College of Gastroenterology; BSG, British Society of Gastroenterology; CCA, cholangiocarcinoma; EASL: European Association for the Study of the Liver.

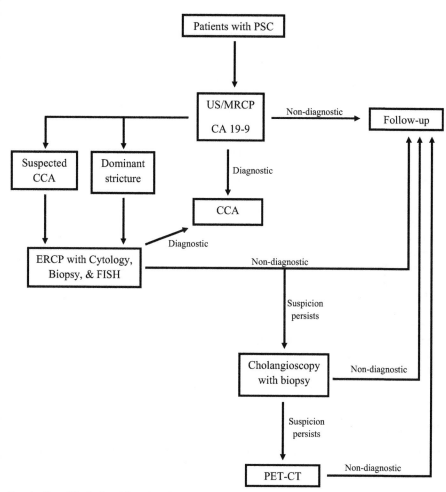

Fig. 1. Simplified algorithm for diagnosis and management of CCA in patients with PSC. CCA, cholangiocarcinoma; CT, computed tomography; ERCP, endoscopic retrograde cholangiopancreatography; FISH, fluorescence in situ hybridization; PSC, primary sclerosing cholangitis; US, ultrasound.

screening for CCA, with significantly higher 5 year survival rates of 68% versus 20% in the surveillance arm (P < .001).[49] CA 19-9 and MRCP in combination should each be performed in asymptomatic patients every 6 to 2 months. Early recognition of CCA hopefully allows for curative radical surgical intervention or liver transplantation.

SUMMARY

PSC is an autoimmune cholangiopathy that can occur at any age and is observed in both men and women. It is frequently, although not always, associated with IBD. Patients with PSC often are asymptomatic and only have a cholestatic liver biochemical profile at presentation. Others have nonspecific symptoms such as fatigue and pruritus. Health care providers must have high vigilance to diagnose patients with PSC because it frequently progresses to end-stage liver disease, is complicated by bacterial cholangitis, and has a higher rate of deadly malignancies such as CCA, gallbladder cancer, colorectal adenocarcinoma, and hepatocellular carcinoma. CCA, in particular, is a feared complication as the onset is unpredictable, is rapidly progressive, has poor treatment options, and has extremely high mortality.

Various tests are available to assess for CCA. The studies generally have high specificity but less optimal sensitivity. These tests include serum tumor markers such as CA 19-9, imaging studies such as MRI/MRCP, and endoscopic-assisted studies such as ERCP. In the setting of PSC, any abrupt change in the serum biochemical profile, development of symptoms such as worsened pruritus, jaundice, abdominal pain, weight loss, fevers, and chills, or identification of a dominant stricture on imaging should prompt an aggressive diagnostic effort to assess for CCA. When there is suspicion for CCA, ERCP with brushings and biopsy, and FISH should be obtained to confirm the diagnosis. Unfortunately, however, when CCA is symptomatic and initially diagnosed, it is often locally advanced and inoperable. Thus, there is an impetus for the surveillance of patients with PSC to identify CCA at an early stage and improve outcomes.

Better outcomes for CCA diagnosed at an early stage have been demonstrated. Yet, at present, there is no universal surveillance program for CCA in asymptomatic patients with PSC, largely because diagnostic testing is imperfect. However, serum CA 19-9 and MRCP every 6 to 12 months is a generally accepted surveillance protocol for CCA in patients with PSC. An algorithm for surveillance for CCA in PSC is outlined in **Fig. 1**.

In the future, advances in understanding the underpinnings of CCA in patients with PSC, including genetic and epigenetic factors that contribute to the development of CCA, will allow for the identification of novel serum tumor biomarkers and diagnostic agents, as well as more informed targeted surveillance strategies, for patients with PSC.

DISCLOSURE

There are no pertinent financial interests or relationships to disclose for either author.

REFERENCES

1. Karlsen TH, Folseraas T, Thorburn D, et al. Primary sclerosing cholangitis – a comprehensive review. J Hepatol 2017;67(6):1298–323.
2. Chapman MH, Webster GJ, Bannoo S, et al. Cholangiocarcinoma and dominant strictures in patients with primary sclerosing cholangitis: a 25-year single-centre experience. Eur J Gastroenterol Hepatol 2012;24(9):1051–8.
3. Boonstra K, Weersma RK, van Erpecum KJ, et al. Population-based epidemiology, malignancy risk, and outcome of primary sclerosing cholangitis. Hepatology 2013;58(6):2045–55.
4. Conrad K, Roggenbuck D, Laass MW. Diagnosis and classification of ulcerative colitis. Autoimmun Rev 2014;13(4–5):463–6.
5. Nakamura K, Ito T, Kotoh K, et al. Hepatopancreatobiliary manifestations of inflammatory bowel disease. Clinical Journal of Gastroenterology 2012;5(1):1–8.
6. Yimam KK, Bowlus CL. Diagnosis and classification of primary sclerosing cholangitis. Autoimmun Rev 2014;13(4–5):445–50.
7. Weismuller TJ, Trivedi PJ, Bergquist A, et al. Patient age, sex, and inflammatory bowel disease phenotype associate with course of primary sclerosing cholangitis. Gastroenterology 2017;152(8):1975–84.

8. Broome U, Olsson R, Loof L, et al. Natural history and prognostic factors in 305 Swedish patients with primary sclerosing cholangitis. Gut 1996;38(4):610–5.
9. Takakura WR, Tabibian JH, Bowlus CL. The evolution of natural history of primary sclerosing cholangitis. Curr Opin Gastroenterol 2017;33(2):71–7.
10. Burak K, Angulo P, Pasha TM, et al. Incidence and risk factors for cholangiocarcinoma in primary sclerosing cholangitis. Am J Gastroenterol 2004;99(3):523–6.
11. Fevery J, Henckaerts L, Van Oirbeek R, et al. Malignancies and mortality in 200 patients with primary sclerosering cholangitis: a long-term single-centre study. Liver Int 2012;32(2):214–22.
12. Liu K, Wang R, Kariyawasam V, et al. Epidemiology and outcomes of primary sclerosing cholangitis with and without inflammatory bowel disease in an Australian cohort. Liver Int 2017;37(3):442–8.
13. de Valle MB, Bjornsson E, Lindkvist B. Mortality and cancer risk related to primary sclerosing cholangitis in a Swedish population-based cohort. Liver Int 2012; 32(3):441–8.
14. Ngu JH, Gearry RB, Frampton CM, et al. Mortality and the risk of malignancy in autoimmune liver diseases: a population-based study in Canterbury, New Zealand. Hepatology 2012;55(2):522–9.
15. Burak K, Angulo P, Pasha TM, et al. Incidence and risk factors for cholangiocarcinoma in primary sclerosing cholangigis. Am J Gastroenterol 2004.
16. Boberg KM, Bergquist A, Mitchell S, et al. Cholangiocarcinoma in primary sclerosing cholangitis: risk factors and clinical presentation. Scand J Gastroenterol 2002;37(10):1205–11.
17. Saadi M, Yu C, Othman MO. A review of the challenges associated with the diagnosis and therapy of primary sclerosing cholangitis. Journal of Clinical and Translational Hepatology 2014;2(1):45–52.
18. Lindor KD, Kowdley KV, Harrison ME. ACG clinical guideline: primary sclerosing cholangitis. Am J Gastroenterol 2015;110(5):646–59.
19. Ponsioen CY. Diagnosis, differential diagnosis, and epidemiology of primary sclerosing cholangitis. Dig Dis 2015;33:134–9.
20. Ehlken H, Schramm C. Primary sclerosing cholangitis and cholangiocarcinoma: pathogenesis and modes of diagnostics. Dig Dis 2013;31(1):118–25.
21. Boyd S, Tenca A, Jokelainen K, et al. Screening primary sclerosing cholangitis and biliary dysplasia with endoscopic retrograde cholangiography and brush cytology: risk factors for biliary neoplasia. Endoscopy 2016;48(5):432–9.
22. Chung BK, Karlsen TH, Folseraas T. Cholangiocytes in the pathogenesis of primary sclerosing cholangitis and development of cholangiocarcinoma. Biochim Biophys Acta 2017. https://doi.org/10.1016/j.bbadis.2017.08.020.
23. Zarski JP, Barange K, Souvignet C, et al. Biliary dysplasia as a marker of cholangiocarcinoma in primary sclerosing cholangitis. J Hepatol 2001;34(3):360–5.
24. Alberts R, de Vries EMG, Goode EC, et al. Genetic association analysis identifies variants associated with disease progression in primary sclerosing cholangitis. Gut 2018;67(8):1517–24.
25. Cheung AC, LaRusso NF, Gores GJ, et al. Epigenetics in the primary biliary cholangitis and primary sclerosing cholangitis. Semin Liver Dis 2017;37(2):159–74.
26. Melum E, Franke A, Schramm C, et al. Genome-wide association analysis in primary sclerosing cholangitis identifies two non-HLA susceptibility loci. Nat Genet 2011;43(1):17–9.
27. Rudolph G, Gotthardt D, Kloters-Plachky P, et al. Influence of dominant bile duct stenoses and biliary infections on outcome in primary sclerosing cholangitis. Journal of hepatology 2009;51(1):149–55.

28. Aabakken L, Karlsen TH, Albert J, et al. Role of endoscopy in primary sclerosing cholangitis: European society of gastrointestinal endoscopy (ESGE) and European association for the study of the liver (EASL) clinical guideline. Endoscopy 2017;49(6):588–608.

29. Morris-Stiff G, Bhati C, Olliff S, et al. Cholangiocarcinoma complicating primary sclerosing cholangitis: a 24-year experience. Dig Surg 2008;25(2):126–32.

30. Rizvi S, Gores GJ. Pathogenesis, diagnosis, and management of cholangiocarcinoma. Gastroenterology 2013;145(6):1215–29.

31. Fevery J, Verslype C. An update on cholangiocarcinoma associated with primary sclerosing cholangitis. Curr Opin Gastroenterol 2010;26(3):236–45.

32. Trilianos P, Agnihotri A, Ucbilek E, et al. Greater biosynthetic liver dysfunction in primary sclerosing cholangitis suggests co-existent or impending cholangiocarcinoma. Journal of Clinical and Translational Hepatology 2016;4(1):1–4.

33. Rizvi S, Eaton JE, Gores GJ. Primary sclerosing cholangitis as a premalignant biliary tract disease: surveillance and management. Clin Gastroenterol Hepatol 2015;13(12):2152–65.

34. Molodecky NA, Kareemi H, Parab R, et al. Incidence of primary sclerosing cholangitis: a systematic review and meta-analysis. Hepatology 2011;53(5):1590–9.

35. Toy E, Balasubramanian S, Selmi C, et al. The prevalence, incidence and natural history of primary sclerosing cholangitis in an ethnically diverse population. BMC Gastroenterol 2011;11.

36. Rosen CB, Heimbach JK, Gores GJ. Liver transplantation for cholangiocarcinoma. Transpl Int 2010;23(7):692–7.

37. Charatcharoenwitthaya P, Enders FB, Halling KC, et al. Utility of serum tumor markers, imaging, and biliary cytology for detecting cholangiocarcinoma in primary sclerosing cholangitis. Hepatology 2008;48(4):1106–17.

38. Sapisochin G, Facciuto M, Rubbia-Brandt L, et al. Liver transplantation for "very early" intrahepatic cholangiocarcinoma: international retrospective study supporting a prospective assessment. Hepatology 2016;64(4):1178–88.

39. Stremitzer S, Jones RP, Quinn LM, et al. Clinical outcome after resection of early-stage hilar cholangiocarcinoma. Eur J Surg Oncol 2018;45:213–7.

40. Boyd S, Mustonen H, Tenca A, et al. Surveillance of primary sclerosing cholangitis with ERC and brush cytology: risk factors for cholangiocarcinoma. Scand J Gastroenterol 2017;52(2):242–9.

41. Banales JM, Inarrairaegui M, Arbelaiz A, et al. Serum metabolites as diagnostic biomarkers for cholangiocarcinoma, hepatocellular carcinoma and primary sclerosing cholangitis. Hepatology 2018. https://doi.org/10.1002/hep.30319.

42. Lee JJ, Schindera ST, Jang HJ, et al. Cholangiocarcinoma and its mimickers in primary sclerosing cholangitis. Abdominal Radiology 2017;42(12):2898–908.

43. Wannhoff A, Gotthardt DN. Recent developments in the research on biomarkers of cholangiocarcinoma in primary sclerosing cholangitis. Clinics and Research in Hepatology and Gastroenterology 2018. https://doi.org/10.1016/j.clinre.2018.08.013.

44. Sinakos E, Saenger AK, Keach J, et al. Many patients with primary sclerosing cholangitis and increased serum levels of carbohydrate antigen 19-9 do not have cholangiocarcinoma. Clin Gastroenterol Hepatol 2011;9(5):434–9.e431.

45. Wannhoff A, Hov JR, Folseraas T, et al. FUT2 and FUT3 genotype determines CA19-9 cut-off values for detection of cholangiocarcinoma in patients with primary sclerosing cholangitis. J Hepatol 2013;59(6):1278–84.

46. Levy C, Lymp J, Angulo P, et al. The value of serum CA 19-9 in predicting chol-angiocarcinomas in patients with primary sclerosing cholangitis. Dig Dis Sci 2005;50(9):1734–40.
47. Taghavi SA, Eshraghian A, Niknam R, et al. Diagnosis of cholangiocarcinoma in primary sclerosing cholangitis. Expet Rev Gastroenterol Hepatol 2018;12(6): 575–84.
48. Wannhoff A, Rupp C, Friedrich K, et al. Carcinoembryonic antigen level in primary sclerosing cholangitis is not influenced by dominant strictures or bacterial chol-angitis. Dig Dis Sci 2017;62(2):510–6.
49. Ali AH, Tabibian JH. Surveillance for hepatobiliary cancers in patients with pri-mary sclerosing cholangitis. Hepatology 2018;67(6):2338–51.
50. Schramm C, Eaton J, Ringe KI, et al. Recommendations on the use of magnetic resonance imaging in PSC-A position statement from the International PSC Study Group. Hepatology 2017;66(5):1675–88.
51. Kuzu UB, Odemis B, Suna N, et al. The detection of cholangiocarcinoma in pri-mary sclerosing cholangitis patients: single center experience. J Gastrointest Cancer 2016;47(1):8–14.
52. Navaneethan U, Njei B, Lourdusamy V, et al. Comparative effectiveness of biliary brush cytology and intraductal biopsy for detection of malignant biliary strictures: a systematic review and meta-analysis. Gastrointest Endosc 2015;81(1):168–76.
53. Trikudanathan G, Navaneethan U, Njei B, et al. Diagnostic yield of bile duct brushings for cholangiocarcinoma in primary sclerosing cholangitis: a systematic review and meta-analysis. Gastrointest Endosc 2014;79(5):783–9.
54. Nanda A, Brown JM, Berger SH, et al. Triple modality testing by endoscopic retro-grade cholangiopancreatography for the diagnosis of cholangiocarcinoma. Ther-apeutic advances in gastroenterology 2015;8(2):56–65.
55. Levy MJ, Baron TH, Clayton AC, Enders FB, Gostout CJ, Halling KC, Kipp BR, Pe-tersen BT, Roberts LR, Rumalla A, Sebo TJ, Clinic Rev Allerg Immunol (2020) 58:134–149 147.
56. Topazian MD, Wiersema MJ, Gores GJ. Prospective evaluation of advanced mo-lecular markers and imaging techniques in patients with indeterminate bile duct strictures. Am J Gastroenterol 2008;103(5):1263–73.
57. Moreno Luna LE, Kipp B, Halling KC, et al. Advanced cytologic techniques for the detection of malignant pancreatobiliary strictures. Gastroenterology 2006;131(4): 1064–72.
58. Quinn KP, Tabibian JH, Lindor KD. Clinical implications of serial versus isolated biliary fluorescence in situ hybridization (FISH) polysomy in primary sclerosing cholangitis. Scand J Gastroenterol 2017;52(4):377–81.
59. Liew ZH, Loh TJ, Lim TKH, et al. Role of fluorescence in situ hybridization in diag-nosing cholangiocarcinoma in indeterminate biliary strictures. J Gastroenterol Hepatol 2018;33(1):315–9.
60. Rizvi S, Eaton J, Yang JD, et al. Emerging technologies for the diagnosis of peri-hilar cholangiocarcinoma. Semin Liver Dis 2018;38(2):160–9.
61. Brooks C, Gausman V, Kokoy-Mondragon C, et al. Role of fluorescent in situ hy-bridization, cholangioscopic biopsies, and EUS-FNA in the evaluation of biliary strictures. Dig Dis Sci 2018;63(3):636–44.
62. Heimbach JK, Sanchez W, Rosen CB, et al. Transperitoneal fine needle aspiration biopsy of hilar cholangiocarcinoma is associated with disease dissemination. HPB: The Official Journal of the International Hepato Pancreato Biliary Associa-tion 2011;13(5):356–60.

63. Chapman R, Fevery J, Kalloo A, et al. Diagnosis and management of primary sclerosing cholangitis. Hepatology 2010;51(2):660–78.
64. Fevery J, Van Steenbergen W, Van Pelt J, et al. Patients with large-duct primary sclerosing cholangitis and Crohn's disease have a better outcome than those with ulcerative colitis, or without IBD. Aliment Pharmacol Ther 2016;43(5):612–20.
65. Halliday JS, Djordjevic J, Lust M, et al. A unique clinical phenotype of primary sclerosing cholangitis associated with Crohn's disease. Journal of Crohn's & Colitis 2012;6(2):174–81.
66. Song J, Yang L, Bowlus C, et al. Cholangiocarcinoma in patients with primary sclerosing cholangitis (PSC); a comprehensive review. Clin Rev Allerg Immunol 2020;58:134–49.
67. Bowlus CL, Arrivé L, Bergquist A, et al. AASLD practice guidance on primary sclerosing cholangitis and cholangiocarcinoma. Hepatology 2023;77(2):659–702.
68. Chazouilleres O, Beuers U, Bergquist A, et al. Easl clinical practice guidelines on sclerosing cholangitis. J Hepatol 2022;77(3):761–806.
69. Chapman MH, Thorburn D, Hirschfield GM, et al. British Society of Gastroenterology and UK-PSC guidelines for the diagnosis and management of primary sclerosing cholangitis. Gut 2019;68(8):1356–78.
70. Horsley-Silva JL, Rodriguez EA, Franco DL, et al. An update on cancer risk and surveillance in primary sclerosing cholangitis. Liver Int 2017;37(8):1103–9.

Post-Transplant Management and Complications of Autoimmune Hepatitis, Primary Biliary Cholangitis, and Primary Sclerosing Cholangitis including Disease Recurrence

Jacqueline B. Henson, MD[a], Lindsay Y. King, MD, MPH[b],*

KEYWORDS

- Liver transplantation • Primary sclerosing cholangitis • Primary biliary cholangitis
- Autoimmune hepatitis • Rejection • Recurrent disease • Immunosuppression

KEY POINTS

- Transplant recipients with autoimmune liver diseases are at increased risk for rejection compared to other indications for transplant.
- Autoimmune liver diseases can recur post-transplant and increase the risk of graft loss and mortality, particularly in primary sclerosing cholangitis.
- These complications have in some cases been linked to immunosuppressive agents, though there is generally insufficient evidence to recommend specific regimens, and this warrants further study.

INTRODUCTION

Autoimmune liver diseases including autoimmune hepatitis (AIH), primary biliary cholangitis (PBC), and primary sclerosing cholangitis (PSC) are the indication for approximately 15% of liver transplants in the US (4% AIH, 4% PSC, 5% PBC) and 25% in Europe.[1–3] These conditions have been increasing in incidence and prevalence, and, in some European countries, autoimmune liver diseases are or are projected to

[a] Division of Gastroenterology, Department of Medicine, Duke University School of Medicine, DUMC Box 3913, Durham, NC 27710, USA; [b] Division of Gastroenterology, Department of Medicine, Duke University School of Medicine, DUMC Box 3923, Durham, NC 27710, USA
* Corresponding author.
E-mail address: lindsay.king@duke.edu

Clin Liver Dis 28 (2024) 193–207
https://doi.org/10.1016/j.cld.2023.07.009
1089-3261/24/© 2023 Elsevier Inc. All rights reserved.
liver.theclinics.com

soon be the leading indication for transplant.[3,4] Understanding the post-transplant care of these patients is therefore important.

The post-transplant outcomes of patients with autoimmune liver diseases are generally good, with survival rates around 90% at 1 year and 70% at 5 years, though the post-transplant course can present some unique complications (**Table 1**).[5] In addition to rejection, which these patients may be at increased risk for, recurrent disease can also occur and adversely impact graft and patient survival. There are also other disease-specific complications that may require management, including persistent symptoms such as fatigue in PBC and inflammatory bowel disease (IBD) in PSC. This review will provide an overview of post-transplant complications in autoimmune liver diseases and the post-transplant management of these patients.

POST-TRANSPLANT COMPLICATIONS: REJECTION

Patients with autoimmune liver disease are generally considered to be at higher risk for rejection, though the reported incidence has varied over time with evolving immunosuppression strategies, practices regarding protocol biopsies, and, to a lesser extent, histologic definitions.[6-14] Several series have reported a higher risk of early T-cell-mediated rejection (TCMR), late TCMR, and chronic rejection in transplant recipients with AIH.[9-11,15] In early studies, the observed risk was as high as over 80% for early TCMR and 30% for late TCMR, though in more recent data these have been more similar to non-immune liver diseases at 20% to 40% and 10%, respectively (see **Table 1**).[2,10,11,13,16] This change over time may reflect recommendations for augmented immunosuppression in these patients due these early data, though this is uncertain.[17,18] The risk of chronic rejection in recipients with AIH (15%) is also higher than other etiologies of liver disease and may be increased in younger recipients.[9]

Transplant recipients with PBC and PSC have also been found to have an increased risk of early (40%–83%) and late (13%–28%) TCMR, while chronic rejection (5%–8%) may be more similar to non-immune liver diseases (see **Table 1**).[2,6-9,15,16,19] In contrast to AIH, no guidelines have recommended increased immunosuppression in these patients, and the increased risk of TCMR has persisted in more recent studies.[2,16] In PSC, younger age and IBD have been associated with a higher risk of TCMR, though the data for IBD is somewhat conflicting.[7,20,21] Further research on

Table 1
Post-transplant complications in autoimmune liver disease

	AIH	PBC	PSC
Rejection	• Early TCMR: 20%–88% • Late TCMR: 10%–33% • Chronic rejection: 15%	• Early TCMR: 59%–83% • Late TCMR: 13%–26% • Chronic rejection: 8%	• Early TCMR: 39%–71% • Late TCMR: 13%–28% • Chronic rejection: 5%–8%
Recurrence	• 20%–30% at 5 y	• 20%–30% at 10 y	• 20%–25% at 5 y
Other Potential Complications	• Early infection, particularly fungal infections	• Persistent fatigue • Persistent sicca symptoms • Osteoporosis (early)	• Inflammatory bowel disease • Colorectal cancer • Pancreatic cancer • Persistent fatigue • Osteoporosis (early)

the clinical factors, including immunosuppression regimens, associated with rejection in patients with autoimmune liver diseases is needed.

No association between antibody-mediated rejection and autoimmune liver disease has been reported.[22,23] The entity previously considered *de novo* AIH though has recently been renamed plasma cell-rich rejection, as this appears to be a manifestation of allograft rejection.[24-26] This occurs in 3% to 5% of adult liver transplant recipients with non-AIH diseases.[24]

POST-TRANSPLANT COMPLICATIONS: RECURRENT DISEASE
Recurrent Autoimmune Hepatitis

Recurrent AIH occurs in 20% to 30% of recipients at 5 years, with some variability depending on whether biopsies were clinically indicated or obtained by protocol.[5,27-29] This is diagnosed similarly to AIH pre-transplant, with positive autoantibodies, elevated immunoglobulin G (IgG), and typical histologic features, including the presence of lymphoplasmacytic portal inflammation with interface hepatitis, pseudorosettes, and lobular collapse and necrosis in severe cases.[27,30,31] Recurrent AIH has been found on protocol biopsies in the absence of abnormal liver tests. It can be difficult to distinguish from alloimmune rejection, though the features typical for rejection, including endotheliitis and bile duct damage, are usually not present.[31] Recurrent AIH is associated with increased mortality and had reduced graft survival of 12.2 years versus 24.0 years in a large multicenter study.[27]

Several risk factors for recurrent AIH have been reported, including younger age, greater inflammation pre-transplant (higher IgG, high transaminases, moderate/severe inflammation in explant), donor-recipient sex mismatch, use of mycophenolate mofetil (MMF), and the discontinuation of steroids (**Table 2**).[27,29,32-37] The role of immunosuppression regimens is controversial. The link to MMF was identified in a large multicenter study, though some have argued that this may reflect an "era effect" in which other factors from the time period in which MMF was used less commonly underlie this finding.[27] Data on prolonged steroids has also been conflicting, and a systematic review did not find conclusive evidence of a protective effect.[38,39]

Recurrent Primary Biliary Cholangitis

Recurrence of PBC occurs in 20% to 30% of recipients at 10 years.[5,28,40] Diagnosis can be challenging as antimitochondrial antibody and immunoglobulin M (IgM) often persist post-transplant, and cholestasis can be seen in other clinical scenarios.[41] Liver biopsy is therefore typically required. Histopathologic findings are consistent with PBC prior to transplant, with mononuclear cell portal tract infiltrate, portal granulomas, bile duct damage and disappearance, and bile ductular proliferation, though this needs to be distinguished from immune-mediated injury of small bile ducts due to rejection. Until recently, recurrent PBC was not thought to have a significant impact on graft or patient survival, accounting for only 1.3% of graft loss.[42] Yet, more recent data from a large cohort with long-term follow-up found that recurrent disease does confer a slightly increased risk of graft failure and mortality.[43,44]

Reported risk factors for recurrent PBC include younger age, early cholestasis post-transplant, tacrolimus, and MMF, while cyclosporine has been associated with a decreased risk (see **Table 2**).[43-50] The role of ursodeoxycholic acid (UDCA) post-transplant had been uncertain, with early studies demonstrating improvement in cholestasis but not other outcomes.[51] More recent data though has shown a role for UDCA in preventing the development of recurrent PBC as well as improving graft and patient survival.[44,47,52,53] In a large cohort, preventative UDCA was associated

Table 2
Risk factors for recurrent disease post-transplant in autoimmune liver diseases

	AIH	PBC	PSC
Patient Factors	• Younger age[27] • Concomitant autoimmune disease[29] • Black race[32] • High IgG[27,29] • High AST, ALT[27] • More severe inflammation in explant[29,34] • HLA-DR3 or -DR4[33]	• Younger age[43] • Elevated IgM[45]	• Younger age[57,62] • Male sex[68] • Recurrent cholangitis[55] • Higher MELD score[63,65,113] • IBD, especially UC[58,62,64-66] • HLA-DR8[108] • Cholangiocarcinoma[54,65,113]
Transplant Factors	• Donor/recipient sex mismatch[27] • HLA locus mismatching[32]	• Donor/recipient sex mismatch[45] • HLA locus mismatching[46] • Older donor age[46]	• Donor/recipient sex mismatch[114] • Older donor age[58,65,71,113] • Extended criteria donor[67] • CMV donor/recipient mismatch[115] • Living donor first-degree relative[63,116]
Post-Transplant Factors	• MMF[27] • Discontinuation of steroids[35,36,38,39] • Lack of antimetabolite[37]	• Increased cholestasis early post-transplant[43] • Tacrolimus[47,48] • Cyclosporine (↓)[43,45,48,49] • Azathioprine (↓)[49] • UDCA (↓)[44,47,52,53] • Antiretroviral therapy (↓)[50]	• IBD activity[69] • Colectomy(↓)[57,65,67,68] • Biliary complication[63,113] • CMV infection[63] • TCMR: any episode,[65,108,115] multiple episodes,[55,65] steroid resistant[19] • Antithymocyte globulin[64] • Tacrolimus[57] • Cyclosporine (mixed)[61,70] • Prolonged steroids[66] • Single agent or no immunosuppression at 1 year[71]

with 2.26 years of life gained over 20 years, and the best outcomes were observed for the combination of UDCA and cyclosporine.[44]

Recurrent Primary Sclerosing Cholangitis

PSC recurs in 20% to 25% of transplant recipients at 5 years.[54–58] It typically presents with cholestasis and multifocal non-anastomotic biliary strictures greater than 90 days post-transplant and must be differentiated from ischemia, ABO incompatibility, and chronic rejection, which can be challenging.[59–61] Histologic findings are similar to PSC pre-transplant and may include fibrous cholangitis and/or fibro-obliterative lesions with or without ductopenia, biliary fibrosis, or biliary cirrhosis.[59] Ductopenia can also be seen in chronic rejection, so the diagnosis of recurrent PSC should be made based on a combination of clinical and histopathologic findings. Recurrent PSC is also associated with increased graft loss and mortality.[56,58,62,63] This is typically more clinically significant than recurrent AIH and PBC, with nearly half progressing to graft failure in some series.[62]

Risk factors for recurrent PSC are shown in **Table 2**. In several studies, the presence of IBD, particularly ulcerative colitis (UC), and increased IBD activity post-transplant have been associated with an increased risk of recurrent PSC, while a colectomy has been protective.[57,58,62,64–69] These findings suggest that intestinal inflammation may increase the risk of recurrent PSC. Immunosuppression regimens have also been linked to recurrent PSC. Use of steroid-free antithymocyte globulin induction protocols, tacrolimus, and prolonged steroids have been associated with recurrent PSC in some studies, while cyclosporine has been mixed.[57,61,64,66,70] Reduced immunosuppression with one agent or no immunosuppression after 1 year has also been linked to recurrent PSC.[71] The seemingly mixed association between both more and less immunosuppression being linked to recurrent PSC may reflect underlying individual differences in recurrence risk and immunosuppression needs.

OTHER POST-TRANSPLANT COMPLICATIONS
Infection

Though all patients post-transplant are at risk for infection, patients with AIH are at higher risk for fatal infections in the early post-transplant period (particularly fungal infections), and this contributes to inferior outcomes relative to PSC and PBC.[13,72,73] Surprisingly, based on limited data, this risk does not appear to be related to immunosuppression strategy either before or after transplant, including prolonged use of steroids, though it could be related to spontaneous immunosuppression in patients with AIH.[13,74,75]

Osteoporosis

All transplant recipients experience accelerated bone loss in the immediate post-transplant period, likely related to high doses of steroids and possibly calcineurin inhibitors.[76,77] Patients with cholestatic liver diseases may have decreased bone density post-transplant relative to other etiologies, but this typically improves after 4 to 6 months.[76–79] In patients maintained on long-term steroids, this risk may persist, though a single-center cohort of patients with AIH found that the proportion who developed osteoporosis was similar to published rates for other transplant recipients.[36,76,80]

Fatigue and Other Symptoms

Fatigue is a burdensome symptom in cholestatic liver disease, especially PBC, and is associated with impaired quality of life.[81] Transplantation may improve fatigue in some patients with PBC, though nearly half still suffer from this symptom 2 years post-transplant, and fatigue may worsen in males.[82–84] In PSC, fatigue persists in one-third of patients, though, in contrast to PBC, improves in males.[85] Sicca symptoms in patients with PBC also persist post-transplant.[40]

Inflammatory Bowel Disease

Most patients with PSC have concomitant IBD, particularly UC. The presence of IBD and its degree of activity may increase the risk of rejection and recurrent PSC, as discussed above, though IBD alone does not appear to impact graft or patient survival.[86] IBD may, however, be associated with an increased risk of CMV infection.[86]

The natural history of IBD post-transplant is variable. The disease course can be quiescent or more aggressive, and de novo IBD develops in 20% at 5 years.[87–90] Up to 25% of recipients require the escalation of IBD therapy despite transplant-related immunosuppression, and immunosuppression regimens have also been linked to IBD outcomes.[88] Tacrolimus and MMF may be associated with increased disease activity, while azathioprine and cyclosporine have been associated with an improved course.[88,90,91] Azathioprine may also protect against the development of de novo IBD, and MMF may increase this risk.[88,91] Combination biologic and antirejection therapy is associated with an increased risk of Clostridium difficile, though the overall rate of serious infections is similar to the general liver transplant population.[92]

Gastrointestinal Malignancy

Patients with PSC are at even higher risk for colorectal cancer (CRC) post-transplant, particularly with longer duration of IBD, extensive colitis, and moderate/severe IBD disease activity.[69,93–96] Recipients with PSC and IBD are more than twice as likely to develop CRC compared to PSC without IBD and four times as likely as IBD without PSC.[93,94] Individuals with prior colectomy and an ileoanal pouch may be at increased risk for dysplasia and malignancy in the pouch, though these data have been conflicting.[97,98] In addition to CRC, transplant recipients with PSC may also have an increased risk of pancreatic cancer.[94]

POST-TRANSPLANT MANAGEMENT

Post-transplant management of recipients with autoimmune liver disease must take into account these complications, including an increased risk of rejection, the potential for disease recurrence, and other disease-specific complications. Rejection and recurrent disease should be monitored for closely, as both have been found to impact graft and patient survival, though the optimal approach to this is uncertain.[2,43,44,56,58,62,63] In most cases, these complications will manifest with abnormal liver tests, though histologic disease can be present in the absence of other indicators.[37]

The role of surveillance biopsies in this population is uncertain, though over 25% of a cohort in a study demonstrating a benefit to an individualized approach to surveillance had autoimmune liver disease.[99] In addition, though some data has suggested links between immunosuppressants and these outcomes, in most cases, there is not convincing evidence to support a preferred regimen.[100] Potential strategies to reduce the risk of disease recurrence are shown in **Table 3**.

Autoimmune Hepatitis

Steroid maintenance therapy post-transplant in AIH is controversial.[101,102] Some data support a reduced risk of recurrent AIH, though the evidence has been

Table 3
Potential strategies to reduce the risk of recurrent disease post-transplant

	AIH	PBC	PSC
Pre-Transplant	• Treatment to reduce IgG, AST, ALT		• Treatment to control IBD • Consider colectomy if difficult to control IBD
Post-Transplant	• Adequate maintenance immunosuppression with the consideration of long-term, low-dose corticosteroids vs withdrawal	• Preventative UDCA • Consideration of switching from tacrolimus to cyclosporine after early post-transplant period	• Maintain IBD remission • Consider colectomy if difficult to control IBD

mixed.[16,35,36,38,39] Earlier guidelines from the American Association for the Study of Liver Diseases suggested the use of long-term, low-dose corticosteroids for recipients with AIH, though the more recent guidelines instead suggest gradual withdrawal be considered given the lack of data.[17,31] The International Liver Transplantation Society suggests considering maintaining low-dose steroids or adding MMF or azathioprine to facilitate steroid weaning.[103] An individualized approach accounting for the patient's risk of recurrent disease and rejection, balanced with the effects of long-term steroids, is likely the optimal approach. In addition, though MMF has also been recently implicated as a potential risk factor for recurrent AIH, further research is needed to confirm this finding.[27]

When recurrent disease does develop, immunosuppression should be increased, with the reintroduction of steroids, followed by the addition of azathioprine or MMF if needed, while continuing the calcineurin inhibitor.[31] If there is a lack of response, the antimetabolite or calcineurin inhibitor can be switched, and rapamycin has also been used in patients who did not respond to these regimens.[31,104] In some cases, recurrent disease may progress to graft failure, and retransplantation was needed in 13% to 50% of patients in small series.[35,105]

Primary Biliary Cholangitis

There are no guideline recommendations on immunosuppression regimens in PBC post-transplant, though some centers report changing from tacrolimus to cyclosporine after 3 months to balance the risk of TCMR with disease recurrence.[100] Use of UDCA post-transplant has also not been specifically recommended, though the published guidelines preceded some of the more recent data supporting reduced recurrent PBC, graft loss, and recipient mortality.[40,44,47,52,53,106] Some centers administer preventative UDCA at 10 to 15 mg/kg/d to reduce the risk of these complications.[100] If recurrent PBC develops, UDCA improves cholestasis and may delay histologic progression.[51] Recurrent PBC is now recognized to slightly increase the risk of graft failure, though this rarely requires retransplantation.[43]

Primary Sclerosing Cholangitis

There is also insufficient evidence to suggest a preferred immunosuppression regimen for PSC based on existing data. The potential relationship between immunosuppressive agents and IBD disease course may influence this decision, particularly as IBD activity is associated with recurrent PSC.[69] If recurrent PSC develops, unfortunately no effective treatment exists to slow progression. Some centers use UDCA, though there are no data supporting improved outcomes.[60,107] Up to one-third with recurrent disease may progress to require retransplantation, and outcomes in selected patients may be similar to first-time transplant.[54,108,109]

With regards to the management of IBD, studies have demonstrated the safety and effectiveness of anti-TNF agents and vedolizumab.[110,111] There are no data on the use of newer IBD agents post-transplant, though the thrombosis risk with JAK inhibitors could be a potential concern.[112]

Patients with PSC remain at higher risk for CRC and should continue to undergo yearly colonoscopies.[69,93–95] Recipients with a pouch should also have yearly surveillance, though data to support this practice has been conflicting.[97,98]

SUMMARY

In conclusion, autoimmune liver diseases have unique post-transplant considerations. These recipients are at increased risk of rejection, and recurrent disease may also develop, which can progress to graft loss and increase mortality. Vigilantly monitoring for and managing these complications is therefore important, though data on associated risk factors and immunosuppression strategies has in most cases been mixed. The immunologic complications must be balanced against the complications of immunosuppressive therapy. There are also other disease-specific complications that require management and may impact these decisions, including IBD in PSC. Further work to better understand the optimal management strategies for these post-transplant complications is needed, and the future may involve a more personalized approach with tailored surveillance and immunosuppression strategies.[99]

CLINICS CARE POINTS

- Transplant recipients with autoimmune liver diseases are more likely to experience rejection.
- Transplant recipients with AIH are at increased risk of early infections, particularly fungal infections.
- Fatigue persists in many patients with PBC and PSC post-transplant.
- Management of IBD in PSC is important as this has been associated with both an increased risk of rejection and recurrent disease post-transplant.

CONFLICTS OF INTEREST

No relevant conflicts of interest.

FINANCIAL SUPPORT

J.B. Henson is supported by NIH grant T32DK007568.

REFERENCES

1. Webb GJ, Rana A, Hodson J, et al. Twenty-year comparative analysis of patients with autoimmune liver diseases on transplant waitlists. Clin Gastroenterol Hepatol 2018;16(2):278–87.
2. Levitsky J, Goldberg D, Smith AR, et al. Acute rejection increases risk of graft failure and death in recent liver transplant recipients. Clin Gastroenterol Hepatol 2017;15(4):584–93.
3. Trivedi PJ, Hirschfield GM. Recent advances in clinical practice: epidemiology of autoimmune liver diseases. Gut 2021;70(10):1989–2003.
4. Fosby B, Melum E, Bjøro K, et al. Liver transplantation in the Nordic countries - an intention to treat and post-transplant analysis from the Nordic Liver Transplant Registry 1982-2013. Scand J Gastroenterol 2015;50(6):797–808.
5. Montano-Loza AJ, Bhanji RA, Wasilenko S, et al. Systematic review: recurrent autoimmune liver diseases after liver transplantation. Aliment Pharmacol Ther 2017;45(4):485–500.
6. Berlakovich GA, Imhof M, Karner-Hanusch J, et al. The importance of the effect of underlying disease on rejection outcomes following orthotopic liver transplantation. Transplantation 1996;61(4):554–60.
7. Graziadei IW, Wiesner RH, Marotta PJ, et al. Long-term results of patients undergoing liver transplantation for primary sclerosing cholangitis. Hepatology 1999;30(5):1121–7.

8. Hayashi M, Keeffe EB, Krams SM, et al. Allograft rejection after liver transplantation for autoimmune liver diseases. Liver Transpl Surg 1998;4(3):208–14.

9. Milkiewicz P, Gunson B, Saksena S, et al. Increased incidence of chronic rejection in adult patients transplanted for autoimmune hepatitis: assessment of risk factors. Transplantation 2000;70(3):477–80.

10. Vogel A, Heinrich E, Bahr MJ, et al. Long-term outcome of liver transplantation for autoimmune hepatitis. Clin Transpl 2004;18(1):62–9.

11. Molmenti EP, Netto GJ, Murray NG, et al. Incidence and recurrence of autoimmune/alloimmune hepatitis in liver transplant recipients. Liver Transpl 2002; 8(6):519–26.

12. Shaked A, Ghobrial RM, Merion RM, et al. Incidence and severity of acute cellular rejection in recipients undergoing adult living donor or deceased donor liver transplantation. Am J Transpl 2009;9(2):301–8.

13. Chouik Y, Francoz C, De Martin E, et al. Liver transplantation for autoimmune hepatitis: pre-transplant does not predict the early post-transplant outcome. Liver Int 2023;43(4):906–16.

14. Duclos-Vallée JC, Sebagh M, Rifai K, et al. A 10 year follow up study of patients transplanted for autoimmune hepatitis: histological recurrence precedes clinical and biochemical recurrence. Gut 2003;52(6):893–7.

15. Uemura T, Ikegami T, Sanchez EQ, et al. Late acute rejection after liver transplantation impacts patient survival. Clin Transpl 2008;22(3):316–23.

16. Thurairajah PH, Carbone M, Bridgestock H, et al. Late acute liver allograft rejection; a study of its natural history and graft survival in the current era. Transplantation 2013;95(7):955–9.

17. Lucey MR, Terrault N, Ojo L, et al. Long-term management of the successful adult liver transplant: 2012 practice guideline by the American Association for the Study of Liver Diseases and the American Society of Transplantation. Liver Transpl 2013;19(1):3–26.

18. Satapathy SK, Jones OD, Vanatta JM, et al. Outcomes of liver transplant recipients with autoimmune liver disease using long-term dual immunosuppression regimen without corticosteroid. Transpl Direct 2017;3(7):e178.

19. Brandsaeter B, Schrumpf E, Bentdal O, et al. Recurrent primary sclerosing cholangitis after liver transplantation: a magnetic resonance cholangiography study with analyses of predictive factors. Liver Transpl 2005;11(11):1361–9.

20. Narumi S, Roberts JP, Emond JC, et al. Liver transplantation for sclerosing cholangitis. Hepatology 1995;22(2):451–7.

21. Miki C, Harrison JD, Gunson BK, et al. Inflammatory bowel disease in primary sclerosing cholangitis: an analysis of patients undergoing liver transplantation. Br J Surg 1995;82(8):1114–7.

22. Tajima T, Hata K, Haga H, et al. Risk factors for antibody-mediated rejection in ABO blood-type incompatible and donor-specific antibody-positive liver transplantation. Liver Transpl 2023.

23. Vandevoorde K, Ducreux S, Bosch A, et al. Prevalence, risk factors, and impact of donor-specific alloantibodies after adult liver transplantation. Liver Transpl 2018;24(8):1091.

24. Demetris AJ, Bellamy C, Hübscher SG, et al. Comprehensive update of the banff working group on liver allograft pathology: introduction of antibody-mediated rejection. Am J Transpl 2016;16(10):2816–35.

25. Lee BT, Fiel MI, Schiano TD. Antibody-mediated rejection of the liver allograft: an update and a clinico-pathological perspective. J Hepatol 2021;75(5):1203–16.

26. Harrington CR, Levitsky J. Alloimmune versus autoimmune hepatitis following liver transplantation. Clin Liver Dis 2022;20(1):21–4.
27. Montano-Loza AJ, Ronca V, Ebadi M, et al. Risk factors and outcomes associated with recurrent autoimmune hepatitis following liver transplantation. J Hepatol 2022;77(1):84–97.
28. Gautam M, Cheruvattath R, Balan V. Recurrence of autoimmune liver disease after liver transplantation: a systematic review. Liver Transpl 2006;12(12):1813–24.
29. Montano-Loza AJ, Mason AL, Ma M, et al. Risk factors for recurrence of autoimmune hepatitis after liver transplantation. Liver Transpl 2009;15(10):1254–61.
30. Hübscher SG. Recurrent autoimmune hepatitis after liver transplantation: diagnostic criteria, risk factors, and outcome. Liver Transpl 2001;7(4):285–91.
31. Mack CL, Adams D, Assis DN, et al. Diagnosis and management of autoimmune hepatitis in adults and children: 2019 practice guidance and guidelines from the American association for the study of liver diseases. Hepatology 2020;72(2):671–722.
32. McCabe M, Rush N, Lammert C, et al. HLA-DR mismatch and black race are associated with recurrent autoimmune hepatitis after liver transplantation. Transpl Direct 2021;7(7):e714.
33. Balan V, Ruppert K, Demetris AJ, et al. Long-term outcome of human leukocyte antigen mismatching in liver transplantation: results of the National institute of diabetes and digestive and kidney diseases liver transplantation database. Hepatology 2008;48(3):878–88.
34. Ayata G, Gordon FD, Lewis WD, et al. Liver transplantation for autoimmune hepatitis: a long-term pathologic study. Hepatology 2000;32(2):185–92.
35. Milkiewicz P, Hubscher SG, Skiba G, et al. Recurrence of autoimmune hepatitis after liver transplantation. Transplantation 1999;68(2):253–6.
36. Krishnamoorthy TL, Miezynska-Kurtycz J, Hodson J, et al. Longterm corticosteroid use after liver transplantation for autoimmune hepatitis is safe and associated with a lower incidence of recurrent disease. Liver Transpl 2016;22(1):34–41.
37. Puustinen L, Boyd S, Arkkila P, et al. Histologic surveillance after liver transplantation due to autoimmune hepatitis. Clin Transpl 2017;31(5).
38. Vierling JM, Kerkar N, Czaja AJ, et al. Immunosuppressive treatment regimens in autoimmune hepatitis: systematic reviews and meta-analyses supporting American association for the study of liver diseases guidelines. Hepatology 2020;72(2):753–69.
39. Campsen J, Zimmerman MA, Trotter JF, et al. Liver transplantation for autoimmune hepatitis and the success of aggressive corticosteroid withdrawal. Liver Transpl 2008;14(9):1281–6.
40. Lindor KD, Bowlus CL, Boyer J, et al. Primary biliary cholangitis: 2018 practice guidance from the American association for the study of liver diseases. Hepatology 2019;69(1):394–419.
41. Neuberger J. Recurrent primary biliary cirrhosis. Liver Transpl 2003;9(6):539–46.
42. Rowe IA, Webb K, Gunson BK, et al. The impact of disease recurrence on graft survival following liver transplantation: a single centre experience. Transpl Int 2008;21(5):459–65.
43. Montano-Loza AJ, Hansen BE, Corpechot C, et al. Factors associated with recurrence of primary biliary cholangitis after liver transplantation and effects on graft and patient survival. Gastroenterology 2019;156(1):96–107.

44. Corpechot C, Chazouillères O, Belnou P, et al. Long-term impact of preventive UDCA therapy after transplantation for primary biliary cholangitis. J Hepatol 2020;73(3):559–65.
45. Egawa H, Sakisaka S, Teramukai S, et al. Long-term outcomes of living-donor liver transplantation for primary biliary cirrhosis: a Japanese multicenter study. Am J Transpl 2016;16(4):1248–57.
46. Morioka D, Egawa H, Kasahara M, et al. Impact of human leukocyte antigen mismatching on outcomes of living donor liver transplantation for primary biliary cirrhosis. Liver Transpl 2007;13(1):80–90.
47. Li X, Peng J, Ouyang R, et al. Risk factors for recurrent primary biliary cirrhosis after liver transplantation: a systematic review and meta-analysis. Dig Liver Dis 2021;53(3):309–17.
48. Neuberger J, Gunson B, Hubscher S, et al. Immunosuppression affects the rate of recurrent primary biliary cirrhosis after liver transplantation. Liver Transpl 2004;10(4):488–91.
49. Manousou P, Arvaniti V, Tsochatzis E, et al. Primary biliary cirrhosis after liver transplantation: influence of immunosuppression and human leukocyte antigen locus disparity. Liver Transpl 2010;16(1):64–73.
50. Lytvyak E, Niazi M, Pai R, et al. Combination antiretroviral therapy improves recurrent primary biliary cholangitis following liver transplantation. Liver Int 2021;41(8):1879–83.
51. Charatcharoenwitthaya P, Pimentel S, Talwalkar JA, et al. Long-term survival and impact of ursodeoxycholic acid treatment for recurrent primary biliary cirrhosis after liver transplantation. Liver Transpl 2007;13(9):1236–45.
52. Bosch A, Dumortier J, Maucort-Boulch D, et al. Preventive administration of UDCA after liver transplantation for primary biliary cirrhosis is associated with a lower risk of disease recurrence. J Hepatol 2015;63(6):1449–58.
53. Pedersen MR, Greenan G, Arora S, et al. Ursodeoxycholic acid decreases incidence of primary biliary cholangitis and biliary complications after liver transplantation: a meta-analysis. Liver Transpl 2021;27(6):866–75.
54. Campsen J, Zimmerman MA, Trotter JF, et al. Clinically recurrent primary sclerosing cholangitis following liver transplantation: a time course. Liver Transpl 2008;14(2):181–5.
55. Visseren T, Erler NS, Heimbach JK, et al. Inflammatory conditions play a role in recurrence of PSC after liver transplantation: an international multicentre study. JHEP Rep 2022;4(12):100599.
56. Visseren T, Erler NS, Polak WG, et al. Recurrence of primary sclerosing cholangitis after liver transplantation - analysing the European Liver Transplant Registry and beyond. Transpl Int 2021;34(8):1455–67.
57. Lindström L, Jørgensen KK, Boberg KM, et al. Risk factors and prognosis for recurrent primary sclerosing cholangitis after liver transplantation: a Nordic Multicentre Study. Scand J Gastroenterol 2018;53(3):297–304.
58. Hildebrand T, Pannicke N, Dechene A, et al. Biliary strictures and recurrence after liver transplantation for primary sclerosing cholangitis: a retrospective multicenter analysis. Liver Transpl 2016;22(1):42–52.
59. Graziadei IW, Wiesner RH, Batts KP, et al. Recurrence of primary sclerosing cholangitis following liver transplantation. Hepatology 1999;29(4):1050–6.
60. Bowlus CL, Arrivé L, Bergquist A, et al. AASLD practice guidance on primary sclerosing cholangitis and cholangiocarcinoma. Hepatology 2023;77(2):659–702.

61. Jeyarajah DR, Netto GJ, Lee SP, et al. Recurrent primary sclerosing cholangitis after orthotopic liver transplantation: is chronic rejection part of the disease process? Transplantation 1998;66(10):1300–6.
62. Ravikumar R, Tsochatzis E, Jose S, et al. Risk factors for recurrent primary sclerosing cholangitis after liver transplantation. J Hepatol 2015;63(5):1139–46.
63. Egawa H, Ueda Y, Ichida T, et al. Risk factors for recurrence of primary sclerosing cholangitis after living donor liver transplantation in Japanese registry. Am J Transpl 2011;11(3):518–27.
64. Kugelmas M, Spiegelman P, Osgood MJ, et al. Different immunosuppressive regimens and recurrence of primary sclerosing cholangitis after liver transplantation. Liver Transpl 2003;9(7):727–32.
65. Steenstraten IC, Sebib Korkmaz K, Trivedi PJ, et al. Systematic review with meta-analysis: risk factors for recurrent primary sclerosing cholangitis after liver transplantation. Aliment Pharmacol Ther 2019;49(6):636–43.
66. Cholongitas E, Shusang V, Papatheodoridis GV, et al. Risk factors for recurrence of primary sclerosing cholangitis after liver transplantation. Liver Transpl 2008; 14(2):138–43.
67. Alabraba E, Nightingale P, Gunson B, et al. A re-evaluation of the risk factors for the recurrence of primary sclerosing cholangitis in liver allografts. Liver Transpl 2009;15(3):330–40.
68. Vera A, Moledina S, Gunson B, et al. Risk factors for recurrence of primary sclerosing cholangitis of liver allograft. Lancet 2002;360(9349):1943–4.
69. Peverelle M, Paleri S, Hughes J, et al. Activity of inflammatory bowel disease after liver transplantation for primary sclerosing cholangitis predicts poorer clinical outcomes. Inflamm Bowel Dis 2020;26(12):1901–8.
70. Chen C, Ke R, Yang F, et al. Risk factors for recurrent autoimmune liver diseases after liver transplantation: a meta-analysis. Medicine 2020;99(20):e20205.
71. Akamatsu N, Hasegawa K, Egawa H, et al. Donor age ($\geq$45 years) and reduced immunosuppression are associated with the recurrent primary sclerosing cholangitis after liver transplantation - a multicenter retrospective study. Transpl Int 2021;34(5):916–29.
72. Heinemann M, Adam R, Berenguer M, et al. Longterm survival after liver transplantation for autoimmune hepatitis: results from the European liver transplant registry. Liver Transpl 2020;26(7):866–77.
73. Schramm C, Bubenheim M, Adam R, et al. Primary liver transplantation for autoimmune hepatitis: a comparative analysis of the European Liver Transplant Registry. Liver Transpl 2010;16(4):461–9.
74. Chouik Y, Chazouillères O, Francoz C, et al. Long-term outcome of liver transplantation for autoimmune hepatitis: a French nationwide study over 30 years. Liver Int 2023;43(5):1068–79.
75. Lohse AW, Kögel M, Meyer zum Büschenfelde KH. Evidence for spontaneous immunosuppression in autoimmune hepatitis. Hepatology 1995;22(2):381–8.
76. Guichelaar MMJ, Kendall R, Malinchoc M, et al. Bone mineral density before and after OLT: long-term follow-up and predictive factors. Liver Transpl 2006; 12(9):1390–402.
77. Maalouf NM, Shane E. Osteoporosis after solid organ transplantation. J Clin Endocrinol Metab 2005;90(4):2456–65.
78. Trautwein C, Possienke M, Schlitt HJ, et al. Bone density and metabolism in patients with viral hepatitis and cholestatic liver diseases before and after liver transplantation. Am J Gastroenterol 2000;95(9):2343–51.

79. Eastell R, Dickson ER, Hodgson SF, et al. Rates of vertebral bone loss before and after liver transplantation in women with primary biliary cirrhosis. Hepatology 1991;14(2):296–300.

80. Guichelaar MMJ, Schmoll J, Malinchoc M, et al. Fractures and avascular necrosis before and after orthotopic liver transplantation: long-term follow-up and predictive factors. Hepatology 2007;46(4):1198–207.

81. Poupon RE, Chrétien Y, Chazouillères O, et al. Quality of life in patients with primary biliary cirrhosis. Hepatology 2004;40(2):489–94.

82. Carbone M, Bufton S, Monaco A, et al. The effect of liver transplantation on fatigue in patients with primary biliary cirrhosis: a prospective study. J Hepatol 2013;59(3):490–4.

83. Krawczyk M, Koźma M, Szymańska A, et al. Effects of liver transplantation on health-related quality of life in patients with primary biliary cholangitis. Clin Transpl 2018;32(12):e13434.

84. Pells G, Mells GF, Carbone M, et al. The impact of liver transplantation on the phenotype of primary biliary cirrhosis patients in the UK-PBC cohort. J Hepatol 2013;59(1):67–73.

85. Wunsch E, Stadnik A, Kruk B, et al. Chronic fatigue persists in a significant proportion of female patients after transplantation for primary sclerosing cholangitis. Liver Transpl 2021;27(7):1032–40.

86. Irlès-Depé M, Roullet S, Neau-Cransac M, et al. Impact of preexisting inflammatory bowel disease on the outcome of liver transplantation for primary sclerosing cholangitis. Liver Transpl 2020;26(11):1477–91.

87. Joshi D, Bjarnason I, Belgaumkar A, et al. The impact of inflammatory bowel disease post-liver transplantation for primary sclerosing cholangitis. Liver Int 2013; 33(1):53–61.

88. Mouchli MA, Singh S, Boardman L, et al. Natural history of established and de novo inflammatory bowel disease after liver transplantation for primary sclerosing cholangitis. Inflamm Bowel Dis 2018;24(5):1074–81.

89. Ribaldone DG, Imperatore N, Le Grazie M, et al. Inflammatory bowel disease course in liver transplant versus non-liver transplant patients for primary sclerosing cholangitis: LIVIBD, an IG-IBD study. Dig Liver Dis 2021;53(6):712–6.

90. Fattahi MR, Malek-Hosseini SA, Sivandzadeh GR, et al. Clinical course of ulcerative colitis after liver transplantation in patients with concomitant primary sclerosing cholangitis and ulcerative colitis. Inflamm Bowel Dis 2017;23(7):1160–7.

91. Jørgensen KK, Lindström L, Cvancarova M, et al. Immunosuppression after liver transplantation for primary sclerosing cholangitis influences activity of inflammatory bowel disease. Clin Gastroenterol Hepatol 2013;11(5):517–23.

92. Al Draiweesh S, Ma C, Alkhattabi M, et al. Safety of combination biologic and antirejection therapy post-liver transplantation in patients with inflammatory bowel disease. Inflamm Bowel Dis 2020;26(6):949–59.

93. Singh S, Edakkanambeth Varayil J, Loftus EV Jr, et al. Incidence of colorectal cancer after liver transplantation for primary sclerosing cholangitis: a systematic review and meta-analysis. Liver Transpl 2013;19(12):1361–9.

94. Nasser-Ghodsi N, Mara K, Watt KD. De novo colorectal and pancreatic cancer in liver-transplant recipients: identifying the higher-risk populations. Hepatology 2021;74(2):1003–13.

95. Rao BB, Lashner B, Kowdley KV. Reviewing the risk of colorectal cancer in inflammatory bowel disease after liver transplantation for primary sclerosing cholangitis. Inflamm Bowel Dis 2018;24(2):269–76.

96. Jørgensen KK, Lindström L, Cvancarova M, et al. Colorectal neoplasia in patients with primary sclerosing cholangitis undergoing liver transplantation: a Nordic multicenter study. Scand J Gastroenterol 2012;47(8–9):1021–9.

97. Marchesa P, Lashner BA, Lavery IC, et al. The risk of cancer and dysplasia among ulcerative colitis patients with primary sclerosing cholangitis. Am J Gastroenterol 1997;92(8):1285–8.

98. Imam MH, Eaton JE, Puckett JS, et al. Neoplasia in the ileoanal pouch following colectomy in patients with ulcerative colitis and primary sclerosing cholangitis. J Crohns Colitis 2014;8(10):1294–9.

99. Saunders EA, Engel B, Höfer A, et al. Outcome and safety of a surveillance biopsy guided personalized immunosuppression program after liver transplantation. Am J Transpl 2022;22(2):519–31.

100. Kelly C, Zen Y, Heneghan MA. Post-transplant immunosuppression in autoimmune liver disease. J Clin Exp Hepatol 2023;13(2):350–9.

101. Theocharidou E, Heneghan MA. Con: steroids should not Be withdrawn in transplant recipients with autoimmune hepatitis. Liver Transpl 2018;24(8):1113–8.

102. Kalra A, Burton JR Jr, Forman LM. Pro: steroids can Be withdrawn after transplant in recipients with autoimmune hepatitis. Liver Transpl 2018;24(8):1109–12.

103. Charlton M, Levitsky J, Aqel B, et al. International liver transplantation society consensus statement on immunosuppression in liver transplant recipients. Transplantation 2018;102(5):727–43.

104. Kerkar N, Dugan C, Rumbo C, et al. Rapamycin successfully treats post-transplant autoimmune hepatitis. Am J Transpl 2005;5(5):1085–9.

105. Reich DJ, Fiel I, Guarrera JV, et al. Liver transplantation for autoimmune hepatitis. Hepatology 2000;32(4 Pt 1):693–700.

106. European Association for the Study of the Liver. EASL Clinical Practice Guidelines: the diagnosis and management of patients with primary biliary cholangitis. J Hepatol 2017;67(1):145–72.

107. Lindor KD, Kowdley KV, Luketic VAC, et al. High-dose ursodeoxycholic acid for the treatment of primary sclerosing cholangitis. Hepatology 2009;50(3): 808–14.

108. Alexander J, Lord JD, Yeh MM, et al. Risk factors for recurrence of primary sclerosing cholangitis after liver transplantation. Liver Transpl 2008;14(2):245–51.

109. Henson JB, Patel YA, King LY, et al. Outcomes of liver retransplantation in patients with primary sclerosing cholangitis. Liver Transpl 2017;23(6):769–80.

110. Altwegg R, Combes R, Laharie D, et al. Effectiveness and safety of anti-TNF therapy for inflammatory bowel disease in liver transplant recipients for primary sclerosing cholangitis: a nationwide case series. Dig Liver Dis 2018;50(7):668–74.

111. Spadaccini M, Aghemo A, Caprioli F, et al. Safety of vedolizumab in liver transplant recipients: a systematic review. United Eur Gastroenterol J 2019;7(7):875–80.

112. Agrawal M, Kim ES, Colombel JF. JAK inhibitors safety in ulcerative colitis: practical implications. J Crohns Colitis 2020;14(Supplement_2):S755–60.

113. Gordon FD, Goldberg DS, Goodrich NP, et al. Recurrent primary sclerosing cholangitis in the Adult-to-Adult Living Donor Liver Transplantation Cohort Study: comparison of risk factors between living and deceased donor recipients. Liver Transpl 2016;22(9):1214–22.

114. Khettry U, Keaveny A, Goldar-Najafi A, et al. Liver transplantation for primary sclerosing cholangitis: a long-term clinicopathologic study. Hum Pathol 2003; 34(11):1127–36.

115. Moncrief KJ, Savu A, Ma MM, et al. The natural history of inflammatory bowel disease and primary sclerosing cholangitis after liver transplantation–a single-centre experience. Can J Gastroenterol 2010;24(1):40–6.
116. Aravinthan AD, Doyle AC, Issachar A, et al. First-degree living-related donor liver transplantation in autoimmune liver diseases. Am J Transpl 2016;16(12): 3512–21.

Moving?

Make sure your subscription moves with you!

To notify us of your new address, find your **Clinics Account Number** (located on your mailing label above your name), and contact customer service at:

Email: journalscustomerservice-usa@elsevier.com

800-654-2452 (subscribers in the U.S. & Canada)
314-447-8871 (subscribers outside of the U.S. & Canada)

Fax number: 314-447-8029

**Elsevier Health Sciences Division
Subscription Customer Service
3251 Riverport Lane
Maryland Heights, MO 63043**

*To ensure uninterrupted delivery of your subscription, please notify us at least 4 weeks in advance of move.

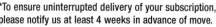

Printed and bound by CPI Group (UK) Ltd, Croydon, CR0 4YY

03/10/2024

01040467-0003